Mitochondria: The Diseases' Cause and Cure

Mitochondria: The Diseases' Cause and Cure

Guest Editors

Susana P. Pereira
Ludgero C. Tavares

MDPI

Basel • Beijing • Wuhan • Barcelona • Belgrade • Novi Sad • Cluj • Manchester

Guest Editors
Susana P. Pereira
UCIBIO - Department of Chemistry
NOVA University Lisbon
Caparica
Portugal

Ludgero C. Tavares
CIVG - Vasco da Gama Research Center
University School Vasco da Gama - EUVG
Coimbra
Portugal

Editorial Office
MDPI AG
Grosspeteranlage 5
4052 Basel, Switzerland

This is a reprint of the Special Issue, published open access by the journal *Biology* (ISSN 2079-7737), freely accessible at: https://www.mdpi.com/journal/biology/special_issues/mitochondria_disease.

For citation purposes, cite each article independently as indicated on the article page online and as indicated below:

Lastname, A.A.; Lastname, B.B. Article Title. *Journal Name* **Year**, *Volume Number*, Page Range.

ISBN 978-3-7258-5715-9 (Hbk)
ISBN 978-3-7258-5716-6 (PDF)
https://doi.org/10.3390/books978-3-7258-5716-6

Contents

About the Editors . . . . **vii**

Susana P. Pereira and Ludgero C. Tavares
Beyond Powerhouses: Roles of Mitochondria, from Development to Therapeutic Potential
Reprinted from: *Biology* **2025**, *14*, 1367, https://doi.org/10.3390/biology14101367 . . . . **1**

José Costa, Patrícia C. Braga, Irene Rebelo, Pedro F. Oliveira and Marco G. Alves
Mitochondria Quality Control and Male Fertility
Reprinted from: *Biology* **2023**, *12*, 827, https://doi.org/10.3390/biology12060827 . . . . **5**

Inês Moniz, Maria Soares, Ana Paula Sousa, João Ramalho-Santos and Ana Branco
The Low Survivability of Transplanted Gonadal Grafts: The Impact of Cryopreservation and Transplantation Conditions on Mitochondrial Function
Reprinted from: *Biology* **2024**, *13*, 542, https://doi.org/10.3390/biology13070542 . . . . **27**

Isabella Bracchi, Juliana Morais, João Almeida Coelho, Ana Filipa Ferreira, Inês Alves, Cláudia Mendes, et al.
The Cardiometabolic Impact of Rebaudioside A Exposure during the Reproductive Stage
Reprinted from: *Biology* **2025**, *14*, 163, https://doi.org/10.3390/biology13030163 . . . . **46**

Consuelo Lomas-Soria, Guadalupe L. Rodríguez-González, Carlos A. Ibáñez, Luis A. Reyes-Castro, Peter W. Nathanielsz and Elena Zambrano
Maternal Obesity Programs the Premature Aging of Rat Offspring Liver Mitochondrial Electron Transport Chain Genes in a Sex-Dependent Manner
Reprinted from: *Biology* **2023**, *12*, 1166, https://doi.org/10.3390/biology12091166 . . . . **63**

Xu Yan, Carolina Tocantins, Mei-Jun Zhu, Susana P. Pereira and Min Du
Maternal Nutrient Excess Induces Stress Signaling and Decreases Mitochondrial Number in Term Fetal Baboon Skeletal Muscle
Reprinted from: *Biology* **2025**, *14*, 868, https://doi.org/10.3390/biology14070868 . . . . **85**

Azra Kulovic-Sissawo, Carolina Tocantins, Mariana S. Diniz, Elisa Weiss, Andreas Steiner, Silvija Tokic, et al.
Mitochondrial Dysfunction in Endothelial Progenitor Cells: Unraveling Insights from Vascular Endothelial Cells
Reprinted from: *Biology* **2024**, *13*, 70, https://doi.org/10.3390/biology13020070 . . . . **103**

Ricardo Amorim, Carina C. Magalhães, Fernanda Borges, Paulo J. Oliveira and José Teixeira
From Non-Alcoholic Fatty Liver to Hepatocellular Carcinoma: A Story of (Mal)Adapted Mitochondria
Reprinted from: *Biology* **2023**, *12*, 595, https://doi.org/10.3390/biology12040595 . . . . **137**

Michelle V. Tomczewski, John Z. Chan, Duaa M. Al-Majmaie, Ming Rong Liu, Alex D. Cocco, Ken D. Stark, et al.
Phenotypic Characterization of Female Carrier Mice Heterozygous for Tafazzin Deletion
Reprinted from: *Biology* **2023**, *12*, 1238, https://doi.org/10.3390/biology12091238 . . . . **158**

Jui-Chih Chang, Huei-Shin Chang, Yi-Chun Chao, Ching-Shan Huang, Chin-Hsien Lin, Zhong-Sheng Wu, et al.
Formoterol Acting via β2-Adrenoreceptor Restores Mitochondrial Dysfunction Caused by Parkinson's Disease-Related UQCRC1 Mutation and Improves Mitochondrial Homeostasis Including Dynamic and Transport
Reprinted from: *Biology* **2024**, *13*, 231, https://doi.org/10.3390/biology13040231 . . . . **181**

Jingfei (Carly) Lin, Sinwoo (Wendy) Hwang, Honglin Luo and Yasir Mohamud
Double-Edged Sword: Exploring the Mitochondria–Complement Bidirectional Connection in Cellular Response and Disease
Reprinted from: *Biology* **2024**, *13*, 431, https://doi.org/10.3390/biology13060431 . . . . **200**

About the Editors

Susana P. Pereira

Susana P. Pereira is a biomedical scientist and an Assistant Researcher at UCIBIO – Applied Molecular Biosciences Unit and the Associate Laboratory i4HB – Institute for Health and Bioeconomy at the Department of Chemistry, NOVA University Lisbon. Susana's research explores how early-life environments shape lifelong health, with a special focus on mitochondria, metabolism, and cardiovascular disease.

Susana leads and collaborates on national and international projects that explore how gestational exposures shape mitochondrial function and disease risk across the lifespan. Susana has published extensively in the fields of perinatal metabolism and mitochondrial dysfunction and has received multiple awards for her scientific and outreach work. Passionate about science communication, Susana is equally committed to mentoring young scientists and engaging the public in meaningful dialogues between research and health. Susana works toward a single vision: a world where no life is cut short by silent damage that began before birth, because the first heartbeat echoes for LIFE.

Ludgero C. Tavares

Ludgero C. Tavares is a biochemist and is an Assistant Professor at EUVG – University School Vasco da Gama, and an Invited Professor at IPL – Polytechnic University of Leiria. Ludgero also currently serves as director of the CIVG – Vasco da Gama Research Center and his research spans diverse areas including toxicology, mitochondrial bioenergetics and nutrition in metabolic and inflammatory diseases. Ludgero is specialized in flux analysis of core metabolic pathways using stable isotope tracers and NMR spectroscopy and is currently focused in the modulation of carbohydrate and lipid metabolism, from cancer research to feed optimization in aquaculture. He is actively involved in managing zebrafish animal facilities, coordinating new degree programs, supervising students and is an advocate for scientific outreach and dissemination. With over 35 peer-reviewed publications and several international collaborations, he hopes that such integrative approaches may help us better understand the mitochondrial roles in health, development, and aging.

biology

MDPI

Editorial

Beyond Powerhouses: Roles of Mitochondria, from Development to Therapeutic Potential

Susana P. Pereira [1,2,*] and Ludgero C. Tavares [3]

1 UCIBIO—Applied Molecular Biosciences Unit, Department of Chemistry, NOVA School of Science and Technology, Universidade NOVA de Lisboa, 2829-516 Caparica, Portugal
2 Associate Laboratory i4HB—Institute for Health and Bioeconomy, NOVA School of Science and Technology, Universidade NOVA de Lisboa, 2829-516 Caparica, Portugal
3 CIVG—Vasco da Gama Research Center, University School Vasco da Gama—EUVG, 3020-210 Coimbra, Portugal
* Correspondence: sps.pereira@fct.unl.pt

Mitochondria, long recognized as the powerhouse of the cell, have emerged as master regulators of cellular fate and therapeutic potential through a broad range of signaling pathways and metabolic modulation. This Special Issue of Biology brings together ten original research and review articles that collectively trace a compelling arc, from the role of mitochondria in reproduction and early-life programming to their dysfunction in pathophysiology and emergence as novel therapeutic targets.

This Special Issue begins by focusing on the reproductive lifespan, as mitochondrial quality control is essential in fertility and gamete viability. Costa et al. [1] contribute a comprehensive review of mitochondrial quality control mechanisms in male fertility, highlighting how disruptions in mitophagy, biogenesis, and dynamics can impair spermatogenesis and sperm function. Their work underlines the importance of mitochondrial surveillance systems in maintaining reproductive health and suggests that mitochondrial dysfunction may underlie idiopathic male infertility.

Complementing this topic, Moniz et al. [2] explore the impact of cryopreservation and transplantation on mitochondrial function in gonadal grafts. Employing a rodent model, they demonstrate that both procedures significantly compromise mitochondrial membrane potential and respiratory capacity, contributing to the low survivability of transplanted tissue. Their findings emphasize the need for improved preservation protocols that safeguard mitochondrial integrity to enhance reproductive outcomes.

Bracchi et al. [3] extend the reproductive theme by investigating the cardiometabolic consequences of Rebaudioside A exposure during the reproductive stage. Their experimental research in female rats reveals that a chronic intake of this non-caloric sweetener alters mitochondrial function in cardiac tissue, leading to increased oxidative stress and impaired energy metabolism. These results raise important questions about the long-term metabolic effects of dietary additives during sensitive reproductive windows.

In the Guest Editor's experience [4–16], a large body of research has focused on how the maternal environment shifts early-life mitochondrial programming, exerting lasting effects on offspring health. In this Special Issue, this theme is further explored; Lomas-Soria et al. [17] show that maternal obesity induces premature aging in mitochondrial electron transport chain genes in the liver of rat offspring, with sex-specific differences. Their transcriptomic analysis reveals the downregulation of key mitochondrial genes in male offspring, suggesting that maternal metabolic status can epigenetically reprogram mitochondrial function in a sex-dependent manner.

Similarly, Yan et al. [18] report that maternal nutrient excess reduces the number of mitochondria and activates stress signaling in fetal baboon skeletal muscle. Using a non-human primate model, they demonstrate that overnutrition during pregnancy leads to mitochondrial depletion and increased expression of unfolded protein response markers, potentially predisposing offspring to metabolic dysfunction. These findings reinforce the concept that mitochondrial health is shaped in utero and may influence disease susceptibility later in life.

Metabolic programming is currently a research hotspot, and as we learn more, increasing attention is being given to the mitochondrial contribution to the onset of pathophysiological processes and the progression of chronic diseases. Mitochondrial dysfunction can not only reflect underlying metabolic disturbances but also actively contribute to pathophysiological mechanisms across various organ systems. For instance, Kulovic-Sissawo et al. [19] investigated mitochondrial dysfunction in endothelial progenitor cells (EPCs), revealing that EPCs exhibit impaired mitochondrial respiration and increased oxidative stress compared to mature endothelial cells. Their study suggests that mitochondrial deficits in EPCs may compromise vascular repair capacity, with implications for cardiovascular disease and aging, highlighting a potential mechanistic link between mitochondrial dysfunction and cardiovascular aging.

Similarly, Amorim et al. [20] explore the progression of non-alcoholic fatty liver disease (NAFLD/MASLD) to hepatocellular carcinoma, as a paradigm of maladaptive mitochondrial responses. Their review demonstrates how impaired β-oxidation, excess ROS production, and disrupted mitochondrial dynamics drive a cascade from steatosis to fibrosis and ultimately to malignancy, positioning mitochondria as both biomarkers and active players in liver disease progression.

Extending this perspective to genetic mitochondrial disorders, Tomczewski et al. [21] provide a phenotypic characterization of female mice heterozygous for Tafazzin deletion, a model of Barth syndrome. They report subtle but significant alterations in cardiac and skeletal muscle mitochondrial function, even in the absence of overt pathology. This study underscores the importance of considering carrier status and sex-specific effects in mitochondrial diseases, and it adds to our understanding of how partial gene deletions can manifest subclinically.

Together, these studies illustrate that mitochondrial dysfunction, whether developmentally programmed, environmentally induced, or genetically inherited, serves as a critical nexus in disease pathogenesis and warrants further investigation as both a target and indicator in the context of aging and chronic disease progression.

Thus, the final arc of this Special Issue explores therapeutic strategies targeting mitochondrial dysfunction. Chang et al. [22] demonstrate that Formoterol, a β2-adrenoreceptor agonist, restores mitochondrial function in cells harboring a Parkinson's disease-related UQCRC1 mutation. Their data show improved mitochondrial dynamics, transport, and bioenergetics, suggesting that β2-agonists may offer neuroprotective benefits by modulating mitochondrial homeostasis.

Closing this Special Issue, Lin et al. [23] explore the bidirectional relationship between mitochondria and the complement system. Their review synthesizes evidence that mitochondrial damage can activate complement pathways while complement proteins can localize to mitochondria and influence their function. This "double-edged sword" highlights the complex interplay between innate immunity and mitochondrial signaling in health and disease.

Collectively, these ten manuscripts offer a panoramic view of mitochondrial biology, from its foundational role in reproduction and development to its critical involvement in disease and its potential as a therapeutic target. Far from being mere energy factories, mitochondria emerge here as dynamic regulators of cellular fate, often exhibiting sex-specific idiosyncrasies. As our mechanistic understanding deepens, so too does the potential of mitochondria-centered strategies to diagnose, treat, and prevent a wide array of complex diseases.

The Guest Editors would like to gratefully acknowledge the Biology Editorial Office for their continued support, as well as the peer reviewers, authors, and respective research units for their valuable contributions. We hope that this Special Issue will provide both insight and inspiration, to enable continued development in this rapidly advancing field.

Funding: This work was financed by national funds from FCT—Fundação para a Ciência e a Tecnologia, I.P., in the scope of the project UIDP/04378/2020 (DOI: 10.54499/UIDP/04378/2020) and UIDB/04378/2020 (DOI: 10.54499/UIDB/04378/2020) of the Research Unit on Applied Molecular Biosciences—UCIBIO and the project LA/P/0140/2020 (DOI: 10.54499/LA/P/0140/2020) of the Associate Laboratory Institute for Health and Bioeconomy—i4HB.

Conflicts of Interest: The authors declare no conflict of interest.

References

1. Costa, J.; Braga, P.C.; Rebelo, I.; Oliveira, P.F.; Alves, M.G. Mitochondria Quality Control and Male Fertility. *Biology* **2023**, *12*, 827. [CrossRef] [PubMed]
2. Moniz, I.; Soares, M.; Sousa, A.P.; Ramalho-Santos, J.; Branco, A. The Low Survivability of Transplanted Gonadal Grafts: The Impact of Cryopreservation and Transplantation Conditions on Mitochondrial Function. *Biology* **2024**, *13*, 542. [CrossRef] [PubMed]
3. Bracchi, I.; Morais, J.; Coelho, J.A.; Ferreira, A.F.; Alves, I.; Mendes, C.; Correia, B.; Gonçalves, A.; Guimarães, J.T.; Falcão-Pires, I.; et al. The Cardiometabolic Impact of Rebaudioside A Exposure during the Reproductive Stage. *Biology* **2024**, *13*, 163. [CrossRef]
4. Pereira, S.P.; Oliveira, P.J.; Tavares, L.C.; Moreno, A.J.; Cox, L.A.; Nathanielsz, P.W.; Nijland, M.J. Effects of moderate global maternal nutrient reduction on fetal baboon renal mitochondrial gene expression at 0.9 gestation. *Am. J. Physiol.-Ren. Physiol.* **2015**, *308*, F1217–F1228. [CrossRef]
5. Pereira, S.P.; Tavares, L.C.; Duarte, A.I.; Baldeiras, I.; Cunha-Oliveira, T.; Martins, J.D.; Santos, M.S.; Maloyan, A.; Moreno, A.J.; Cox, L.A.; et al. Sex-dependent vulnerability of fetal nonhuman primate cardiac mitochondria to moderate maternal nutrient reduction. *Clin. Sci.* **2021**, *135*, 1103–1126. [CrossRef]
6. Pereira, S.P.; Diniz, M.S.; Tavares, L.C.; Cunha-Oliveira, T.; Li, C.; Cox, L.A.; Nijland, M.J.; Nathanielsz, P.W.; Oliveira, P.J. Characterizing Early Cardiac Metabolic Programming via 30% Maternal Nutrient Reduction during Fetal Development in a Non-Human Primate Model. *Int. J. Mol. Sci.* **2023**, *24*, 15192. [CrossRef]
7. Diniz, M.S.; Hiden, U.; Falcão-Pires, I.; Oliveira, P.J.; Sobrevia, L.; Pereira, S.P. Fetoplacental endothelial dysfunction in gestational diabetes mellitus and maternal obesity: A potential threat for programming cardiovascular disease. *Biochim. Biophys. Acta Mol. Basis Dis.* **2023**, *1869*, 166834. [CrossRef]
8. Sousa, D.; Rocha, M.; Amaro, A.; Ferreira-Junior, M.D.; Cavalcante, K.V.N.; Monteiro-Alfredo, T.; Barra, C.; Rosendo-Silva, D.; Saavedra, L.P.J.; Magalhães, J.; et al. Exposure to Obesogenic Environments during Perinatal Development Modulates Offspring Energy Balance Pathways in Adipose Tissue and Liver of Rodent Models. *Nutrients* **2023**, *15*, 1281. [CrossRef]
9. Grilo, L.F.; Tocantins, C.; Diniz, M.S.; Gomes, R.M.; Oliveira, P.J.; Matafome, P.; Pereira, S.P. Metabolic Disease Programming: From Mitochondria to Epigenetics, Glucocorticoid Signalling and Beyond. *Eur. J. Clin. Investig.* **2021**, *51*, e13625. [CrossRef]
10. Stevanović-Silva, J.; Beleza, J.; Coxito, P.; Pereira, S.; Rocha, H.; Gaspar, T.B.; Gärtner, F.; Correia, R.; Martins, M.J.; Guimarães, T.; et al. Maternal high-fat high-sucrose diet and gestational exercise modulate hepatic fat accumulation and liver mitochondrial respiratory capacity in mothers and male offspring. *Metabolism* **2021**, *116*, 154704. [CrossRef] [PubMed]
11. Tocantins, C.; Diniz, M.S.; Grilo, L.F.; Pereira, S.P. The birth of cardiac disease: Mechanisms linking gestational diabetes mellitus and early onset of cardiovascular disease in offspring. *WIREs Mech. Dis.* **2022**, *14*, e1555. [CrossRef]
12. Diniz, M.S.; Magalhães, C.C.; Tocantins, C.; Grilo, L.F.; Teixeira, J.; Pereira, S.P. Nurturing through Nutrition: Exploring the Role of Antioxidants in Maternal Diet during Pregnancy to Mitigate Developmental Programming of Chronic Diseases. *Nutrients* **2023**, *15*, 4623. [CrossRef]
13. Diniz, M.S.; Tocantins, C.; Grilo, L.F.; Pereira, S.P. The Bitter Side of Sugar Consumption: A Mitochondrial Perspective on Diabetes Development. *Diabetology* **2022**, *3*, 583–595. [CrossRef]
14. Grilo, L.F.; Diniz, M.S.; Tocantins, C.; Areia, A.L.; Pereira, S.P. The Endocrine–Metabolic Axis Regulation in Offspring Exposed to Maternal Obesity—Cause or Consequence in Metabolic Disease Programming? *Obesities* **2022**, *2*, 236–255. [CrossRef]

15. Pereira, S.P.; Grilo, L.F.; Tavares, R.S.; Gomes, R.M.; Ramalho-Santos, J.; Ozanne, S.E.; Matafome, P. Chapter 16—Programming of early aging. In *Aging;* Oliveira, P.J., Malva, J.O., Eds.; Academic Press: Cambridge, MA, USA, 2023; pp. 407–431. [CrossRef]
16. Diniz, M.S.; Grilo, L.F.; Tocantins, C.; Falcão-Pires, I.; Pereira, S.P. Made in the Womb: Maternal Programming of Offspring Cardiovascular Function by an Obesogenic Womb. *Metabolites* **2023**, *13*, 845. [CrossRef]
17. Lomas-Soria, C.; Rodríguez-González, G.L.; Ibáñez, C.A.; Reyes-Castro, L.A.; Nathanielsz, P.W.; Zambrano, E. Maternal Obesity Programs the Premature Aging of Rat Offspring Liver Mitochondrial Electron Transport Chain Genes in a Sex-Dependent Manner. *Biology* **2023**, *12*, 1166. [CrossRef]
18. Yan, X.; Tocantins, C.; Zhu, M.-J.; Pereira, S.P.; Du, M. Maternal Nutrient Excess Induces Stress Signaling and Decreases Mitochondrial Number in Term Fetal Baboon Skeletal Muscle. *Biology* **2025**, *14*, 868. [CrossRef]
19. Kulovic-Sissawo, A.; Tocantins, C.; Diniz, M.S.; Weiss, E.; Steiner, A.; Tokic, S.; Madreiter-Sokolowski, C.T.; Pereira, S.P.; Hiden, U. Mitochondrial Dysfunction in Endothelial Progenitor Cells: Unraveling Insights from Vascular Endothelial Cells. *Biology* **2024**, *13*, 70. [CrossRef] [PubMed]
20. Amorim, R.; Magalhães, C.C.; Borges, F.; Oliveira, P.J.; Teixeira, J. From Non-Alcoholic Fatty Liver to Hepatocellular Carcinoma: A Story of (Mal)Adapted Mitochondria. *Biology* **2023**, *12*, 595. [CrossRef]
21. Tomczewski, M.V.; Chan, J.Z.; Al-Majmaie, D.M.; Liu, M.R.; Cocco, A.D.; Stark, K.D.; Strathdee, D.; Duncan, R.E. Phenotypic Characterization of Female Carrier Mice Heterozygous for Tafazzin Deletion. *Biology* **2023**, *12*, 1238. [CrossRef]
22. Chang, J.-C.; Chang, H.-S.; Chao, Y.-C.; Huang, C.-S.; Lin, C.-H.; Wu, Z.-S.; Chang, H.-J.; Liu, C.-S.; Chuang, C.-S. Formoterol Acting via β2-Adrenoreceptor Restores Mitochondrial Dysfunction Caused by Parkinson's Disease-Related UQCRC1 Mutation and Improves Mitochondrial Homeostasis Including Dynamic and Transport. *Biology* **2024**, *13*, 231. [CrossRef] [PubMed]
23. Lin, J.; Hwang, S.; Luo, H.; Mohamud, Y. Double-Edged Sword: Exploring the Mitochondria–Complement Bidirectional Connection in Cellular Response and Disease. *Biology* **2024**, *13*, 431. [CrossRef] [PubMed]

biology

MDPI

Review

Mitochondria Quality Control and Male Fertility

José Costa [1,2,†], Patrícia C. Braga [1,2,3,†], Irene Rebelo [4,5], Pedro F. Oliveira [6] and Marco G. Alves [1,2,3,*]

1 Unit for Multidisciplinary Research in Biomedicine (UMIB), Institute of Biomedical Sciences Abel Salazar (ICBAS), University of Porto, 4050-313 Porto, Portugal; jliuze@gmail.com (J.C.); patriciacbraga.1096@gmail.com (P.C.B.)
2 ITR-Laboratory for Integrative and Translational Research in Population Health, 4050-600 Porto, Portugal
3 Laboratory of Physiology, Department of Imuno-Physiology and Pharmacology, ICBAS-School of Medicine and Biomedical Sciences, University of Porto, 4050-313 Porto, Portugal
4 UCIBIO-REQUIMTE, Laboratory of Biochemistry, Department of Biologic Sciences, Pharmaceutical Faculty, University of Porto, 4050-313 Porto, Portugal; irebelo@ff.up.pt
5 Associate Laboratory i4HB-Institute for Health and Bioeconomy, Laboratory of Biochemistry, Department of Biologic Sciences, Pharmaceutical Faculty, University of Porto, 4050-313 Porto, Portugal
6 LAQV-REQUIMTE, Department of Chemistry, University of Aveiro, 3810-193 Aveiro, Portugal; pfobox@gmail.com
* Correspondence: alvesmarc@gmail.com; Tel.: +351-220428000
† These authors contributed equally to the manuscript.

Simple Summary: Mitochondria play a crucial role in numerous cellular processes, including energy production, apoptosis, and calcium homeostasis. In the male reproductive system, mitochondria are particularly important for the development and maintenance of germ cells, which ultimately lead to the production of healthy sperm. Dysfunction in mitochondrial physiology can lead to an imbalance in reactive oxygen species, which can have detrimental effects on sperm quality. Thus, mitochondrial quality control can ultimately define male reproductive capacity. Studies have shown that non-communicable diseases such as obesity, diabetes, and cardiovascular disease can have a negative impact on mitochondrial function in sperm, leading to decreased sperm motility, concentration, and viability. Therefore, understanding and managing mitochondrial quality control could be a valuable approach to developing new strategies to combat male infertility. Herein we discuss the relevance of mitochondria quality control to male fertility, particularly the role of oxidative stress and the parameters needed to be evaluated.

Abstract: Mitochondria are pivotal to cellular homeostasis, performing vital functions such as bioenergetics, biosynthesis, and cell signalling. Proper maintenance of these processes is crucial to prevent disease development and ensure optimal cell function. Mitochondrial dynamics, including fission, fusion, biogenesis, mitophagy, and apoptosis, maintain mitochondrial quality control, which is essential for overall cell health. In male reproduction, mitochondria play a pivotal role in germ cell development and any defects in mitochondrial quality can have serious consequences on male fertility. Reactive oxygen species (ROS) also play a crucial role in sperm capacitation, but excessive ROS levels can trigger oxidative damage. Any imbalance between ROS and sperm quality control, caused by non-communicable diseases or environmental factors, can lead to an increase in oxidative stress, cell damage, and apoptosis, which in turn affect sperm concentration, quality, and motility. Therefore, assessing mitochondrial functionality and quality control is essential to gain valuable insights into male infertility. In sum, proper mitochondrial functionality is essential for overall health, and particularly important for male fertility. The assessment of mitochondrial functionality and quality control can provide crucial information for the study and management of male infertility and may lead to the development of new strategies for its management.

Keywords: male fertility; mitochondrial quality control; non-communicable diseases; spermatozoa

1. Introduction

Mitochondria, commonly known as the "powerhouses of the cell", are intricate organelles present in all eukaryotic cells. They consist of two membranes, the outer mitochondrial membrane (OMM) and the inner mitochondrial membrane (IMM), which separate the mitochondrial matrix from the cytoplasm of the cell and define the intermembrane space and mitochondrial matrix [1]. While OMM is highly permeable, IMM is selectively impermeable to most substances. This property is essential for the development of specific transport systems that regulate the movement of molecules to and from mitochondria [1]. The IMM can be further divided into two subdomains, an inner boundary membrane which is in contact with the OMM and the cristae membrane [2]. The cristae membrane is responsible for enclosing the oxidative phosphorylation (OXPHOS) respiratory chain complexes, including complexes I, II, III, and IV [3].

Mitochondria play a critical role in maintaining cellular homeostasis, by facilitating distinct and essential physiological processes such as bioenergetics, biosynthesis, and cell signalling. One of its primary functions is the synthesis of ATP, which occurs through cellular respiration and involves the conversion of ADP and phosphate ions into ATP by the mitochondrial ATP synthase. ATP is the primary energy currency of the cell and is required for various cellular processes, including muscle contraction, protein synthesis, and signal transmission [2]. ATP is also used in a variety of cellular functions, including biosynthesis and degradation of proteins, maintenance of membrane potentials [4] and also to many other physiological functions. Furthermore, mitochondria are known to be a major source of reactive oxygen species (ROS). Specifically, ROS are primarily generated in the respiratory complexes I and III of the electron transport chain (ETC) [5]. Mitochondria regulate the production of ROS through several mechanisms, including the modulation of mitochondrial membrane potential (MMP), the redox state of the ETC complexes, and the availability of oxygen [2,6]. These organelles are considered cell signalling centres and may participate in stress responses [7]. In addition to their primary functions, mitochondria are also involved in several other biological processes. They play a role in aging, thermogenesis, and calcium storage, thereby contributing to the maintenance of cellular calcium homeostasis [2]. Mitochondria use fission and fusion as the primary processes to regulate multiple aspects, including their distribution in the cytoplasm, as well as their size, shape, and number [2]. Mitochondrial quality control is maintained through various processes, including mitochondrial fission and fusion, biogenesis, mitophagy and apoptosis [8]. All these processes are essential for several physiological functions, including male reproduction.

Mitochondria play a crucial role in the male reproductive tract, contributing to the occurrence of spermatogenesis (sperm production) and oocyte fertilization. Spermatogenesis occurs in the seminiferous tubules, where germ cell proliferation and differentiation processes lead to the production of a high quantity of spermatozoa, which heavily rely on mitochondrial function [9]. It can be divided into three phases—spermatogonia mitosis (amplification of spermatogonial stem cells (SSCs)), spermatocytes meiosis (reduction in the chromosome number), and spermiogenesis where the round shaped spermatids are transformed into a more elongated shape [10]. Mitochondria found in spermatogonia and early spermatocytes are small and conventional, exhibiting limited OXPHOS activity. As spermatogenesis progresses to later stages, such as spermatocytes, spermatids, and spermatozoa, the mitochondria undergo a transformation to become more condensed, elongated, and efficient in their OXPHOS activity [11].

Changes in mitochondria morphology depicted in Figure 1 appear to occur prior to their structural association with the sperm flagellum. While most mitochondria are lost during spermiogenesis, some are arranged within the developing spermatid tail [12] and are metabolically more efficient [13] (Figure 1).

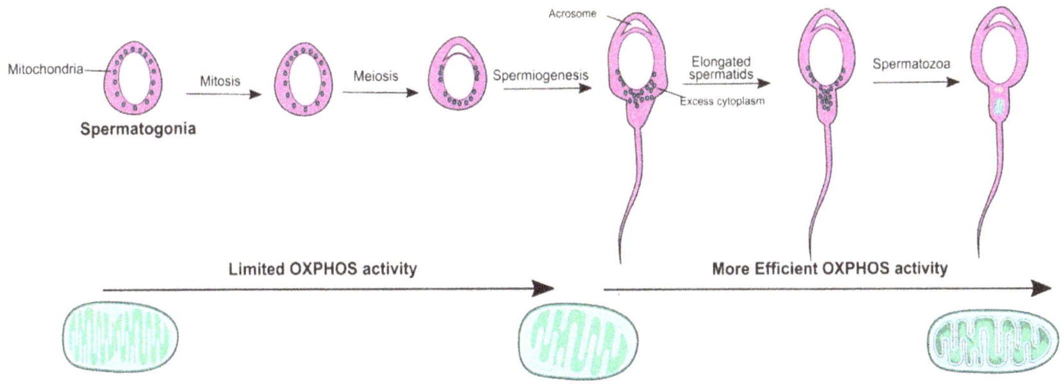

Figure 1. Schematic representation of the stages of spermatogenesis and the corresponding alterations in mitochondrial morphology. Mitochondria has a more orthodox shape in the early stages and become increasingly elongated and condensed as spermatogenesis progresses exhibiting a more efficient Oxidative Phosphorylation (OXPHOS) activity.

In testicular tissue, mitochondria have multiple functions that include energy production [14], steroid hormones production in the testis [15], the maintenance of cell proliferation [16] and cell death [17]. Moreover, in spermatozoa, mitochondria-generated ROS play a vital role in the physiological processes that enable these cells to fertilize an oocyte. These processes include biochemical changes linked to tyrosine phosphorylation, cholesterol release, and the interaction between sperm and egg. However, excessive ROS production can lead to oxidative stress (OS) and contribute to several deleterious events [18]. Human spermatozoa contain only one copy of mtDNA per mitochondrion [19] and their mtDNA sequence is identical to that found in somatic cells. However, the absence or weakness of DNA repair mechanisms in sperm mtDNA leads to a higher mutation rate [2]. Mitochondria in spermatozoa play a crucial role in ATP production, which is essential for promoting sperm motility [20], thus human spermatozoa motility depends on the correct performance of the OXPHOS [21]. Overall, the appropriate functionality of the ETC is inexorable to mitochondrial performance which, in turn, is associated with sperm function [2]. Any alterations that affect mitochondrial quality and performance in sperm have the potential to cause male infertility. Therefore, this review aims to explore the role of mitochondria throughout the male reproductive tract and how their quality control, including dysfunction in response to various metabolic cues such as metabolic disorders and environmental pollutants, may affect male fertility.

2. Mitochondria Physiology throughout the Male Reproductive Tract

As stated, spermatogenesis is an event that can be divided in three phases to transform spermatogonial stem cells (SSCs) into spermatozoa and occurs in the seminiferous tubules of the testis [13]. In the spermatozoa, there are between 70–80 mitochondria located in the midpiece [12,13]. Notably, there are metabolic and morphological changes in mitochondria physiology along the different cellular microenvironment of the testis which encloses SSCs, spermatocytes and spermatids [13]. Sertoli cells play a vital role in maintaining the homeostasis of the testis by forming the blood–testis barrier (BTB), which creates a specialized microenvironment in the adluminal space of the seminiferous epithelium [22]. The BTB is a highly specialized tight junction located in the adluminal compartment of the seminiferous epithelium. Its main function is to prevent autoantigens present in spermatogenic cells from being recognized by immune cells of the host [22,23]. The SSCs are located at the base of the BTB, which enables them to utilize nutrients and glucose from the blood supply to produce ATP [24]. Mitochondria in SSCs are immature and highly vacuolated, with a spherical shape and a low electron-lucid matrix and few cristae. In contrast, spermatocytes and spermatids possess a large number of mature mitochondria [25]. Throughout spermatogenesis, germ cells go through several microenvironments with varying concentrations of glucose and metabolites as SSCs are turned into mature sperm [26]. During this process, the mitochondria not only increase in number but also change shape, particularly in meiotic prophase I [26]. These variations in mitochondrial size and shape depend on the proper functioning of fusion/fission and mitophagy, which are essential for maintaining intracellular homeostasis [27], as it will be explained further in detail. Moreover, as spermatogonia and SSCs are located in the basal compartment, they have direct contact with blood and interstitial fluid, providing them with access to glucose and other metabolites. However, spermatocytes and spermatids have limited access to these nutrients [26]. The differential access to metabolites between the basal compartment and adluminal compartment reflects the changing metabolic needs of male germ cells during the various stages of spermatogenesis. It appears that spermatogonia primarily rely on glucose to produce energy through glycolysis [28], while spermatocytes and spermatids rely on lactate provided by Sertoli cells, as well as pyruvate, as their main energy sources [29]. The lactate produced by Sertoli cells is converted to pyruvate by lactate dehydrogenase. Pyruvate is then utilized in mitochondria to produce ATP, indicating that spermatocytes and spermatids in the adluminal compartment are dependent on mitochondrial OXPHOS activity for energy generation [26]. The high energy demand of meiotic spermatocytes, particularly during the meiotic prophase I (MPI), requires a substantial supply of lactate and pyruvate. This demand is expected given the significant energy needed to complete meiosis, including DNA replication, recombination, and chromosomal segregation [26]. This phase represents approximately 90% of meiosis, a quarter of the spermatogenic process, and can be further divided into four different stages (leptotene, zygotene, pachytene, and diplotene) [30]. Electron microscopy studies conducted in rodent testes have shown that there is an increase in OXPHOS activity during the MPI stage of meiosis. Specifically, during pachytene, mitochondria present in the spermatocytes assume a more elongated shape while the cristae are more compact [31]. This type of mitochondrial organization has been shown to be associated with increased OXPHOS activity [32]. Conversely, in spermatids that have completed the meiosis process, the mitochondria are fragmented, and the cristae do not have either an orthodox or a condensed shape, indicating a return to reliance on glycolysis [31].

Sertoli cells play a crucial role in regulating the number of germ cells in the testis. They do this by modulating apoptosis during mitosis, which prevents the overproduction of germ cells and maintains the homeostasis of the testis [33]. After phagocytosis of apoptotic spermatogenic cells, the lipids from these cells are degraded into fatty acids which undergo β-oxidation to generate ATP in Sertoli cells. The degradation of the apoptotic cells into lipids results in a significant increase in long-chain acyl-CoA dehydrogenase, an enzyme involved in β-oxidation, in the mitochondria of Sertoli cells. This process of utilizing lipids from apoptotic germ cells for energy production is an important mechanism for maintaining the metabolic activity of Sertoli cells and for supporting the development of germ cells [34]. In addition to promoting β-oxidation of lipids, Sertoli cells also play a role in regulating mitochondrial biogenesis and OXPHOS activity in germ cells. Activin A, a protein secreted by Sertoli cells, has been shown to promote mitochondrial biogenesis and the formation of elongated cristae-rich mitochondria in spermatocytes and spermatids. This is achieved through transcriptional regulation of key genes involved in mitochondrial biogenesis, including peroxisome proliferator-activated receptor-γ coactivator 1α, nuclear respiratory factor (NRF) 1, and NRF2 [24,31]. These transcription factors activate the expression of genes involved in mitochondrial DNA replication, transcription, and translation, as well as those encoding components of the electron transport chain, leading to increased OXPHOS activity in germ cell [35].

Leydig cells are another crucial somatic cell type found in the testis. Their role in male germ cell differentiation is less well studied than that of Sertoli cells [13]. Leydig cells are in the interstitial tissue of the testis and are responsible for the production and secretion of steroid hormones, particularly androgens such as testosterone. These hormones are synthesized and released into the bloodstream in response to the stimulation of luteinizing hormone (LH) from the pituitary gland [36]. While the exact role of Leydig cells in male germ cell differentiation is not fully understood, it is known that androgens play an important role in the regulation of spermatogenesis and male fertility. Testosterone plays an essential role in spermatogenesis as it is required for the development of spermatogonia and the initiation of meiosis. It also regulates the release of spermatids from Sertoli cells into the lumen of the seminiferous tubules [37]. When circulating LH binds to its receptor on Leydig cells, it triggers a signalling cascade that increases the production of cyclic AMP (cAMP). This increase in cAMP promotes the transport of cholesterol to the inner mitochondrial membrane (IMM) and initiates the first step of testosterone production. This step involves the conversion of cholesterol into pregnenolone by the P450 cholesterol side-chain cleavage enzyme (P450scc). Pregnenolone then undergoes further enzymatic reactions to eventually produce testosterone [38]. When referring to cholesterol in mitochondria, its typical functions are biogenesis, membrane maintenance and the production of steroids [39]. Although the primary function of mitochondria is to produce ATP, this is not the case for Leydig cells. The morphology of the cristae in Leydig cells does not allow the connection between the F1 complexes of ATP synthase in the mitochondrial matrix when they are close to the mitochondrial membrane [40]. Therefore, Leydig cells produce less ATP, and their mitochondria are mainly responsible for the production of steroid hormones, such as testosterone, through the steroidogenesis pathway.

After leaving the testicular seminiferous tubules, spermatozoa have to mature in the epididymis where they gain the capacity to reach and fertilize the oocyte [41]. Epididymal cells create a unique microenvironment in the epididymal lumen to support sperm maturation. This microenvironment is maintained by epithelial cells, which keep the pH acidic and the bicarbonate concentration low. This ensures that the spermatozoa do not become prematurely activated while they are maturing in the epididymis [41]. The acidic pH is supported by proton secretion by V-ATPases, which are abundant in the apical membrane and intracellular vesicles of the narrow and clear cells in the epididymis [41]. The narrow and clear cells present in the epididymis are considered mitochondria-rich cells and these abundant mitochondria are linked to the acidification of the lumen due to their carbonic anhydrase activity, endocytic activity and most importantly, proton secretion through V-ATPase [42].

It is important to mention the importance of ROS in spermatozoa capacitation, since protein tyrosine phosphorylation is regulated by ROS production [43]. The presence of ROS triggers a cascade of biochemical reactions that enhance sperm motility. First, ROS induces the conversion of ATP to cAMP by the enzyme adenylyl cyclase. Next, cAMP activates protein kinase A (PKA), which further stimulates ROS production and the enzyme NADPH oxidase. PKA also phosphorylates serine and tyrosine residues, leading to activation of protein tyrosine kinase (PTK). Finally, PTK triggers phosphorylation of tyrosine residues in the sperm flagellum axoneme, resulting in increased motility [43]. Another key event during capacitation is the mobilization of calcium ions, which is also triggered by ROS. This increase in calcium ions leads to the cleavage of PIP2 (phosphatidylinositol-4,5-biphosphate), producing DAG (diacylglycerol). The presence of DAG and PKC (protein kinase C) induces the phosphorylation of phospholipase A2, a membrane enzyme that plays a critical role in sperm function. This phosphorylation event increases the fluidity of the spermatozoa membrane, enabling it to fuse with the oocyte. This membrane fusion is a crucial step in fertilization and requires precise coordination between sperm and oocyte. [44]. Overall, the interplay between ROS, calcium ions, PKC, and phospholipase A2 during capacitation is a finely tuned process that ensures successful fertilization.

Spermatozoa are highly vulnerable to the harmful effects of ROS, which include superoxide anion, hydrogen peroxide, hydroxyl radical, nitric oxide, and peroxynitrite. Elevated levels of ROS can lead to oxidative damage, impairing sperm function [45]. This impairment translates into a loss of sperm motility and mitochondrial activity and also the possibility of losing the ability to fertilize oocytes [46]. Spermatozoa have limited capacity to repair oxidative damage, as their chromatin is highly compacted and lacks the necessary machinery to synthesize new proteins. Therefore, they rely on antioxidant enzymes that are produced during spermatogenesis and epididymal maturation to provide some degree of protection [46]. During epididymal maturation, the plasma membrane of spermatozoa becomes enriched with polyunsaturated fatty acids (PUFAs) [13]. While PUFAs contribute to the integrity of the sperm membrane and improve its ability to fuse with the oocyte during fertilization, they also increase the sperm susceptibility to OS. Therefore, the balance between ROS and antioxidants is critical for maintaining proper sperm function and fertility [47].

As discussed above, to fertilize an oocyte, spermatozoa must be prepared through morphological alterations, such as the remodelling of the plasma membrane. Those changes will assist the penetration of the oocyte and the survival of sperm in the female reproductive tract. This process, known as capacitation, is mainly characterized by the activation of tyrosine kinase via cAMP [13]. Capacitation is related to the improvement of sperm characteristics such as membrane fluidity, motility, and calcium inflow, facilitating spermatozoa to penetrate the oocyte [48]. Glycolysis and mitochondrial OXPHOS are the main metabolic pathways that support capacitation, as ATP is required for this process to occur [49]. In a study by Carrageta and colleagues, human spermatozoa were incubated under in vitro capacitation conditions with varying glucose concentrations. Spermatozoa incubated without glucose exhibited a lower viability, while those incubated with glucose maintained viability over time [49]. The study also revealed that the sperm cells incubated with glucose exhibited higher levels of tyrosine residue phosphorylation, which is a commonly used biomarker for sperm capacitation. This finding demonstrates the importance of glucose in promoting human sperm capacitation [49]. ATP production via OXPHOS occurs in the midpiece of spermatozoa, primarily supporting sperm motility. However, it is also crucial for maintaining chromatin structure and regulating the acrosome reaction in spermatozoa [50]. Zhang and colleagues investigated sperm MMP in young college students, using the N-α-benzoyl-DL-arginine-para-nitroanilide HCl (BAPNA) substrate method to measure acrosin activity and DNA fragmentation index (DFI) to assess chromatin integrity. Their findings indicated that individuals with low MMP had reduced acrosin activity and lower DFI when compared to those with high or moderate MMP [50]. This study also found that sperm MMP dissipation led to ROS overproduction and reduced ATP content [50]. Overall, mitochondria play a vital role throughout the male reproductive tract, and their dysfunction can cause errors during spermatogenesis, sperm capacitation and oocyte fertilization, leading to male infertility.

3. Relevance of Mitochondrial (Dys)function to Male Fertility

Mitochondrial activity plays a crucial role in all stages of male reproductive potential, from spermatogenesis to oocyte fecundation. In spermatozoa, mitochondria are located in the midpiece and form the mitochondrial sheath that surrounds the axoneme [51]. This structure is connected to the axoneme by a reticulum of filaments and synthesizes ATP, which is necessary for the proper sperm function [52,53]. Recent comparative studies have shown that the amount of mitochondria in the sheath is directly related to sperm velocity and ATP production. For instance, Gu and colleagues studied sperm morphology and mitochondrial functions in 10 mammalian species, including humans, and found that a higher number of mitochondria in the sheath was positively correlated with increased sperm motility and ATP production [54]. In humans, studies have shown that low sperm motility is associated with smaller midpieces, abnormally assembled mitochondria, and mitochondrial membranes with structural defects [51]. These findings suggest a direct correlation between the correct mitochondrial structure and fertilization rates [55].

Sperm quality is closely linked to proper mitochondrial function, and disruptions in the ETC pathway can adversely affect sperm quality [51]. In humans, the MMP, which serves as an indicator of energy and mitochondrial functions, has been found to be associated with sperm viability [56] and the ability to perform acrosome reaction [57] as well as the capacity to fertilize oocytes naturally or in vitro [58]. When measuring the enzymatic activity of the respiratory chain complexes, Ruiz-Pesini and colleagues used specific modulators of the ETC complexes and found that their correct functioning influenced sperm parameters such as motility and vitality [21]. They were also able to demonstrate a direct correlation between mitochondrial enrichment of complex II and more efficient spermatogenesis, leading to a higher number of ejaculated spermatozoa [21]. Lastly, mitochondrial respiration and oxygen consumption have been linked to higher sperm motility and capacitation [59], further highlighting the direct relationship between mitochondrial function and healthy sperm physiology, as we summarized in Table 1.

Mitochondria are also involved in other processes that can affect sperm quality, such as generation of ROS, calcium control and cell signalling [51] (Figure 2). The overproduction of ROS by leukocytes, immature germ cells, and defective spermatozoa can exceed the physiological threshold leading to oxidative stress, which is very deleterious for the sperm [51]. Therefore, it is crucial to maintain a delicate balance of ROS levels in the male reproductive system. Oxidative stress can have a negative impact on sperm quality and function, including reducing sperm motility, affecting mitochondrial activity, and ultimately, reducing the ability of sperm to successfully fertilize the oocyte [60]. The high levels of PUFAs in the sperm membrane make them highly susceptible to lipid peroxidation caused by ROS. This peroxidation of lipids can also trigger the generation of ROS by sperm mitochondria. PUFAs penetrate the IMM and inhibit the proper flow of electrons in the ETC, leading to the production of superoxide anions, oxidative DNA damage [61] and DNA base oxidation [62]. When OS is present, there is increased amount of ROS that stimulates more generation of ROS [2]. This is due to the formation of aldehyde–protein adducts, which are by-products of lipid peroxidation and bind to proteins in the mitochondrial ETC, causing the generation of more ROS in the mitochondria [63] (Figure 2). This perpetuates a cycle of ROS generation and the resulting OS, which ultimately leads to apoptosis of spermatozoa. This occurs because sperm mitochondria are extremely sensitive to oxidative stress, despite being the main intracellular ROS generator [51]. Therefore, the maintenance of ROS levels within the physiological range is crucial for preserving sperm quality and function.

Koppers and colleagues demonstrated that mitochondrial ROS generated from complex III can cause the release of hydrogen peroxide into the extracellular space without detectable peroxidative damage. In contrast, the induction of mitochondrial ROS from complex I results in leakage into the mitochondrial matrix, leading to peroxidative damage to the IMM [61]. This damage to the IMM caused by mitochondrial ROS from complex I may result in the opening of the mitochondrial permeability transition pores and fragmentation of the IMM, leading to activation of the mitochondrial intrinsic apoptotic pathway [64]. Since the chemical triggers for apoptosis that exist in somatic cells are not present in the spermatozoa, these will automatically undergo truncated apoptosis unless pro-survival factors are able to prevent this process [65]. However, the specific signalling pathways that mediate these processes in spermatozoa are not well understood. An important signalling molecule is calcium, which plays a crucial role in sperm function. Calcium is a messenger that participates in a variety of cellular processes. In humans, it has been demonstrated to be crucial in sperm function, being involved in the movement of the flagellum, capacitation, acrosome reaction and chemotaxis [66]. Calcium-dependent pores in the sperm IMM open in response to high intracellular calcium levels, allowing calcium to enter mitochondria and reduce MMP [67], activating the apoptotic pathway [51].

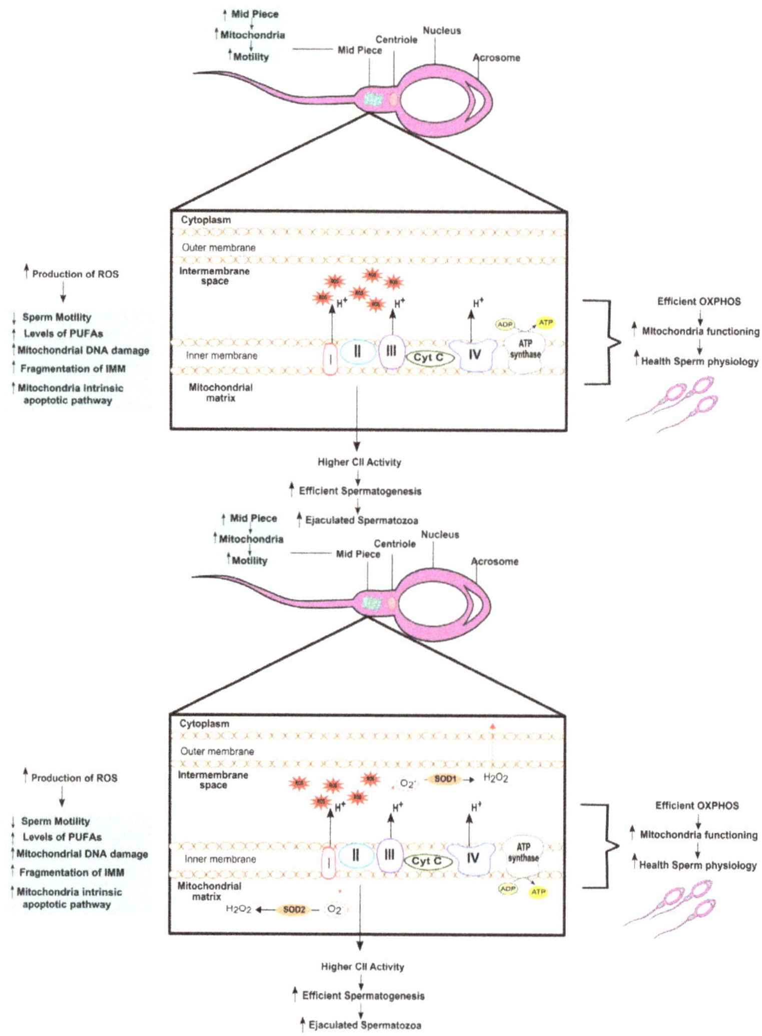

Figure 2. Schematic summary of the complex relationship between mitochondrial quality and spermatozoa health. An efficient oxidative phosphorylation (OXPHOS), particularly at the complex II (CII) level in the electron transport chain, will lead to more ejaculated spermatozoa presenting a better health sperm physiology. Furthermore, a higher mid piece of the spermatozoon is directly linked with a higher motility. However, an imbalance between reactive oxygen species (ROS), will lead to lower sperm motility as well as an increase in mitochondrial DNA damage, an increase in polyunsaturated fatty acids (PUFAs) and increase in the mitochondrial apoptotic pathway. The enzymes superoxide dismutase 1 and 2 (SOD1 and SOD2, respectively) composed the metabolic machinery that handles reactive oxygen species (ROS) in the mitochondrial matrix. Specifically, these enzymes are able to convert superoxide radical anion ($O_2^{\bullet-}$) into hydrogen peroxide (H_2O_2).

Research on sperm apoptosis has demonstrated that apoptotic markers in sperm are similar to those found in somatic cells. In both cases, phosphatidylserine is externalized in the plasma membrane, mitochondrial integrity is compromised, caspase is activated, and DNA damage occurs [68–71]. Despite the similarities, understanding and explaining the apoptotic process in spermatozoa remains a challenge due to the unique physiological conditions of these cells [51]. Apoptotic markers of immature sperm, such as blebbing of the plasma membrane, formation of apoptotic bodies, impaired mitochondrial integrity, defects of the nuclear envelope, and fragmentation of the nucleus, have been associated with infertility in men with reproductive issues [72]. Conversely, these markers are not present in fertile men and mature sperm [73]. The mitochondria, responsible for the intrinsic apoptotic pathway, are thought to play a crucial role in triggering apoptosis in spermatozoa. For example, a study conducted on infertile men with spermatic alterations showed a direct positive correlation among ROS, cytochrome c outside the mitochondria, and the induction of caspases 9 and 3. In another study by Paasch and collaborators it was shown that inducing apoptosis in human sperm leads to higher activity of caspase 9 and 3, along with lower MMP and sperm motility [74]. Activation of caspases 9 and 3 is associated with low sperm quality, higher DNA fragmentation, and reduced fertilization capabilities. Furthermore, when caspase 3 is activated together with disrupted MMP, it leads to the release of phosphatidylserine in spermatozoa [75]. These findings are consistent with the notion that the intrinsic apoptotic pathway involving mitochondria plays a role in regulating sperm apoptosis.

The phosphatidylinositol 3-kinase (PI3K)/AKT signalling pathway plays a crucial role in regulating cell cycle progression, growth, proliferation, survival, and migration [2]. Under stress, the activation of AKT promotes cell survival [76]. Activation of the PI3K enzyme leads to the phosphorylation of AKT1, which, in turn, silences apoptotic pathway promoters, helping to maintain the functionality of spermatozoa. [65]. Inhibition of the PI3K enzyme in this pathway results in the dephosphorylation of AKT1, leading to the initiation of the intrinsic apoptotic pathway in spermatozoa [2]. Consequently, this leads to caspase activation, increased production of mitochondrial ROS, oxidative DNA damage, and reduced sperm motility [77]. Due to the unique architecture of the sperm head, which separates the nucleus from the mitochondria and cytoplasm in the sperm midpiece, endonucleases that are activated during apoptosis are unable to cleave nuclear DNA. As a result, DNA fragmentation in nuclear DNA is not a consequence of apoptosis [77].

Multiple changes can occur in mtDNA at the molecular level, including deletions, substitutions, and other point mutations. These changes can result in poor sperm quality and subsequently male infertility [14]. Mouse models have been used to study the role of OXPHOS in spermatogenesis. Specifically, mice with error-prone mtDNA replication and a mutation in the subunit of the mtDNA polymerase γ have been found to have infertility issues [78]. The "mtDNA mutator" mice presented early degradation in multiple organ systems, particularly the testes, where severely degenerated seminiferous tubes and germ cell depletion were observed at 10 months of age [78]. Jiang and colleagues demonstrated that altering the expression levels of the mtDNA regulator, mitochondrial transcription factor A (Tfam), could affect infertility in mtDNA mutant mice. Increasing Tfam expression levels mitigated the infertility phenotype, while decreasing levels worsened the phenotype [79]. Additionally, mitochondrial dysfunction has been shown to affect MPI in mice. Mice with a high level (4696 bp) pathogenic deletion in mtDNA had low OXPHOS activity, which resulted in meiotic arrests at the transition between zygotene and pachytene [15]. In mice lacking the testis-specific adenine nucleotide translocator 4 (Ant4), a genetic ablation caused spermatogenic arrest in the leptotene phase of MPI [80].

In humans, it has been reported that males with poor sperm quality have a higher prevalence of sperm mitochondrial DNA deletions compared to normozoospermic males [81]. Large-scale mtDNA deletions have been reported to occur more frequently in males with obstructive azoospermia compared to fertile and infertile men with non-obstructive azoospermia [2]. This can be attributed to blockage in the reproductive tract, which creates a higher level of OS and mitochondrial dysfunction. These deletions can affect the OXPHOS system, causing a decrease in ATP production, which can lead to poor sperm motility and decreased fertilization capacity. In addition, these deletions can also cause oxidative damage to sperm DNA, leading to increased levels of sperm DNA fragmentation and subsequent infertility. Additionally, large deletions or a high number of deletions can lead to disruption of ETC, reducing the efficiency of oxidative phosphorylation and impairing ATP synthesis [82]. This mitochondrial dysfunction can affect sperm quality and motility. Indeed, one of the most sensitive biomarkers of male fertility is sperm mtDNA copy number [83]. When the copy number of human mtDNA is altered, both sperm motility and fertilization capacity are be affected [84]. It has been demonstrated that infertile males or those with abnormal semen parameters have a decline in mtDNA integrity when copy number increases [85]. Conversely, a decrease in mtDNA copy number in spermatozoa has been associated with lower sperm motility [86]. The regulation of proteins in sperm has been shown to be differentially affected in patients with decreased sperm motility [87], particularly proteins involved in the fibrous sheath and energy production [88], as well as those involved in spermatogenesis, sperm maturation, sperm tail structure and motility, and mitochondrial quality control [89]. In samples from patients with reduced sperm motility, it has been shown differential protein expression of several proteins. Proteins involved in energy and metabolism, such as triose-phosphate isomerase, glycerol kinase 2, and succinyl-CoA:3-ketoacid co-enzyme A transferase 1, are expressed at higher levels compared to those involved in sperm motility and structure, as well as stress response [90]. This suggests a possible shift in energy production towards glycolysis rather than OXPHOS, which may be a compensatory mechanism to maintain ATP levels and reduce OS in spermatozoa with impaired motility. Additionally, proteins involved in mitochondrial quality control, such as Lon peptidase 1 and prohibitin, were downregulated, suggesting a possible role of mitochondrial dysfunction in reduced sperm motility. In many cases, mitochondrial dysfunction leading to errors in spermatogenesis, sperm capacitation, and oocyte fertilization, which affect sperm quality, motility, and fertilization capacity, are caused by external factors such as metabolic diseases. Thus, a deeper understanding of the impact of metabolic diseases on mitochondrial quality control is imperative to manage and ensure adequate spermatogenesis and prevent male infertility. Appropriate management of metabolic diseases may include lifestyle modifications, pharmacological interventions, or other treatments aimed at reducing mitochondrial dysfunction and improving overall metabolic health. By doing so, we can improve male fertility outcomes and reduce the incidence of infertility caused by metabolic diseases.

Table 1. Spermatozoa fitness alterations due to mitochondrial dysfunction.

Mitochondrial Associated Mechanism	Spermatozoa Outcomes	References
↓ MMP	↓ sperm viability ↓ Acrosome reaction	[57]
↓ ETC	↓ sperm motility ↓ sperm vitality	[21]
↑ amount of mitochondria in the sheath	↑ sperm morphology ↑ ATP production	[53]
Enrichment of complex II	More efficient spermatogenesis ↑ ejaculated spermatozoa	[21]
↑ Oxidative stress	↓ sperm motility ↓ fertilization capacity	[59]
Damage in IMM	↑ apoptotic pathway ↓ MMP ↓ sperm motility	[63]
↓ mtDNA integrity	Poor sperm quality	[14,83,85]

4. Non-Communicable Diseases and Environmental Impact on Mitochondrial Quality of Testicular Cells and Sperm

When analysing mitochondrial quality in male fertility, it is crucial to take into account both internal mitochondrial parameters and cues that may alter the mitochondria's proper operation. Indeed, non-communicable diseases (NCDs) are an example of a condition that can impact male fertility by altering mitochondrial function. NCDs refer to chronic, non-infectious and non-transmissible diseases that can have a significant impact on overall health and well-being [91]. By studying the relationship between NCDs and mitochondrial function, we can gain a deeper understanding of how these diseases can affect male fertility and develop targeted strategies to mitigate their negative effects. Among the most common NCDs are cardiovascular and neurological diseases, as well as cancer and diabetes. Obesity, which is associated with a group of other NCDs including diabetes mellitus (DM), hypertension, metabolic syndrome, non-alcoholic fatty liver disease, and cardiovascular diseases, is also a major risk factor [91]. In addition, recent studies have linked obesity to some types of cancer such as colorectal, liver, and prostate [92].

Obesity is associated with mitochondrial dysfunction, which results in lower energy metabolism. When nutrient supply is abundant, cells produce more mitochondria. However, if nutrient supply remains excessive, the mitochondrial system becomes overloaded, leading to dysfunction and accumulation of non-oxidized lipid products. This causes accumulation of fat and OS, which leads to mitochondrial damage and a further decline in energy metabolism [91]. Excess adipose tissue is known to increase aromatase activity, which converts testosterone to oestradiol, leading to decreased testosterone levels in men [93]. Since testosterone is crucial for regulating spermatogenesis, this reduction in testosterone levels can significantly reduce sperm production [94]. Moreover, decreased testosterone levels are also accompanied by mitochondrial dysfunction in Leydig cells, resulting in oxidative damage to lipids, proteins, and mtDNA, promoting the production of ROS and reduced ATP levels [95]. Obesity is often correlated with a diet rich in saturated fats (SFA) and low in PUFAs [96]. In humans, a direct correlation between increased amounts of SFA and decreased sperm count and concentration has been described [97]. Conversely, a higher intake of omega-3 PUFAs has been linked to better sperm quality. These findings highlight the importance of a balanced and healthy diet in maintaining mitochondrial function and male fertility, as described in Figure 3.

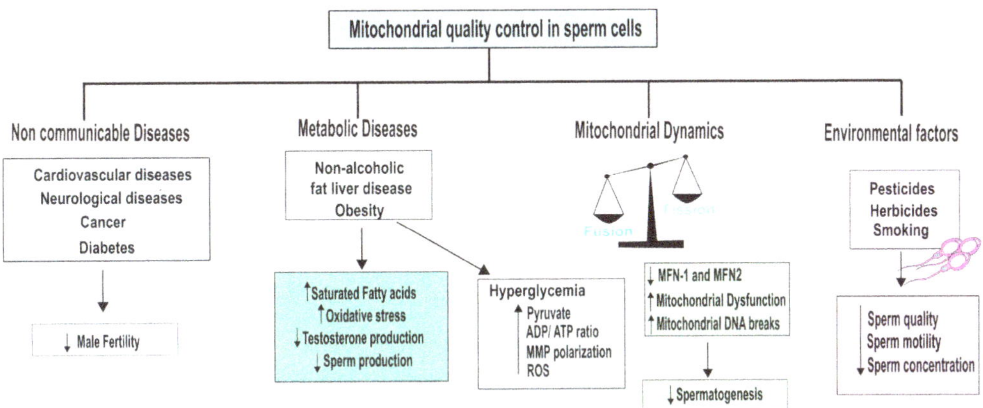

Figure 3. Overview of the interconnected homeodynamics of sperm cells and mitochondrial quality control. Various factors can influence this delicate balance, including non-communicable diseases, metabolic diseases, mitochondrial dynamics, and environmental factors. An imbalance in any of these conditions can result in unhealthy spermatozoa, compromising male fertility. Abbreviations: ROS- Reactive oxygen species; MMP—mitochondrial membrane potential; MFN-1—mitofusin 1 and MFN-2—mitofusin 2.

Regarding PUFAs, it has been suggested to play a role in modulating sperm bioenergetic pathways. Indeed, PUFAs are important components of cell membranes and play a role in regulating mitochondrial function, oxidative stress, and inflammation [98]. There is a isoenzyme form of sperm lactate dehydrogenase (LDH-C4) that is crucial for the nutritional regulation of omega-3 PUFA [98]. This enzyme is present in both the mitochondrial matrix and the cytosol of spermatozoa, and plays a crucial role in the energy metabolism of spermatozoa by catalysing the conversion of pyruvate to lactate and the adjuvant oxidation of NADH [20,99]. LDH-C4 also enables the concurrent advancement of OXPHOS and glycolysis transporting reducing equivalents from the cytosol into the mitochondria and by regenerating NAD+, respectively [94]. It has also shown that a that a diet rich in omega-3 PUFAs can reduce OS in sperm cells by increasing the ratio of aconitase to fumarase activity [98]. The activity ratio of these two Krebs cycle enzymes is considered a marker for mitochondrial production of ROS [100]. On the other hand, a diet high in SFA and low in PUFA has been linked to decreased activity of LDH-C4, pyruvate dehydrogenase, and respiratory enzymes [100].

Despite growing interest in the relationship between diet and reproductive health, the potential effects of dietary carbohydrates on sperm quality remain largely unexplored by scientific research [94]. Glucose is the main fuel for glycolysis in sperm cells, where it is metabolized to pyruvate and/or lactate to produce ATP, the essential energy source for sperm motility. Thus, any reduction in glucose uptake and metabolism by sperm can lead to a decrease in ATP levels, impairing their ability to swim and fertilize an egg [94]. Elevated blood glucose levels have been associated with decreased testosterone production and increased OS in the body [101]. These factors can negatively impact sperm health by impairing mitochondrial function, which is crucial for generating energy and maintaining motility [102]. As a result, high blood glucose levels may lead to reduced sperm motility, highlighting the importance of controlling blood glucose levels for optimal reproductive health. Diabetes mellitus (DM) refers to a group of metabolic disorders characterized by chronic hyperglycaemia resulting from defects in insulin secretion, insulin action, or both. It is a complex and heterogeneous condition, with multiple subtypes and underlying mechanisms, but chronic hyperglycaemia is the defining feature of all forms of DM [103]. The pathogenesis of DM involves a complex interplay of various factors, including an imbalance between free radical formation and the antioxidant defence mechanisms in the body. This OS can result in damage to cellular components, leading to impaired insulin signalling and glucose metabolism [104]. Hence, the dysregulation of the redox balance, characterized by increased free radical formation and/or decreased antioxidant defences, plays a crucial role in the development and progression of DM. DM is associated with a range of vascular and organ-related complications that arise due to overproduction of ROS induced by hyperglycaemia. ROS can cause oxidative damage to various tissues and organs, leading to inflammation, cell injury, and impaired organ function [105]. Mitochondrial dysfunction is a critical factor in the pathogenesis of diabetes, as evidenced by the lower rates of ATP synthesis observed in individuals with a family history of the disease, even before the onset of poor glucose tolerance [106]. Hyperglycaemia promotes the synthesis of pyruvate and increases the flow of reducing equivalents into the ETC [105], resulting in a higher increased ATP/ADP ratio and MMP polarization. However, the significant electrochemical potential difference created by the proton gradient can partially inhibit complex III of the ETC, leading to coenzyme Q accumulation in its reduced form and subsequent generation of superoxide [106]. This increased reduction in coenzyme Q and the resulting production of ROS is suggested to be responsible for mitochondrial dysfunction, which is a key factor in the metabolic abnormalities and tissue histopathology associated with DM [106]. Normally, mitochondria maintain a slightly reduced MMP that generates less ROS, but in hyperglycaemia, hyperpolarization of the MMP leads to increased production of ROS [105].

It was found that exposure to high glucose concentrations causes rapid fragmentation of mitochondria, leading to increased production of ROS [107]. Incubating sperm with high glucose concentrations prevented periodic fluctuations in ROS production by inhibiting mitochondrial fission [107]. This suggests that hyperglycaemic conditions induce dynamic changes in mitochondrial morphology that contribute to the overproduction of ROS. Thus, the mitochondrial fission/fusion machinery represents a potential target for monitoring and regulating acute and chronic ROS production in hyperglycaemia-related disorders [105].

Taken together, these findings indicate that one of the main complications of obesity and DM is the overproduction of ROS and the resulting OS. Understanding the mechanisms underlying ROS production and regulation is critical for developing effective interventions to mitigate the negative consequences of hyperglycaemia and OS. As discussed above, both spermatozoa and germ cells are vulnerable to oxidative stress (OS), which can negatively impact sperm quality by reducing sperm count, motility, and increasing the incidence of abnormalities [108]. Furthermore, oxidative damage to mitochondrial DNA can increase the frequency of large-scale deletions and DNA strand breaks, accelerating germ cell apoptosis and reducing sperm quantity, which is associated with male infertility and lower semen quality [86]. The importance of mitochondrial respiratory activity in mammalian spermatogenesis has also been highlighted by studies linking defects in mitochondrial respiration to meiotic arrest and abnormal sperm morphology [15]. These findings emphasize the crucial role of mitochondrial function and OS regulation in maintaining sperm quality and male reproductive health.

In recent years, there has been an increase in life expectancy, leading to an increase in the age of parents and a corresponding rise in infertility issues. However, there is still limited research on the effects of aging on male fertility and how advanced paternal age affects offspring [109]. Aging in males is associated with changes in the hypothalamic–pituitary–gonadal axis and alterations in the testis, penis, and prostate [12]. Testosterone levels decrease, sperm motility slows, and erectile dysfunction becomes more common in older men [12]. In addition, there is an increase in chromosomal defects and DNA damage, which may have consequences for the offspring [110]. In cells, mitochondrial dysfunction also has a direct correlation with age, where respiratory chain function is affected with advancing age [12]. Studies in mice expressing defective polymerase gamma (POLG), which is essential in mitochondrial DNA replication, have shown premature aging [111]. Using nuclear magnetic resonance (NMR) spectroscopy, Jarak and colleagues were able to identify metabolic changes associated with different stages of reproductive maturity in mice. A notable finding was a significant decrease in testicular creatine content in older mice, indicating changes in the conditions required for male germ cell development [112]. Creatine is a crucial component in the energy metabolism of tissues with high energy demands, including the testis, and assists in ATP replenishment. Therefore, alterations in creatine levels may suggest metabolic changes associated with aging in the testis. In addition, the study showed that advanced age in mice was associated with increased levels of complex I protein, which is linked to ROS overproduction, as well as increased expression levels in the other OXPHOS complexes [112]. However, when comparing 24-month-old mice to 12-month-old mice, there was a significant decrease in the expression levels of the OXPHOS complexes with age, suggesting a decline in mitochondrial function [112].

While NCDs and aging can contribute to mitochondrial dysfunction in the male reproductive tract, there are several environmental factors that can also impact male fertility. In particular, there is growing interest in the potential impact of toxicants, such as herbicides on sperm quality [113]. Despite increased research in this area, our understanding of how these chemicals affect the molecular processes that influence sperm quality remains limited [114]. Anifandis and colleagues demonstrated the negative impact of herbicides on human sperm motility and mitochondrial function by treating spermatozoa with 1 mg/L of Roundup, whose primary active component is glyphosate (GLY) [113]. Using mitochondrial staining, the researchers observed a decrease in sperm motility and mitochondrial staining after one hour of exposure to Roundup, compared to control cells. This suggests that GLY may cause reduced sperm motility by inducing oxidative stress in mitochondria and increasing the production of mitochondrial apoptotic signals [113]. In a more recent study, Ferramosca and colleagues investigated the effects of GLY and glufosinate ammonium (GA) on the efficacy of mitochondrial respiration in human sperm mitochondria. Their findings showed that GLY significantly reduces mitochondrial functionality by lowering oxygen in both the active and passive stages of mitochondrial respiration. In addition, GA may induce mitochondrial permeability by altering the PI3K/AKT complex phosphorylation status, resulting in the loss of motility in human sperm mitochondria [114]. These examples underscore the impact of environmental factors such as pesticides and herbicides on mitochondrial quality control in sperm, which can compromise male fertility.

Cigarette smoking is one of the major health concerns in people of fertile age, and nicotine is its main component. [115]. Detection of nicotine and its major metabolite, cotinine, in the seminal plasma of smokers has demonstrated that tobacco chemicals can penetrate the blood–testis barrier and cause harm to spermatozoa [116]. Components of cigarette smoke are known to be toxic and their intake can lead to testicular microcirculation, DNA, and chromosomal damage in germ cells [117]. Numerous studies have shown that cigarette smoking reduces semen volume, sperm concentration, motility, and normal physiology [118–120], while also decreasing the sperm's ability to fertilize [121,122]. Additionally, sperm from smokers have higher levels of oxidative DNA damage and aneuploidy compared to non-smokers [123]. Chohan and Badawy used phosphorescent analysis to measure oxygen concentrations in sperm suspensions and compared sperm respiration rates in smokers and non-smokers. Their findings revealed that cigarette smoking significantly influences sperm respiration by reducing mitochondrial oxygen consumption [115]. Overall, cigarette smoking has a detrimental effect on male fertility, and its negative impact on sperm motility, morphology, and DNA integrity is well-established. It is important for individuals of reproductive age to avoid cigarette smoking to protect their reproductive health.

While the health advantages of physical activity have been extensively studied for a variety of medical conditions, the impact of exercise on male fertility remains unclear [95]. Several studies indicate that the type, duration, and intensity of exercise have varying impacts on male fertility [95]. Vigorous exercise has been found to reduce male reproductive capacity [124], whereas aerobic, resistance, or combined exercises have been shown to improve male fertility [125]. Although the effects of physical exercise on sperm quality are well established, the underlying mechanisms remain unclear [95]. However, some compelling evidence suggests that high-intensity exercise can induce OS [126,127], which may play a role on impacting male fertility. Aerobic exercise leads to increased oxygen consumption, which is associated with a higher rate of electrons passing through the mitochondrial respiratory chain complexes, possibly causing OS [128,129]. Additionally, catecholamines released during exercise, prostanoid metabolism, xanthine oxidase, and NAD(P)H oxidase are sources of ROS [95]. Regular exercise or chronic anaerobic training can enhance endogenous antioxidant defence mechanisms, reducing oxidative damage [129,130]. However, it has been suggested that rigorous training or prolonged competition periods may increase OS [131]. This is because ROS release can dysregulate the inflammatory and neuroendocrine systems, which may exceed the capacity of the antioxidant system to protect against damage [132]. In healthy young adults who do not exercise regularly, any type of exercise can increase free testosterone concentrations. However, for athletes, only high-intensity exercise appears to lead to an increase in testosterone levels [95]. Recent studies among elite athletes have revealed that their testosterone levels are significantly lower than the physiologically normal range, which could be a consequence of chronic exposure to high levels of aerobic exercise volume and intensity [133,134]. This puts athletes at risk of overtraining and persistent fatigue [95]. Unfortunately, low testosterone levels have been associated with OS, which can result in a decline in sperm quality, thus affecting male fertility [18].

5. Mitochondria Quality Control Parameters Essential to Evaluate

Mitochondria play a crucial role in male fertility, contributing to spermiogenesis, capacitation of the spermatozoa, and oocyte fecundation [13]. Therefore, when assessing the quality of mitochondrial functions as a biomarker or sentinel for sperm quality, several factors should be considered along the male reproductive tract. As already explored, mitochondria morphology differs significantly along spermatogenesis. Specifically, mitochondria in SSCs are heavily vacuolated, spherical, and lack cristae. Furthermore, fusion of OMM and IMM is regulated by proteins anchored to the membrane, including mitofusin

(MFN)-1,2 and optic atrophy (OPA)-1. These proteins facilitate the fusion of the OMM and IMM, and when they are non-functional, they can lead to the disintegration of the mitochondria [135]. On the other hand, fission is controlled by proteins such as cytosolic dynamin, Fission1 protein (Fis-1), mitochondrial fission factor (MFF), and dynamin-related protein 1 (Drp1). Drp1 is transported from the cytosol to the mitochondria, and a Drp1 deficiency can result in mitochondria hyperfusion [136]. A recent study conducted by Varuzhanyan and colleagues aimed to investigate the significance of mitochondrial fusion in mouse spermatogenesis. They found that double mutants for MFN-1 and MFN-2 were unable to produce any sperm, indicating that mitochondrial fusion is necessary for proper spermatogenesis functioning [137]. In Drosophila melanogaster, a mutation in the mitofusin homolog (Marf) has been associated to male sterility, being essential for the maintenance of male germline stem cells [138]. Therefore, it is evident that mitochondrial fusion/fission is essential for the correct functioning of spermatogenesis and these mechanisms could pointed as a possible biomarker on mitochondrial fitness that can be correlated with spermatozoa health (Figure 3). Additionally, recent findings have highlighted the critical role of autophagy in post-meiotic spermatids for cellular remodelling [139]. Although excess mitochondria are removed during spermatogenesis, the involvement of mitophagy in maintaining mitochondrial quality in the male reproductive tract is still under intense debate and requires further understanding [26].

Throughout the male reproductive tract, a significant amount of energy is required to complete the complex processes involved in spermatogenesis and oocyte fertilization. The primary source of energy is derived from OXPHOS [140]. Sperm contains substrates such as glutamic acid (GLU) [141], pyruvate, and lactate that serve as potential energy sources [142]. GLU can be converted into α-ketoglutarate through reactions involving alanine aminotransferase (ALT) and aspartate aminotransferase (AST). In this process, pyruvate and oxaloacetate are transformed into alanine and aspartate, respectively, which contribute to OXPHOS [141]. Alternatively, pyruvate can be reduced to L-lactate by lactate dehydrogenase, generating NAD+ for glycolysis. Pyruvate can also enter the Krebs cycle to support OXPHOS [99]. LDH activity in the mitochondrial matrix of sperm was first discovered in rabbit epididymal spermatozoa and has since been reported in several species, including humans [143]. In humans, LDH-C4 is present in the sperm mitochondrial matrix and facilitates the conversion of lactate to pyruvate, thereby aiding in mitochondrial energy production [144]. Studies have shown that supplementation of sperm media with lactate and pyruvate improves mitochondrial function compared to media containing only glucose [145]. However, this finding has sparked debate over the preferred metabolic pathway for maintaining optimal sperm function [146]. Both oxidative and glycolytic energy metabolism pathways work in tandem to generate energy [145]. Despite the ongoing debate, the crucial question remains whether sperm mitochondria should operate at their maximum capacity, as increased mitochondrial activity leads to increased ROS production [145]. As previously mentioned, ROS are considered harmful by-products of mitochondrial metabolism. When the level of ROS exceeds the antioxidant defences of the cell, it leads to cell damage and oxidative stress [147]. However, mild oxidative stress is necessary for sperm functions such as fertilization, motility, and capacitation, despite causing damage to sperm structure and function [148]. For example, ROS can promote capacitation by regulating tyrosine phosphorylation through redox, which enhances the sperm's ability to bind to the zona pellucida [149]. Research on stallion spermatozoa has associated increased ROS production with rapid mitochondrial activity in sperm [142]. In another study, higher ROS levels were observed in stallion spermatozoa with good freezability after cryopreservation, compared to those with poor freezability, indicating increased mitochondrial activity [150]. Therefore, while excessive ROS production can cause OS and impair sperm function, a moderate amount of ROS is required for proper sperm function. The optimal balance between ROS generation and antioxidant defence should be maintained to support healthy sperm function [145]. In conclusion, mitochondria play a vital role in male fertility, and their quality and proper functioning in sperm are maintained not only through biogenesis mechanisms, but also by balancing oxidative and glycolytic metabolic pathways and by balancing the overproduction and underproduction of ROS. The goal is to prevent cell damage, oxidative stress, and apoptosis, and to enable all phases of the male reproductive tract to function properly. Maintaining optimal mitochondrial function is essential for healthy sperm and successful fertilization. Therefore, future research should focus on understanding the precise mechanisms that regulate mitochondrial metabolism and identifying potential therapeutic targets to enhance mitochondrial function and improve male fertility.

6. Conclusions

Mitochondria are essential organelles for male fertility, and their correct functioning is critical for the success of the reproductive process. Mitochondria play an essential role in generating ATP, the energy required for the physiological mechanisms involved in spermatogenesis and fertilization. However, mitochondria also produce ROS, which can lead to cellular damage, oxidative stress, and apoptosis if not properly maintained. One of the crucial functions of mitochondria in sperm is to produce ATP, which is necessary for various sperm processes, including motility, hyperactivation, capacitation, and acrosome reaction. The correct functioning of mitochondria in sperm is directly related to sperm quality, and defects in mitochondrial function can lead to male infertility. Mitochondria are susceptible to damage from both internal and external factors. Internal factors include overproduction of ROS by leucocytes, immature germ cells, and defective spermatozoa, which can cause oxidative stress and damage mitochondria. External factors that can damage mitochondria include NCDs, such as obesity and diabetes, aging, and poor health habits such as lack of exercise and smoking. Mitochondria have quality control mechanisms to prevent malfunctions. One such mechanism is biogenesis, which ensures that only functional mitochondria are retained, and dysfunctional ones are eliminated. Metabolic pathways in sperm also play a crucial role in maintaining mitochondrial function, by balancing oxidative and glycolysis metabolic pathways and maintaining a physiological equilibrium in the production of ROS. Assessing mitochondrial functionality and quality control is crucial to understanding and managing male infertility. Measuring mitochondrial DNA quality and assessing mitochondrial function in sperm can provide valuable information for diagnosing and treating male infertility. Additionally, developing interventions that target the mitochondrial pathways involved in sperm function may lead to improved treatments for male infertility. In conclusion, mitochondria play a critical role in male fertility, and their correct functioning is essential for the success of the reproductive process. Maintaining a balance between ATP generation and ROS production is necessary to prevent damage to the sperm and maintain sperm quality. By understanding the mechanisms involved in mitochondrial function and quality control, we can develop effective interventions for the treatment of male infertility.

Author Contributions: Conceptualization, methodology, writing—original draft preparation, J.C.; Conceptualization, methodology, Writing—original draft preparation, funding acquisition, P.C.B.; Writing-review and editing, I.R.; Conceptualization, methodology, writing—review and editing, funding acquisition P.F.O.; Conceptualization, methodology, writing—review and editing, supervision, project administration, funding acquisition, M.G.A. All authors have read and agreed to the published version of the manuscript.

Funding: This work was supported by the Portuguese Foundation for Science and Technology: D M.G. Alves (2021.03439.CEECIND), UMIB (UIDB/00215/2020 and UIDP/00215/2020), ITR (LA/P/0064/2020) and LAQVREQUIMTE (UIDB/50006/2020), the post-graduation student Patrícia C. Braga (UI/BD/150750/2020), and co-funded by FEDER funds through the COMPETE/ QREN, FSE/POPH, and POCI—COMPETE 2020 (POCI-01-0145-FEDER-007491) funds.

Institutional Review Board Statement: Not applicable.

Informed Consent Statement: Not applicable.

Data Availability Statement: Not applicable.

Conflicts of Interest: The authors declare no conflict of interest.

References

1. Turcotte, L.P. Mitochondria: Biogenesis, structure, and function—Symposium introduction. *Med. Sci. Sports Exerc.* **2003**, *35*, 82–85. [CrossRef] [PubMed]
2. Durairajanayagam, D.; Singh, D.; Agarwal, A.; Henkel, R. Causes and consequences of sperm mitochondrial dysfunction. *Andrologia* **2021**, *53*, e13666. [CrossRef] [PubMed]
3. Kuhlbrandt, W. Structure and function of mitochondrial membrane protein complexes. *BMC Biol.* **2015**, *13*, 89. [CrossRef] [PubMed]
4. Bonora, M.; Patergnani, S.; Rimessi, A.; De Marchi, E.; Suski, J.M.; Bononi, A.; Giorgi, C.; Marchi, S.; Missiroli, S.; Poletti, F.; et al. ATP synthesis and storage. *Purinergic Signal.* **2012**, *8*, 343–357. [CrossRef] [PubMed]
5. Quinlan, C.L.; Perevoshchikova, I.V.; Hey-Mogensen, M.; Orr, A.L.; Brand, M.D. Sites of reactive oxygen species generation by mitochondria oxidizing different substrates. *Redox Biol.* **2013**, *1*, 304–312. [CrossRef]
6. Murphy, M.P. How mitochondria produce reactive oxygen species. *Biochem. J.* **2009**, *417*, 1–13. [CrossRef]
7. Pellegrino, M.W.; Haynes, C.M. Mitophagy and the mitochondrial unfolded protein response in neurodegeneration and bacterial infection. *BMC Biol.* **2015**, *13*, 22. [CrossRef]
8. Huang, M.L.; Chiang, S.; Kalinowski, D.S.; Bae, D.H.; Sahni, S.; Richardson, D.R. The Role of the Antioxidant Response in Mitochondrial Dysfunction in Degenerative Diseases: Cross-Talk between Antioxidant Defense, Autophagy, and Apoptosis. *Oxid. Med. Cell. Longev.* **2019**, *2019*, 6392763. [CrossRef]
9. Lv, C.; Wang, X.; Guo, Y.; Yuan, S. Role of Selective Autophagy in Spermatogenesis and Male Fertility. *Cells* **2020**, *9*, 2523. [CrossRef]
10. Staub, C.; Johnson, L. Review: Spermatogenesis in the bull. *Animal* **2018**, *12*, s27–s35. [CrossRef]
11. De Martino, C.; Floridi, A.; Marcante, M.L.; Malorni, W.; Scorza Barcellona, P.; Bellocci, M.; Silvestrini, B. Morphological, histochemical and biochemical studies on germ cell mitochondria of normal rats. *Cell Tissue Res.* **1979**, *196*, 1–22. [CrossRef] [PubMed]
12. Vertika, S.; Singh, K.K.; Rajender, S. Mitochondria, spermatogenesis, and male infertility—An update. *Mitochondrion* **2020**, *54*, 26–40. [CrossRef] [PubMed]
13. Park, Y.J.; Pang, M.G. Mitochondrial Functionality in Male Fertility: From Spermatogenesis to Fertilization. *Antioxidants* **2021**, *10*, 98. [CrossRef] [PubMed]
14. St John, J.C.; Jokhi, R.P.; Barratt, C.L. The impact of mitochondrial genetics on male infertility. *Int. J. Androl.* **2005**, *28*, 65–73. [CrossRef]
15. Nakada, K.; Sato, A.; Yoshida, K.; Morita, T.; Tanaka, H.; Inoue, S.; Yonekawa, H.; Hayashi, J. Mitochondria-related male infertility. *Proc. Natl. Acad. Sci. USA* **2006**, *103*, 15148–15153. [CrossRef]
16. Ramalho-Santos, J.; Varum, S.; Amaral, S.; Mota, P.C.; Sousa, A.P.; Amaral, A. Mitochondrial functionality in reproduction: From gonads and gametes to embryos and embryonic stem cells. *Hum. Reprod. Update* **2009**, *15*, 553–572. [CrossRef]
17. Friedman, J.R.; Nunnari, J. Mitochondrial form and function. *Nature* **2014**, *505*, 335–343. [CrossRef]
18. Aitken, R.J.; Drevet, J.R. The Importance of Oxidative Stress in Determining the Functionality of Mammalian Spermatozoa: A Two-Edged Sword. *Antioxidants* **2020**, *9*, 111. [CrossRef]
19. Ankel-Simons, F.; Cummins, J.M. Misconceptions about mitochondria and mammalian fertilization: Implications for theories on human evolution. *Proc. Natl. Acad. Sci. USA* **1996**, *93*, 13859–13863. [CrossRef]
20. Piomboni, P.; Focarelli, R.; Stendardi, A.; Ferramosca, A.; Zara, V. The role of mitochondria in energy production for human sperm motility. *Int. J. Androl.* **2012**, *35*, 109–124. [CrossRef]
21. Ruiz-Pesini, E.; Lapena, A.C.; Diez-Sanchez, C.; Perez-Martos, A.; Montoya, J.; Alvarez, E.; Diaz, M.; Urries, A.; Montoro, L.; Lopez-Perez, M.J.; et al. Human mtDNA haplogroups associated with high or reduced spermatozoa motility. *Am. J. Hum. Genet.* **2000**, *67*, 682–696. [CrossRef] [PubMed]
22. Naito, M.; Itoh, M. Patterns of infiltration of lymphocytes into the testis under normal and pathological conditions in mice. *Am. J. Reprod. Immunol.* **2008**, *59*, 55–61. [CrossRef] [PubMed]
23. Meinhardt, A.; Hedger, M.P. Immunological, paracrine and endocrine aspects of testicular immune privilege. *Mol. Cell. Endocrinol.* **2011**, *335*, 60–68. [CrossRef]
24. Boussouar, F.; Benahmed, M. Lactate and energy metabolism in male germ cells. *Trends Endocrinol. Metab.* **2004**, *15*, 345–350. [CrossRef] [PubMed]
25. Cho, Y.M.; Kwon, S.; Pak, Y.K.; Seol, H.W.; Choi, Y.M.; Park, D.J.; Park, K.S.; Lee, H.K. Dynamic changes in mitochondrial biogenesis and antioxidant enzymes during the spontaneous differentiation of human embryonic stem cells. *Biochem. Biophys. Res. Commun.* **2006**, *348*, 1472–1478. [CrossRef] [PubMed]
26. Varuzhanyan, G.; Chan, D.C. Mitochondrial dynamics during spermatogenesis. *J. Cell. Sci.* **2020**, *133*, jcs235937. [CrossRef]
27. Hara, H.; Kuwano, K.; Araya, J. Mitochondrial Quality Control in COPD and IPF. *Cells* **2018**, *7*, 86. [CrossRef]
28. Rato, L.; Alves, M.G.; Socorro, S.; Duarte, A.I.; Cavaco, J.E.; Oliveira, P.F. Metabolic regulation is important for spermatogenesis. *Nat. Rev. Urol.* **2012**, *9*, 330–338. [CrossRef]

29. Bajpai, M.; Gupta, G.; Setty, B.S. Changes in carbohydrate metabolism of testicular germ cells during meiosis in the rat. *Eur. J. Endocrinol.* **1998**, *138*, 322–327. [CrossRef]
30. Handel, M.A.; Schimenti, J.C. Genetics of mammalian meiosis: Regulation, dynamics and impact on fertility. *Nat. Rev. Genet.* **2010**, *11*, 124–136. [CrossRef]
31. Meinhardt, A.; McFarlane, J.R.; Seitz, J.; de Kretser, D.M. Activin maintains the condensed type of mitochondria in germ cells. *Mol. Cell. Endocrinol.* **2000**, *168*, 111–117. [CrossRef] [PubMed]
32. Mannella, C.A. The relevance of mitochondrial membrane topology to mitochondrial function. *Biochim. Biophys. Acta* **2006**, *1762*, 140–147. [CrossRef] [PubMed]
33. Lee, J.; Richburg, J.H.; Younkin, S.C.; Boekelheide, K. The Fas system is a key regulator of germ cell apoptosis in the testis. *Endocrinology* **1997**, *138*, 2081–2088. [CrossRef]
34. Xiong, W.; Wang, H.; Wu, H.; Chen, Y.; Han, D. Apoptotic spermatogenic cells can be energy sources for Sertoli cells. *Reproduction* **2009**, *137*, 469–479. [CrossRef] [PubMed]
35. Li, L.; Shen, J.J.; Bournat, J.C.; Huang, L.; Chattopadhyay, A.; Li, Z.; Shaw, C.; Graham, B.H.; Brown, C.W. Activin signaling: Effects on body composition and mitochondrial energy metabolism. *Endocrinology* **2009**, *150*, 3521–3529. [CrossRef] [PubMed]
36. O'Shaughnessy, P.J. Hormonal control of germ cell development and spermatogenesis. *Semin. Cell Dev. Biol.* **2014**, *29*, 55–65. [CrossRef]
37. McLachlan, R.I.; O'Donnell, L.; Meachem, S.J.; Stanton, P.G.; de Kretser, D.M.; Pratis, K.; Robertson, D.M. Identification of specific sites of hormonal regulation in spermatogenesis in rats, monkeys, and man. *Recent. Prog. Horm. Res.* **2002**, *57*, 149–179. [CrossRef]
38. Flück, C.E.; Miller, W.L.; Auchus, R.J. The 17, 20-lyase activity of cytochrome p450c17 from human fetal testis favors the delta5 steroidogenic pathway. *J. Clin. Endocrinol. Metab.* **2003**, *88*, 3762–3766. [CrossRef]
39. Martin, L.A.; Kennedy, B.E.; Karten, B. Mitochondrial cholesterol: Mechanisms of import and effects on mitochondrial function. *J. Bioenerg. Biomembr.* **2016**, *48*, 137–151. [CrossRef]
40. Prince, F.P. Lamellar and tubular associations of the mitochondrial cristae: Unique forms of the cristae present in steroid-producing cells. *Mitochondrion* **2002**, *1*, 381–389. [CrossRef]
41. Breton, S.; Ruan, Y.C.; Park, Y.J.; Kim, B. Regulation of epithelial function, differentiation, and remodeling in the epididymis. *Asian J. Androl.* **2016**, *18*, 3–9. [CrossRef] [PubMed]
42. Brown, D.; Breton, S. Mitochondria-rich, proton-secreting epithelial cells. *J. Exp. Biol.* **1996**, *199*, 2345–2358. [CrossRef] [PubMed]
43. Leclerc, P.; de Lamirande, E.; Gagnon, C. Cyclic adenosine 3′,5′monophosphate-dependent regulation of protein tyrosine phosphorylation in relation to human sperm capacitation and motility. *Biol. Reprod.* **1996**, *55*, 684–692. [CrossRef] [PubMed]
44. de Lamirande, E.; Gagnon, C. Impact of reactive oxygen species on spermatozoa: A balancing act between beneficial and detrimental effects. *Hum. Reprod.* **1995**, *10* (Suppl. 1), 15–21. [CrossRef] [PubMed]
45. O'Flaherty, C. Peroxiredoxins: Hidden players in the antioxidant defence of human spermatozoa. *Basic. Clin. Androl.* **2014**, *24*, 4. [CrossRef]
46. O'Flaherty, C. Orchestrating the antioxidant defenses in the epididymis. *Andrology* **2019**, *7*, 662–668. [CrossRef]
47. Vernet, P.; Aitken, R.J.; Drevet, J.R. Antioxidant strategies in the epididymis. *Mol. Cell. Endocrinol.* **2004**, *216*, 31–39. [CrossRef]
48. Galantino-Homer, H.L.; Visconti, P.E.; Kopf, G.S. Regulation of protein tyrosine phosphorylation during bovine sperm capacitation by a cyclic adenosine 3′5′-monophosphate-dependent pathway. *Biol. Reprod.* **1997**, *56*, 707–719. [CrossRef]
49. Carrageta, D.F.; Guerra-Carvalho, B.; Sousa, M.; Barros, A.; Oliveira, P.F.; Monteiro, M.P.; Alves, M.G. Mitochondrial Activation and Reactive Oxygen-Species Overproduction during Sperm Capacitation are Independent of Glucose Stimuli. *Antioxidants* **2020**, *9*, 750. [CrossRef]
50. Zhang, G.; Yang, W.; Zou, P.; Jiang, F.; Zeng, Y.; Chen, Q.; Sun, L.; Yang, H.; Zhou, N.; Wang, X.; et al. Mitochondrial functionality modifies human sperm acrosin activity, acrosome reaction capability and chromatin integrity. *Hum. Reprod.* **2019**, *34*, 3–11. [CrossRef]
51. Boguenet, M.; Bouet, P.E.; Spiers, A.; Reynier, P.; May-Panloup, P. Mitochondria: Their role in spermatozoa and in male infertility. *Hum. Reprod. Update* **2021**, *27*, 697–719. [CrossRef] [PubMed]
52. Olson, G.E.; Winfrey, V.P. Mitochondria-cytoskeleton interactions in the sperm midpiece. *J. Struct. Biol.* **1990**, *103*, 13–22. [CrossRef] [PubMed]
53. Schmidt, H.; Carter, A.P. Review: Structure and mechanism of the dynein motor ATPase. *Biopolymers* **2016**, *105*, 557–567. [CrossRef]
54. Gu, N.H.; Zhao, W.L.; Wang, G.S.; Sun, F. Comparative analysis of mammalian sperm ultrastructure reveals relationships between sperm morphology, mitochondrial functions and motility. *Reprod. Biol. Endocrinol.* **2019**, *17*, 66. [CrossRef] [PubMed]
55. Baccetti, B.; Capitani, S.; Collodel, G.; Strehler, E.; Piomboni, P. Recent advances in human sperm pathology. *Contraception* **2002**, *65*, 283–287. [CrossRef] [PubMed]
56. Barbagallo, F.; La Vignera, S.; Cannarella, R.; Aversa, A.; Calogero, A.E.; Condorelli, R.A. Evaluation of Sperm Mitochondrial Function: A Key Organelle for Sperm Motility. *J. Clin. Med.* **2020**, *9*, 363. [CrossRef] [PubMed]
57. Gallon, F.; Marchetti, C.; Jouy, N.; Marchetti, P. The functionality of mitochondria differentiates human spermatozoa with high and low fertilizing capability. *Fertil. Steril.* **2006**, *86*, 1526–1530. [CrossRef] [PubMed]
58. Marchetti, P.; Ballot, C.; Jouy, N.; Thomas, P.; Marchetti, C. Influence of mitochondrial membrane potential of spermatozoa on in vitro fertilisation outcome. *Andrologia* **2012**, *44*, 136–141. [CrossRef]

59. Stendardi, A.; Focarelli, R.; Piomboni, P.; Palumberi, D.; Serafini, F.; Ferramosca, A.; Zara, V. Evaluation of mitochondrial respiratory efficiency during in vitro capacitation of human spermatozoa. *Int. J. Androl.* **2011**, *34*, 247–255. [CrossRef]
60. Nowicka-Bauer, K.; Nixon, B. Molecular Changes Induced by Oxidative Stress that Impair Human Sperm Motility. *Antioxidants* **2020**, *9*, 134. [CrossRef]
61. Koppers, A.J.; De Iuliis, G.N.; Finnie, J.M.; McLaughlin, E.A.; Aitken, R.J. Significance of mitochondrial reactive oxygen species in the generation of oxidative stress in spermatozoa. *J. Clin. Endocrinol. Metab.* **2008**, *93*, 3199–3207. [CrossRef] [PubMed]
62. O'Flaherty, C.; Matsushita-Fournier, D. Reactive oxygen species and protein modifications in spermatozoa. *Biol. Reprod.* **2017**, *97*, 577–585. [CrossRef] [PubMed]
63. Aitken, R.J.; Whiting, S.; De Iuliis, G.N.; McClymont, S.; Mitchell, L.A.; Baker, M.A. Electrophilic aldehydes generated by sperm metabolism activate mitochondrial reactive oxygen species generation and apoptosis by targeting succinate dehydrogenase. *J. Biol. Chem.* **2012**, *287*, 33048–33060. [CrossRef] [PubMed]
64. Aitken, R.J. Reactive oxygen species as mediators of sperm capacitation and pathological damage. *Mol. Reprod. Dev.* **2017**, *84*, 1039–1052. [CrossRef]
65. Aitken, R.J. Not every sperm is sacred; a perspective on male infertility. *Mol. Hum. Reprod.* **2018**, *24*, 287–298. [CrossRef]
66. Espino, J.; Mediero, M.; Lozano, G.M.; Bejarano, I.; Ortiz, A.; Garcia, J.F.; Pariente, J.A.; Rodriguez, A.B. Reduced levels of intracellular calcium releasing in spermatozoa from asthenozoospermic patients. *Reprod. Biol. Endocrinol.* **2009**, *7*, 11. [CrossRef]
67. Treulen, F.; Uribe, P.; Boguen, R.; Villegas, J.V. Mitochondrial permeability transition increases reactive oxygen species production and induces DNA fragmentation in human spermatozoa. *Hum. Reprod.* **2015**, *30*, 767–776. [CrossRef]
68. Barroso, G.; Taylor, S.; Morshedi, M.; Manzur, F.; Gavino, F.; Oehninger, S. Mitochondrial membrane potential integrity and plasma membrane translocation of phosphatidylserine as early apoptotic markers: A comparison of two different sperm subpopulations. *Fertil. Steril.* **2006**, *85*, 149–154. [CrossRef]
69. Espinoza, J.A.; Paasch, U.; Villegas, J.V. Mitochondrial membrane potential disruption pattern in human sperm. *Hum. Reprod.* **2009**, *24*, 2079–2085. [CrossRef]
70. Grunewald, S.; Sharma, R.; Paasch, U.; Glander, H.J.; Agarwal, A. Impact of caspase activation in human spermatozoa. *Microsc. Res. Tech.* **2009**, *72*, 878–888. [CrossRef]
71. Aitken, R.J.; Koppers, A.J. Apoptosis and DNA damage in human spermatozoa. *Asian J. Androl.* **2011**, *13*, 36–42. [CrossRef] [PubMed]
72. Wang, X.; Sharma, R.K.; Sikka, S.C.; Thomas, A.J., Jr.; Falcone, T.; Agarwal, A. Oxidative stress is associated with increased apoptosis leading to spermatozoa DNA damage in patients with male factor infertility. *Fertil. Steril.* **2003**, *80*, 531–535. [CrossRef] [PubMed]
73. Grunewald, S.; Fitzl, G.; Springsguth, C. Induction of ultra-morphological features of apoptosis in mature and immature sperm. *Asian J. Androl.* **2017**, *19*, 533–537. [CrossRef] [PubMed]
74. Paasch, U.; Grunewald, S.; Dathe, S.; Glander, H.J. Mitochondria of human spermatozoa are preferentially susceptible to apoptosis. *Ann. N. Y. Acad. Sci.* **2004**, *1030*, 403–409. [CrossRef] [PubMed]
75. Sakkas, D.; Ramalingam, M.; Garrido, N.; Barratt, C.L. Sperm selection in natural conception: What can we learn from Mother Nature to improve assisted reproduction outcomes? *Hum. Reprod. Update* **2015**, *21*, 711–726. [CrossRef]
76. Szymonowicz, K.; Oeck, S.; Malewicz, N.M.; Jendrossek, V. New Insights into Protein Kinase B/Akt Signaling: Role of Localized Akt Activation and Compartment-Specific Target Proteins for the Cellular Radiation Response. *Cancers* **2018**, *10*, 78. [CrossRef]
77. Koppers, A.J.; Mitchell, L.A.; Wang, P.; Lin, M.; Aitken, R.J. Phosphoinositide 3-kinase signalling pathway involvement in a truncated apoptotic cascade associated with motility loss and oxidative DNA damage in human spermatozoa. *Biochem. J.* **2011**, *436*, 687–698. [CrossRef]
78. Kujoth, G.C.; Hiona, A.; Pugh, T.D.; Someya, S.; Panzer, K.; Wohlgemuth, S.E.; Hofer, T.; Seo, A.Y.; Sullivan, R.; Jobling, W.A.; et al. Mitochondrial DNA mutations, oxidative stress, and apoptosis in mammalian aging. *Science* **2005**, *309*, 481–484. [CrossRef]
79. Jiang, M.; Kauppila, T.E.S.; Motori, E.; Li, X.; Atanassov, I.; Folz-Donahue, K.; Bonekamp, N.A.; Albarran-Gutierrez, S.; Stewart, J.B.; Larsson, N.G. Increased Total mtDNA Copy Number Cures Male Infertility Despite Unaltered mtDNA Mutation Load. *Cell. Metab.* **2017**, *26*, 429–436.e424. [CrossRef]
80. Brower, J.V.; Lim, C.H.; Jorgensen, M.; Oh, S.P.; Terada, N. Adenine nucleotide translocase 4 deficiency leads to early meiotic arrest of murine male germ cells. *Reproduction* **2009**, *138*, 463–470. [CrossRef]
81. Ieremiadou, F.; Rodakis, G.C. Correlation of the 4977 bp mitochondrial DNA deletion with human sperm dysfunction. *BMC Res. Notes* **2009**, *2*, 18. [CrossRef] [PubMed]
82. O'Connell, M.; McClure, N.; Lewis, S.E. A comparison of mitochondrial and nuclear DNA status in testicular sperm from fertile men and those with obstructive azoospermia. *Hum. Reprod.* **2002**, *17*, 1571–1577. [CrossRef] [PubMed]
83. Rajender, S.; Rahul, P.; Mahdi, A.A. Mitochondria, spermatogenesis and male infertility. *Mitochondrion* **2010**, *10*, 419–428. [CrossRef] [PubMed]
84. Faja, F.; Carlini, T.; Coltrinari, G.; Finocchi, F.; Nespoli, M.; Pallotti, F.; Lenzi, A.; Lombardo, F.; Paoli, D. Human sperm motility: A molecular study of mitochondrial DNA, mitochondrial transcription factor A gene and DNA fragmentation. *Mol. Biol. Rep.* **2019**, *46*, 4113–4121. [CrossRef]
85. Song, G.J.; Lewis, V. Mitochondrial DNA integrity and copy number in sperm from infertile men. *Fertil. Steril.* **2008**, *90*, 2238–2244. [CrossRef]

86. Wei, Y.-H.; Kao, S.-H. Mitochondrial DNA mutation and depletion are associated with decline of fertility and motility of human sperm. *Zool. Stud.* **2000**, *39*, 1–12.
87. Martinez-Heredia, J.; de Mateo, S.; Vidal-Taboada, J.M.; Ballesca, J.L.; Oliva, R. Identification of proteomic differences in asthenozoospermic sperm samples. *Hum. Reprod.* **2008**, *23*, 783–791. [CrossRef]
88. Parte, P.P.; Rao, P.; Redij, S.; Lobo, V.; D'Souza, S.J.; Gajbhiye, R.; Kulkarni, V. Sperm phosphoproteome profiling by ultra performance liquid chromatography followed by data independent analysis (LC-MS(E)) reveals altered proteomic signatures in asthenozoospermia. *J. Proteomics* **2012**, *75*, 5861–5871. [CrossRef]
89. Nowicka-Bauer, K.; Lepczynski, A.; Ozgo, M.; Kamieniczna, M.; Fraczek, M.; Stanski, L.; Olszewska, M.; Malcher, A.; Skrzypczak, W.; Kurpisz, M.K. Sperm mitochondrial dysfunction and oxidative stress as possible reasons for isolated asthenozoospermia. *J. Physiol. Pharmacol.* **2018**, *69*, 403–417. [CrossRef]
90. Siva, A.B.; Kameshwari, D.B.; Singh, V.; Pavani, K.; Sundaram, C.S.; Rangaraj, N.; Deenadayal, M.; Shivaji, S. Proteomics-based study on asthenozoospermia: Differential expression of proteasome alpha complex. *Mol. Hum. Reprod.* **2010**, *16*, 452–462. [CrossRef]
91. Camps, J.; Garcia-Heredia, A.; Hernandez-Aguilera, A.; Joven, J. Paraoxonases, mitochondrial dysfunction and non-communicable diseases. *Chem. Biol. Interact.* **2016**, *259*, 382–387. [CrossRef] [PubMed]
92. Cerda, C.; Sanchez, C.; Climent, B.; Vazquez, A.; Iradi, A.; El Amrani, F.; Bediaga, A.; Saez, G.T. Oxidative stress and DNA damage in obesity-related tumorigenesis. *Adv. Exp. Med. Biol.* **2014**, *824*, 5–17. [CrossRef] [PubMed]
93. Zhao, J.; Zhai, L.; Liu, Z.; Wu, S.; Xu, L. Leptin level and oxidative stress contribute to obesity-induced low testosterone in murine testicular tissue. *Oxid. Med. Cell. Longev.* **2014**, *2014*, 190945. [CrossRef] [PubMed]
94. Ferramosca, A.; Zara, V. Diet and Male Fertility: The Impact of Nutrients and Antioxidants on Sperm Energetic Metabolism. *Int. J. Mol. Sci.* **2022**, *23*, 2542. [CrossRef]
95. Lunetti, P.; Capobianco, L.; Zara, V.; Ferramosca, A. Physical Activity and Male Reproductive Function: A New Role for Gamete Mitochondria. *Exerc. Sport. Sci. Rev.* **2021**, *49*, 99–106. [CrossRef] [PubMed]
96. Siri-Tarino, P.W.; Sun, Q.; Hu, F.B.; Krauss, R.M. Saturated fat, carbohydrate, and cardiovascular disease. *Am. J. Clin. Nutr.* **2010**, *91*, 502–509. [CrossRef]
97. Saez, F.; Drevet, J.R. Dietary Cholesterol and Lipid Overload: Impact on Male Fertility. *Oxid. Med. Cell. Longev.* **2019**, *2019*, 4521786. [CrossRef]
98. Ferramosca, A.; Moscatelli, N.; Di Giacomo, M.; Zara, V. Dietary fatty acids influence sperm quality and function. *Andrology* **2017**, *5*, 423–430. [CrossRef]
99. Ferramosca, A.; Zara, V. Bioenergetics of mammalian sperm capacitation. *Biomed. Res. Int.* **2014**, *2014*, 902953. [CrossRef]
100. Ferramosca, A.; Conte, A.; Moscatelli, N.; Zara, V. A high-fat diet negatively affects rat sperm mitochondrial respiration. *Andrology* **2016**, *4*, 520–525. [CrossRef]
101. La Vignera, S.; Condorelli, R.; Vicari, E.; D'Agata, R.; Calogero, A.E. Diabetes mellitus and sperm parameters. *J. Androl.* **2012**, *33*, 145–153. [CrossRef] [PubMed]
102. Ferramosca, A.; Pinto Provenzano, S.; Montagna, D.D.; Coppola, L.; Zara, V. Oxidative stress negatively affects human sperm mitochondrial respiration. *Urology* **2013**, *82*, 78–83. [CrossRef] [PubMed]
103. Schleicher, E.; Gerdes, C.; Petersmann, A.; Muller-Wieland, D.; Muller, U.A.; Freckmann, G.; Heinemann, L.; Nauck, M.; Landgraf, R. Definition, Classification and Diagnosis of Diabetes Mellitus. *Exp. Clin. Endocrinol. Diabetes* **2022**, *130*, S1–S8. [CrossRef] [PubMed]
104. Ahmed, R.G. The Physiological and Biochemical Effects of Diabetes on The Balance between Oxidative Stress and Antioxidant Defense System. *Med. J. Islam. World Acad. Sci.* **2005**, *15*, 31–42.
105. Yu, T.; Robotham, J.L.; Yoon, Y. Increased production of reactive oxygen species in hyperglycemic conditions requires dynamic change of mitochondrial morphology. *Proc. Natl. Acad. Sci. USA* **2006**, *103*, 2653–2658. [CrossRef]
106. Rolo, A.P.; Palmeira, C.M. Diabetes and mitochondrial function: Role of hyperglycemia and oxidative stress. *Toxicol. Appl. Pharmacol.* **2006**, *212*, 167–178. [CrossRef]
107. Amaral, S.; Oliveira, P.J.; Ramalho-Santos, J. Diabetes and the impairment of reproductive function: Possible role of mitochondria and reactive oxygen species. *Curr. Diabetes Rev.* **2008**, *4*, 46–54. [CrossRef]
108. Saez Lancellotti, T.E.; Boarelli, P.V.; Monclus, M.A.; Cabrillana, M.E.; Clementi, M.A.; Espinola, L.S.; Cid Barria, J.L.; Vincenti, A.E.; Santi, A.G.; Fornes, M.W. Hypercholesterolemia impaired sperm functionality in rabbits. *PLoS ONE* **2010**, *5*, e13457. [CrossRef]
109. Carrageta, D.F.; Guerra-Carvalho, B.; Spadella, M.A.; Yeste, M.; Oliveira, P.F.; Alves, M.G. Animal models of male reproductive ageing to study testosterone production and spermatogenesis. *Rev. Endocr. Metab. Disord.* **2022**, *23*, 1341–1360. [CrossRef]
110. Sharma, R.; Agarwal, A.; Rohra, V.K.; Assidi, M.; Abu-Elmagd, M.; Turki, R.F. Effects of increased paternal age on sperm quality, reproductive outcome and associated epigenetic risks to offspring. *Reprod. Biol. Endocrinol.* **2015**, *13*, 35. [CrossRef]
111. Trifunovic, A.; Wredenberg, A.; Falkenberg, M.; Spelbrink, J.N.; Rovio, A.T.; Bruder, C.E.; Bohlooly, Y.M.; Gidlof, S.; Oldfors, A.; Wibom, R.; et al. Premature ageing in mice expressing defective mitochondrial DNA polymerase. *Nature* **2004**, *429*, 417–423. [CrossRef] [PubMed]
112. Jarak, I.; Almeida, S.; Carvalho, R.A.; Sousa, M.; Barros, A.; Alves, M.G.; Oliveira, P.F. Senescence and declining reproductive potential: Insight into molecular mechanisms through testicular metabolomics. *Biochim. Biophys. Acta Mol. Basis Dis.* **2018**, *1864*, 3388–3396. [CrossRef] [PubMed]

113. Anifandis, G.; Amiridis, G.; Dafopoulos, K.; Daponte, A.; Dovolou, E.; Gavriil, E.; Gorgogietas, V.; Kachpani, E.; Mamuris, Z.; Messini, C.I.; et al. The In Vitro Impact of the Herbicide Roundup on Human Sperm Motility and Sperm Mitochondria. *Toxics* **2017**, *6*, 2. [CrossRef] [PubMed]
114. Ferramosca, A.; Lorenzetti, S.; Di Giacomo, M.; Murrieri, F.; Coppola, L.; Zara, V. Herbicides glyphosate and glufosinate ammonium negatively affect human sperm mitochondria respiration efficiency. *Reprod. Toxicol.* **2021**, *99*, 48–55. [CrossRef] [PubMed]
115. Chohan, K.R.; Badawy, S.Z. Cigarette smoking impairs sperm bioenergetics. *Int. Braz. J. Urol.* **2010**, *36*, 60–65. [CrossRef] [PubMed]
116. Pacifici, R.; Altieri, I.; Gandini, L.; Lenzi, A.; Pichini, S.; Rosa, M.; Zuccaro, P.; Dondero, F. Nicotine, cotinine, and trans-3-hydroxycotinine levels in seminal plasma of smokers: Effects on sperm parameters. *Ther. Drug. Monit.* **1993**, *15*, 358–363. [CrossRef] [PubMed]
117. Collin, O.; Kilter, S.; Bergh, A. Tobacco smoke disrupts testicular microcirculation in the rat. *Int. J. Androl.* **1995**, *18*, 141–145. [CrossRef]
118. Evans, H.J.; Fletcher, J.; Torrance, M.; Hargreave, T.B. Sperm abnormalities and cigarette smoking. *Lancet* **1981**, *1*, 627–629. [CrossRef]
119. Vogt, H.J.; Heller, W.D.; Borelli, S. Sperm quality of healthy smokers, ex-smokers, and never-smokers. *Fertil. Steril.* **1986**, *45*, 106–110. [CrossRef]
120. Rantala, M.L.; Koskimies, A.I. Semen quality of infertile couples—Comparison between smokers and non-smokers. *Andrologia* **1987**, *19*, 42–46. [CrossRef]
121. Sofikitis, N.; Takenaka, M.; Kanakas, N.; Papadopoulos, H.; Yamamoto, Y.; Drakakis, P.; Miyagawa, I. Effects of cotinine on sperm motility, membrane function, and fertilizing capacity in vitro. *Urol. Res.* **2000**, *28*, 370–375. [CrossRef] [PubMed]
122. Zitzmann, M.; Rolf, C.; Nordhoff, V.; Schrader, G.; Rickert-Fohring, M.; Gassner, P.; Behre, H.M.; Greb, R.R.; Kiesel, L.; Nieschlag, E. Male smokers have a decreased success rate for in vitro fertilization and intracytoplasmic sperm injection. *Fertil. Steril.* **2003**, *79* (Suppl. 3), 1550–1554. [CrossRef] [PubMed]
123. Shi, Q.; Ko, E.; Barclay, L.; Hoang, T.; Rademaker, A.; Martin, R. Cigarette smoking and aneuploidy in human sperm. *Mol. Reprod. Dev.* **2001**, *59*, 417–421. [CrossRef] [PubMed]
124. Jozkow, P.; Rossato, M. The Impact of Intense Exercise on Semen Quality. *Am. J. Mens. Health* **2017**, *11*, 654–662. [CrossRef] [PubMed]
125. Hajizadeh Maleki, B.; Tartibian, B.; Chehrazi, M. Effects of Aerobic, Resistance, and Combined Exercise on Markers of Male Reproduction in Healthy Human Subjects: A Randomized Controlled Trial. *J. Strength Cond. Res.* **2019**, *33*, 1130–1145. [CrossRef]
126. Finkler, M.; Lichtenberg, D.; Pinchuk, I. The relationship between oxidative stress and exercise. *J. Basic Clin. Physiol. Pharmacol.* **2014**, *25*, 1–11. [CrossRef]
127. Powers, S.K.; Radak, Z.; Ji, L.L. Exercise-induced oxidative stress: Past, present and future. *J. Physiol.* **2016**, *594*, 5081–5092. [CrossRef]
128. Bloomer, R.J.; Goldfarb, A.H.; McKenzie, M.J. Oxidative stress response to aerobic exercise: Comparison of antioxidant supplements. *Med. Sci. Sports Exerc.* **2006**, *38*, 1098–1105. [CrossRef]
129. Finaud, J.; Lac, G.; Filaire, E. Oxidative stress: Relationship with exercise and training. *Sports Med.* **2006**, *36*, 327–358. [CrossRef]
130. Kocabas, R.; Namiduru, E.S.; Bagceci, A.M.; Erenler, A.K.; Karakoc, O.; Orkmez, M.; Akan, M.; Erdemli, H.K.; Taysi, S.; Tarakcioglu, M. The acute effects of interval exercise on oxidative stress and antioxidant status in volleyball players. *J. Sports Med. Phys. Fit.* **2018**, *58*, 421–427. [CrossRef]
131. Sharifi, G.; Najafabadi, A.B.; Ghashghaei, F.E. Oxidative stress and total antioxidant capacity in handball players. *Adv. Biomed. Res.* **2014**, *3*, 181. [CrossRef] [PubMed]
132. Slattery, K.; Bentley, D.; Coutts, A.J. The role of oxidative, inflammatory and neuroendocrinological systems during exercise stress in athletes: Implications of antioxidant supplementation on physiological adaptation during intensified physical training. *Sports Med.* **2015**, *45*, 453–471. [CrossRef] [PubMed]
133. Kraemer, W.J.; Fragala, M.S.; Watson, G.; Volek, J.S.; Rubin, M.R.; French, D.N.; Maresh, C.M.; Vingren, J.L.; Hatfield, D.L.; Spiering, B.A.; et al. Hormonal responses to a 160-km race across frozen Alaska. *Br. J. Sports Med.* **2008**, *42*, 116–120. [CrossRef] [PubMed]
134. Hooper, D.R.; Kraemer, W.J.; Stearns, R.L.; Kupchak, B.R.; Volk, B.M.; DuPont, W.H.; Maresh, C.M.; Casa, D.J. Evidence of the Exercise-Hypogonadal Male Condition at the 2011 Kona Ironman World Championships. *Int. J. Sports Physiol. Perform.* **2019**, *14*, 170–175. [CrossRef]
135. Song, Z.; Ghochani, M.; McCaffery, J.M.; Frey, T.G.; Chan, D.C. Mitofusins and OPA1 mediate sequential steps in mitochondrial membrane fusion. *Mol. Biol. Cell.* **2009**, *20*, 3525–3532. [CrossRef]
136. Smirnova, E.; Griparic, L.; Shurland, D.L.; van der Bliek, A.M. Dynamin-related protein Drp1 is required for mitochondrial division in mammalian cells. *Mol. Biol. Cell.* **2001**, *12*, 2245–2256. [CrossRef]
137. Varuzhanyan, G.; Rojansky, R.; Sweredoski, M.J.; Graham, R.L.J.; Hess, S.; Ladinsky, M.S.; Chan, D.C. Mitochondrial fusion is required for spermatogonial differentiation and meiosis. *eLife* **2019**, *8*, e51601. [CrossRef]
138. Senos Demarco, R.; Jones, D.L. Mitochondrial fission regulates germ cell differentiation by suppressing ROS-mediated activation of Epidermal Growth Factor Signaling in the Drosophila larval testis. *Sci. Rep.* **2019**, *9*, 19695. [CrossRef]

139. Shang, Y.; Wang, H.; Jia, P.; Zhao, H.; Liu, C.; Liu, W.; Song, Z.; Xu, Z.; Yang, L.; Wang, Y.; et al. Autophagy regulates spermatid differentiation via degradation of PDLIM1. *Autophagy* **2016**, *12*, 1575–1592. [CrossRef]
140. Kausar, S.; Wang, F.; Cui, H. The Role of Mitochondria in Reactive Oxygen Species Generation and Its Implications for Neurodegenerative Diseases. *Cells* **2018**, *7*, 274. [CrossRef]
141. Holecek, M. Why Are Branched-Chain Amino Acids Increased in Starvation and Diabetes? *Nutrients* **2020**, *12*, 3087. [CrossRef] [PubMed]
142. Darr, C.R.; Varner, D.D.; Teague, S.; Cortopassi, G.A.; Datta, S.; Meyers, S.A. Lactate and Pyruvate Are Major Sources of Energy for Stallion Sperm with Dose Effects on Mitochondrial Function, Motility, and ROS Production. *Biol. Reprod.* **2016**, *95*, 34. [CrossRef] [PubMed]
143. Storey, B.T.; Kayne, F.J. Energy metabolism of spermatozoa. VI. Direct intramitochondrial lactate oxidation by rabbit sperm mitochondria. *Biol. Reprod.* **1977**, *16*, 549–556. [PubMed]
144. Storey, B.T. Mammalian sperm metabolism: Oxygen and sugar, friend and foe. *Int. J. Dev. Biol.* **2008**, *52*, 427–437. [CrossRef] [PubMed]
145. Moraes, C.R.; Meyers, S. The sperm mitochondrion: Organelle of many functions. *Anim. Reprod. Sci.* **2018**, *194*, 71–80. [CrossRef]
146. Rodriguez-Gil, J.E.; Bonet, S. Current knowledge on boar sperm metabolism: Comparison with other mammalian species. *Theriogenology* **2016**, *85*, 4–11. [CrossRef]
147. Meyers, S.A. Cryostorage and Oxidative Stress in Mammalian Spermatozoa. In *Studies on Men's Health and Fertility*; Agarwal, A., Aitken, R.J., Alvarez, J.G., Eds.; Humana Press: Totowa, NJ, USA, 2012; pp. 41–56. [CrossRef]
148. Gibb, Z.; Lambourne, S.R.; Aitken, R.J. The paradoxical relationship between stallion fertility and oxidative stress. *Biol. Reprod.* **2014**, *91*, 77. [CrossRef]
149. Aitken, R.J.; Jones, K.T.; Robertson, S.A. Reactive oxygen species and sperm function—In sickness and in health. *J. Androl.* **2012**, *33*, 1096–1106. [CrossRef]
150. Yeste, M.; Estrada, E.; Rocha, L.G.; Marin, H.; Rodriguez-Gil, J.E.; Miro, J. Cryotolerance of stallion spermatozoa is related to ROS production and mitochondrial membrane potential rather than to the integrity of sperm nucleus. *Andrology* **2015**, *3*, 395–407. [CrossRef]

biology

MDPI

Review

The Low Survivability of Transplanted Gonadal Grafts: The Impact of Cryopreservation and Transplantation Conditions on Mitochondrial Function

Inês Moniz [1,2], Maria Soares [1,2], Ana Paula Sousa [2,3,4], João Ramalho-Santos [2,5] and Ana Branco [2,*]

1 Doctoral Programme in Experimental Biology and Biomedicine (PDBEB), Institute for Interdisciplinary Research, University of Coimbra, 3030-789 Coimbra, Portugal; inescmoniz@hotmail.com (I.M.)
2 CNC—Centre for Neuroscience and Cell Biology, CIBB—Centre for Innovative Biomedicine and Biotechnology, University of Coimbra, Azinhaga de Santa Comba, Polo 3, 3000-548 Coimbra, Portugal
3 Reproductive Medicine Unit, Unidade Local de Saúde de Coimbra, Praceta Prof. Mota Pinto, 3000-075 Coimbra, Portugal
4 Eugin Coimbra, Rua Filipe Hodart, 3000-185 Coimbra, Portugal
5 Department of Live Sciences, University of Coimbra, Calçada Martim de Freitas, 3000-456 Coimbra, Portugal
* Correspondence: abranco@fmed.uc.pt

Simple Summary: Gonadal tissue transplantation as a fertility preservation technique is highly conditioned by our current knowledge of functionality following transplantation, tissue cryodamage, and ischemia–reperfusion injury. This paper presents an updated review of the literature on mitochondrial dysfunction and oxidative stress in the context of gonadal tissue cryopreservation and transplantation.

Abstract: Advances in tissue preservation techniques have allowed reproductive medicine and assisted reproductive technologies (ARTs) to flourish in recent years. Because radio- and chemotherapy procedures are often gonadotoxic, irreversible damage can preclude future gamete production and endocrine support. Accordingly, in recent years, the freezing and storage of gonadal tissue fragments prior to the first oncological treatment appointment and autologous transplantation post-recovery have been considered improved solutions for fertility recovery in cancer survivors. Nevertheless, the cryopreservation and transplantation of thawed tissues is still very limited, and positive outcomes are relatively low. This review aims to discuss the limitations of oncofertility protocols with a focus on the impacts of mitochondrial dysfunction, oxidative stress, and the loss of antioxidant defense in graft integrity.

Keywords: oncofertility; cryopreservation; transplantation; mitochondrial dysfunction; oxidative stress; fertility preservation

1. Fertility Preservation in Oncological Patients

Fertility preservation has evolved considerably in the past two decades. Young patients with cancer undergoing radiotherapy, systemic chemotherapy, and/or oncological gonadectomy can have their fertility severely compromised, as most of these therapeutic approaches target not only malignant cells, but also a wide variety of healthy cells. With chemotherapy, the loss of reproductive function can occur in a cell-cycle-dependent manner—with the usage of antimetabolites (e.g., Cytarabine)—or in a cell-cycle-independent manner—with anthracyclins, alkylating, and/or platinum agents [1–3]. These highly aggressive drugs can have short- and long-term effects on the ovary, starting with primordial follicle atresia and apoptosis and culminating in inflammation and vascular and stromal injury, permanently disrupting estradiol production and altering the follicular reserve [1,3]. In the testis, these compounds can damage the germinal epithelium and target Leydig and proliferating spermatogonial stem cells (SSCs), disrupting sperm and hormone production and ultimately contributing to infertility [4,5].

Radiotherapy to the head and neck is potentially damaging to the hypothalamus–pituitary axis and to the central nervous system (hindering gonadotropin production), whereas exposure to the pelvic and abdominal regions can directly damage the highly sensitive testes and ovaries [6,7].

In a 2018 survey, more than 60% of all cancer patients monitored reported a strong desire to have children [8], while a 2023 survey involving pediatric patients found that more than 50% of all questionees wished to have children in the future [9]. Therefore, all patients should be counseled about the possible risks of infertility before beginning oncological treatment to guarantee full awareness of all available options.

For post-pubertal men, sperm cryopreservation and banking have been viable options for several decades. Nevertheless, these approaches are unviable for non-sperm-producing pre-pubertal patients with cancer [10]. In such cases, there have been ongoing clinical trials focused on the possibility of cryopreserving testicular tissue (TT) containing SSCs. This experimental protocol encompasses a unilateral orchiectomy or an open testicular biopsy to collect the testicular tissue and carry out its preparation and fragmentation, the embedding in cryoprotectant solution, and its ensuing cryopreservation. After completing all oncological treatments, the preserved tissue is thawed and grafted to homotopic or ectopic sites (e.g., peritoneal space) [5,11,12]. This provides cancer survivors with a tool to recover hormone production and restore spermatogenesis. Fayomi and colleagues recently proved that the autologous transplantation of cryopreserved testicular tissue into a priorly damaged (through chemotherapy) testis could recover the endocrine function and fertility of non-human primates [13]. As of 2023, the cryopreservation of testicular tissue from pre- and post-pubertal patients has been reported in more than 700 patients worldwide [10–14]. Thus, although still mostly experimental, testicular tissue cryopreservation might be a possible method of preserving germ cell lines in pre-pubertal patients [11,12,15].

Contrastingly, the cryopreservation of unfertilized mature oocytes is the most established fertility preservation option for adult women [2,10]. This method allows patients to preserve oocytes in the absence of a reproductive partner, proving an advantage over the cryopreservation of fertilized eggs [2]. However, to complete fertilization, this option requires intracytoplasmic sperm injection (ICSI) and follicular phase controlled ovarian stimulation, which is inconceivable in young patients and many times impractical in adults due to the urgency to begin oncological treatments. Most importantly, oocyte cryopreservation fails to legitimately restore reproductive independence and ovarian and endocrine function to cancer survivors [2]. Instead, patients can opt to cryopreserve ovarian tissue grafts for future autologous transplantation. This protocol encompasses a surgical laparoscopy or laparotomy, followed by the segmentation of the collected tissue into small transplantable fragments, the equilibration of the tissue in a cryoprotectant solution, and, finally, the cryopreservation of the prepared grafts by slow-freezing or vitrification [16–18]. Contrary to testicular tissue cryopreservation, ovarian tissue banking is no longer experimental, and since the first human birth registered in 2004, it has allowed patients—even those unqualified for ovarian stimulation and IVF—to successfully preserve thousands of immature follicles [17–19]. After completing all oncological treatments, the tissues are thawed, cleansed of their cryoprotective media, and transplanted back into the remaining ovary, eventually restoring the patient's fertility and endocrine function. A 2022 meta-analysis that included 735 women throughout 87 distinct studies estimated that this fertility preservation technique summed a pooled success rate of 37% for pregnancies and 28% for life births [13,20]. Endocrine function—indicated by the production of estrogen, follicle-stimulating hormone (FSH), luteinizing hormone (LH), and anti-Müllerian hormone (AMH)—was recovered in most of the cases, validating this protocol as a reasonably reliable tool for cancer survivors [20,21].

Regardless, pregnancy and live birth rates continue to be subpar in patients who undergo these procedures, so it is important to notice that the cryopreservation of human samples for future clinical application—whether cellular or tissue in nature—is still highly conditioned by our current understanding of the mechanisms behind cryodamage and ischemia–reperfusion (I/R) injury.

2. Cryopreservation: Principles of Cryopreservation and Known Limitations

Cryopreservation is the process whereby living cells, tissues, or organs can be stored for an indeterminate amount of time in sub-zero temperatures while maintaining structure, viability, and biological function in a transiently quiescent state [22,23]. Most cryopreservation techniques follow the same core principles, starting with bathing the tissue in a cryoprotectant (CPA) solution, followed by slow-freezing or vitrification, and ending with storage in liquid nitrogen [24]. This first step is essential for the successful banking of biological samples, as it impedes ice crystal formation and physical and osmotic injury that disrupts cellular membranes and intracellular structures [23,25]. Most cryoprotectant solutions can be categorized into permeating CPAs—which include glycerol, dimethyl sulfoxide (DMSO), ethylene glycol (EG), and 1,2-propanediol (PROH)—and non-permeating CPAs—such as sugars (e.g., sucrose and trehalose) and proteins (e.g., human serum albumin (HSA)) [26–29].

The preservation of complex tissues can be an especially arduous process. Whereas with single-cell-line cryopreservation, the main obstacle is to maintain the cell's internal architecture and to suspend all biological function, with complex tissues—many times comprising different cell lines and organized structures and vessels—there is a need to uniformly preserve each cell type, their three-dimensional organization, and biochemical activity, while also taking into account that cells from different natures might respond differently to specific CPAs and cryogenic temperatures [23,30,31]. Diffusion through multicellular structures can be hindered by differing membrane permeabilities and complexities; ergo, each cryopreservation protocol must be designed and optimized according to the particularities of the target tissue [23,30]. Moreover, composite tissues are also susceptible to damage caused by the formation of ice crystals and osmotic injury.

Cryoprotectants can, for the most part, prevent cryodamage by limiting water transport and by stopping ice crystal formation [26–28]. However, CPAs can also contribute to cell toxicity during cryopreservation [28,32,33]. Thus, recent efforts have focused on exploring new techniques that might mitigate the damage caused by the freezing process and by the cytotoxicity inherent to the usage of CPAs [34,35].

2.1. Cryodamage: Mitochondrial Dysfunction and Oxidative Stress

Under homeostatic conditions, mitochondria generate adenosine triphosphate (ATP) via oxidative phosphorylation (OXPHOS), with the passage of electrons being carried out through the electron transport chain (ETC); at the final complex, the electrons are delivered from cytochrome c oxidase to molecular oxygen (O_2), reducing it to water (H_2O) [36–38]. Throughout this process, the leak of electrons from the ETC (0.1–2% of the total electron transport) can, instead, precociously reduce molecular O_2 to the free radical superoxide ($O_2^{\bullet-}$) that, in turn, can be converted into hydrogen peroxide (H_2O_2) by superoxide dismutases (SODs) [36–38]. In normal physiological levels, $O_2^{\bullet-}$ and H_2O_2 can participate in numerous redox pathways to eliminate invading microorganisms [39,40]. Under cryogenic temperatures, however, ROS production can escalate to dangerous levels (Figure 1).

Throughout the freezing protocol, the cell enters a metabolically dormant state, where mitochondrial ATP is not produced. During this time, the mitochondria can undergo a permeability transition, resulting in swelling that, in extreme cases, culminates in the rupture of the mitochondrial membrane [41,42]. The consequent release of proteins from ruptured organelles activates caspases and nucleases to initiate apoptosis. In fact, several reports reveal that cryopreserved samples can suffer mitochondrial dysfunction, concurrent with a great decrease in ATP synthesis and a surge in the generation of mitochondrial ROS (mtROS) [42–45]. Excess $O_2^{\bullet-}$ drives the export of cytochrome c from the mitochondria into the cytosol, where it binds to Apaf-1 to form apoptosomes that, in turn, activate caspase-9 to trigger apoptosis [37,45,46]. Likewise, surplus H_2O_2 can undergo the Fenton reaction—triggered by Fe(II) salts—to generate the highly reactive hydroxyl (•OH); this free radical can cleave the covalent bounds in proteins and carbohydrates to induce DNA damage and disrupt chromosomal alignment and microtubule formation in metaphase II mouse oocytes [40,45,46].

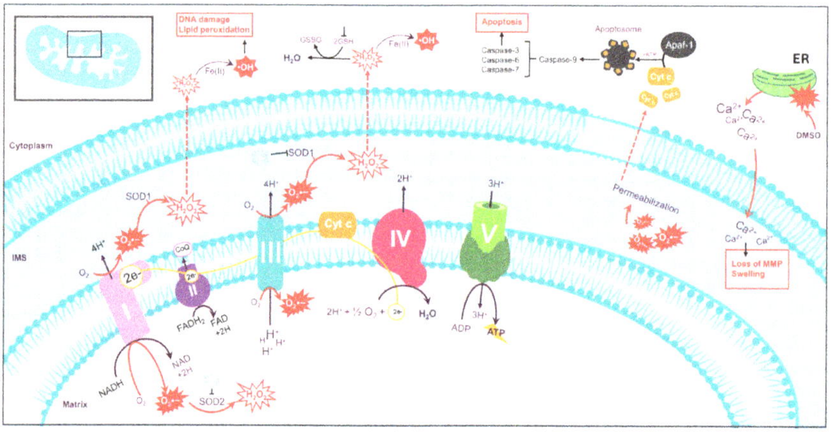

Figure 1. The generation of mitochondrial ROS under cryogenic conditions. The electrons (e-) are transported through the ETC (complex I, complex II, coenzyme Q (CoQ), complex III, cytochrome c (Cyt c), and complex IV) to ultimately produce ATP (complex V). Under cryogenic conditions, the leak of electrons from the ETC reduces O_2 to $O_2^{\bullet-}$. Excess $O_2^{\bullet-}$ alters the mitochondrial membrane's permeability, resulting in the release of cytochrome c (Cyt c) to the cytosol. Cyt c interacts with Apaf-1 to form the apoptosome that, in turn, activates caspase-9 to trigger the caspase cascade and initiate apoptosis. $O_2^{\bullet-}$ is converted to H_2O_2 by superoxide dismutase 1 (SOD1) on the mitochondrial intermembrane space (IMS) and by superoxide dismutase 2 (SOD2) on the mitochondrial matrix. Under cryogenic conditions, the activity of both SODs is inhibited. H_2O_2 can traverse to the outer mitochondrial membrane, where it is converted to the highly damaging •OH. GSH fails to degrade H_2O_2 in cryogenic conditions. DMSO elicits ER stress, resulting in the mass release of Ca^+. The excessive internalization of Ca^+ by the mitochondria results in mitochondrial swelling and the loss of MMP. Abbreviations: NAD (nicotinamide adenine dinucleotide); FAD (flavin adenine dinucleotide); and GSSG (glutathione disulfide).

It is important to note that the freezing–thawing cycle also strongly reduces SOD activity and the expression of intracellular glutathione (GSH) [47,48]. While SOD catalyzes the removal of $O_2^{\bullet-}$, GSH is responsible for degrading H_2O_2 [40]. Thus, by lowering SOD and GSH activity, cryopreservation compromises the cells' antioxidant defenses and leaves them vulnerable to further oxidative damage.

CPAs fail to protect the cell against oxidative stress and, alone, can be a source of ROS. For instance, DMSO is known to illicit endoplasmic reticulum (ER) stress that results in the exacerbated release of Ca^{2+} from the ER. The excess ions are then incorporated by the mitochondria, where they prompt mitochondrial Ca^{2+} overload, swelling, and loss of mitochondrial membrane potential (MMP). In concert, these alterations magnify the generation of ROS in a redundant and vicious cycle [49,50]. Ultimately, there is still a need to develop new strategies that mitigate mitochondrial dysfunction and oxidative damage caused by the currently established cryopreservation techniques.

2.2. Freezing Conditions and the Mitochondrial Health of Reproductive Tissues

With ovarian tissue cryopreservation (OTC), follicle loss begins with the mechanical damage intrinsic to the initial preparation of the tissue. After the ovary is collected, the ovarian medulla is removed so that only a thin section of the cortex remains. This fragmentation facilitates the rapid penetration of the CPAs into the tissue, reducing the formation of ice crystals and effectively minimizing the harm caused by low temperatures. Naturally, during this thinning process, the largest developing follicles, including most of the primary, secondary, and antral follicles, are lost [49]. Following preparation, the tissue is exposed to second and third aggressors, the cytotoxic CPAs, and sub-zero temperatures. Historically, the first report of a human life birth after OTC used DMSO (1.5 mmol/L) and followed a slow-freezing protocol [19]. Most techniques now employ a combination of permeating and non-permeating CPAs. Additionally, given the significant stromal cell damage and follicle loss observed during most slow-freezing protocols, vitrification has emerged as a promising alternative to store OT. This approach involves ultra-swift cooling in the presence of concentrated CPAs, inducing an ice-free, glassy, amorphous state that effectively preserves stromal integrity and safeguards the sample against cellular damage. Vitrification assures a more efficient alternative to slow-freezing, particularly in regard to the preservation of secondary follicles and stromal cells, as it minimizes the damage caused to granulosa cells in secondary follicles (Table 1) [50,51].

Table 1. Most used protocols and CPA concentrations for human OT cryopreservation.

Freezing Technique	CPA	Working Concentration	Reference
Slow-freezing	DMSO	0.0015–1.5 M	[19,50,52,53]
	EG	1.5 M	[32,52]
	PROH	1.26–1.5 M	[21,52,54,55]
	Glycerol	1.5 M	[32,52]
	Sucrose	0.1–0.175 M	[21,54]
Vitrification	DMSO	2 M; 20%	[56,57]
	EG	17–38%	[56,58–60]
	Trehalose	0.2–0.5 M	[57,59]
	Sucrose	0.175–1 M	[55,56,58,60]

It has been hypothesized that primordial follicles are the most resistant to cryogenic conditions since they have lowered metabolic activity. Studies carried out on different animal models confirmed that the mitochondria of oocytes contained within cryopreserved OT exhibited ultrastructural abnormalities, including the loss of cristae, granulated matrixes, swelling, and degeneration [61–63]. Simultaneously, the neighboring stromal cells presented loss of intracellular organelles, vacuolization, and similar mitochondrial abnormalities [62,63]. Other studies identified a significant loss of MMP and a decrease in mitochondrial OXPHOS in oocytes and stromal cells from cryopreserved-thawed OT, respectively [62,64]. In OT grafts, mitochondrial dysfunction is progressively more evident in its inner sections, closer to where the medulla was removed, rather than the outer sections [21]. Coincidently, follicle loss during OTC protocols is more marked in the medullar area [16,21]. In a recent study, Wu and colleagues reported that transplanted cryopreserved OT suffered a higher decline in follicle reserve when compared to transplanted fresh OT [64]. These results are consistent with those obtained by Rodrigues et al., who found that cryopreservation markedly decreased the tissues' global oxygen consumption rates and the number of morphologically intact follicles—especially in tissues undergoing transplantation after being previously cryopreserved (transplanted-cryopreserved) [65]. Conjointly, these studies confirm that OTC directly impacts the graft's ability to survive transplantation with its initial follicle pool intact, probably due to a decline in mitochondrial function and a reduced ability to meet the required energetic demands to survive transplantation. As described in the previous section, in frozen samples, mitochondrial dysfunction is accompanied by a corresponding increase in the generation of ROS. Studies show that slow frozen OT displays abnormally high levels of ROS, known to interact and damage lipids, proteins, and nucleic acids, prompting phospholipidic membrane disruption and DNA double-strand breakage [58,64,65]. Such alterations potentiate telomere shortening and the occurrence of spindle malformations and chromosomal abnormalities that not only contribute to tissue injury and stromal death, but also to a decline in oocyte quality [58,64,65] (Figure 1).

As a mostly experimental procedure, there is still no consensus regarding the freezing conditions, the type and concentration of CPAs used, or the thawing/warming protocols followed when cryopreserving testicular tissue. The few trials conducted with humans used a combination of permeating and non-permeating CPAs at varying concentrations to minimize individual cytotoxicity (Table 2).

Table 2. Most used protocols and CPA concentrations for human TT cryopreservation.

Freezing Technique	CPA	Working Concentration	Reference
Slow-freezing	DMSO	0.7 M; 5%	[5,11,66,67]
	EG	1.5 M	[68,69]
	PROH	1.5 M	[5]
	HSA	5%; 10 mg/mL	[11,66]
	Glycerol	6%	[5]
	Sucrose	0.1 M	[5,67–69]
Vitrification	DMSO	2.8 M; 15%	[67,70]
	EG	2.8 M; 15%	[67,70]
	HSA	25 mg/mL	[67,70]
	Sucrose	0.5 M	[67]

Nevertheless, these few studies demonstrated that these storing conditions contribute to structural damage to the seminiferous tubes and ultrastructural changes to spermatogonia and SCs, as evidenced by increased vacuolization and dilated mitochondrial cristae [5,66]. In animal models, different reports also attest to mitochondrial damage connected to a wide variety of testicular tissue cryopreservation (TTC) conditions. In fact, studies demonstrated that most CPAs promote the formation of free radicals and lipid peroxides [71,72]. As with OTC, TT slow-freezing protocols lead to intracellular ice crystal formation and high levels of ROS that damage sperm cell integrity, membranes, DNA structure, and mitochondrial function [73]. After thawing, TT samples can also exhibit germ cell DNA fragmentation, mitochondrial dysfunction, a lowered MMP, and increased ROS levels concurrent to a decrease in cell viability, cytolysis, and tissue disintegration [71,74–76]. Moreover, by severely decreasing the GSH content and SOD and CAT activity, TTC also contributes to the loss of antioxidant capacity, increasing the potential damage to these structures [75,77].

3. The Transplantation of Cryopreserved Gonadal Tissues: The Effects of Ischemia/Reperfusion (I/R) on Reproductive Cells, Mitochondrial Function, and Tissue Integrity

Although cryopreservation damages gonadal tissues, it is important to stress that mass gamete loss occurs primarily after the transplantation of the preserved graft. Indeed, several studies report that follicle loss in ovarian grafts occurs essentially after autotransplantation [49,78]. Some estimate that transplantation is responsible for the loss of 26%

of the primordial follicle reserve and up to 75% of all follicle loss during these fertility preservation protocols; this is mostly attributed to I/R injury (IRI) [49,52].

The ovarian graft is first exposed to ischemia when it is removed from the ovary and separated from its original nutrient and oxygen supply. Without vascular anastomosis, the tissue remains ischemic since angiogenesis and revascularization are only complete after an average of 10 days [78]. During this ischemic period, the OT is susceptible to hypoxic damage. Deprived of O_2, ATP production through OXPHOs is interrupted, and a more glycolytic anaerobic metabolism is induced. This causes the ATP levels to plummet and results in the reduction in redox-active enzymes and ETC carriers (e.g., NADH and coenzyme Q) [79,80]. Hypoxic cells are unable to meet the energetic demands required to keep the tissue healthy, although primordial follicles are marginally more resistant to hypoxic injury and can remain intact even when surrounded by damaged cortical stromal cells [81]. Nevertheless, hypoxic injury triggers the production of ROS and the release of cytokines and growth factors (e.g., TGF-β and TNF-α) that promote apoptosis and the recruitment of immune cells to initiate an inflammatory response [82]. Meanwhile, there is a build-up of metabolic products (such as lactate and succinate)—which cause metabolic acidosis—and a rise in the production of hypoxanthine and lipid peroxides [83–86]. With revascularization, the reestablishment of blood vessels sends a rush of said products to the tissue; succinate is quickly oxidized, causing the mass production of $O_2^{\bullet-}$ via reverse electron transport, whereas xanthine oxidase catalyzes the oxidation of the produced hypoxanthine to xanthine in a reaction that reduces O_2 to form $O_2^{\bullet-}$ and H_2O_2 [79,84,85,87]. This burst of ROS causes damage to proteins and nucleic acids and leads to the peroxidation of lipids that disrupts cell membrane integrity; these ROS are also responsible for the activation of the mitochondrial permeability transition pore (MPTP), which allows for the release of mitochondrial apoptotic and inflammatory cytokines—such as cytochrome c and TNF-α, respectively—which trigger apoptotic and inflammatory pathways [80,83,85,88,89].

Regardless, primordial follicle loss post-transplantation is not exclusively caused by cell death and tissue injury. Numerous reports confirm that after surgery, a great number of inactive follicles undergo premature activation as early as 3 days post-transplantation. With ischemia and oxidative stress, there is a corresponding release of insulin-like growth factor-1 (IGF-1) and hypoxia-inducible factor-1 (HIF-1) that stimulate the rise in granulosa cell proliferation and follicle growth, concurrent to early primordial follicle activation [50,89,90]. This "follicle burnout" depletes the pool of dormant follicles and compromises the long-term reproductive function of the patient [91]. In concert, ischemia and reperfusion provoke mitochondrial alterations that can be directly connected to OT inflammation, degeneration, edema, vascular congestion, and early follicle activation, and can thus be considered greatly responsible for the decline in ovarian reserve observed in transplanted ovarian grafts (Figure 2) [80].

Similar results have been reported in the limited studies focused on TT transplantation. Accordingly, transplantation, rather than cryopreservation, is also to blame for the significant loss of spermatogonia observed in grafted TT. After the removal of the testicular strips from the testis, and during the ischemic period before revascularization, ATP production through the ETC declines, and the levels of hypoxanthine rise [92]. This is consistent with a recent report that attested to a significant loss of SSCs during the ischemic period, concurrent with tubule degeneration at the center of the graft [12]. The angiogenesis of testicular grafts can be completed within 7 days after transplantation; the reestablishment of the blood supply to the transplant causes a burst in ROS production that increases oxidative stress. This, in turn, activates mitogen-activated protein kinases and furthers lipid peroxidation, protein and DNA damage, and the initiation of apoptotic pathways [92,93].

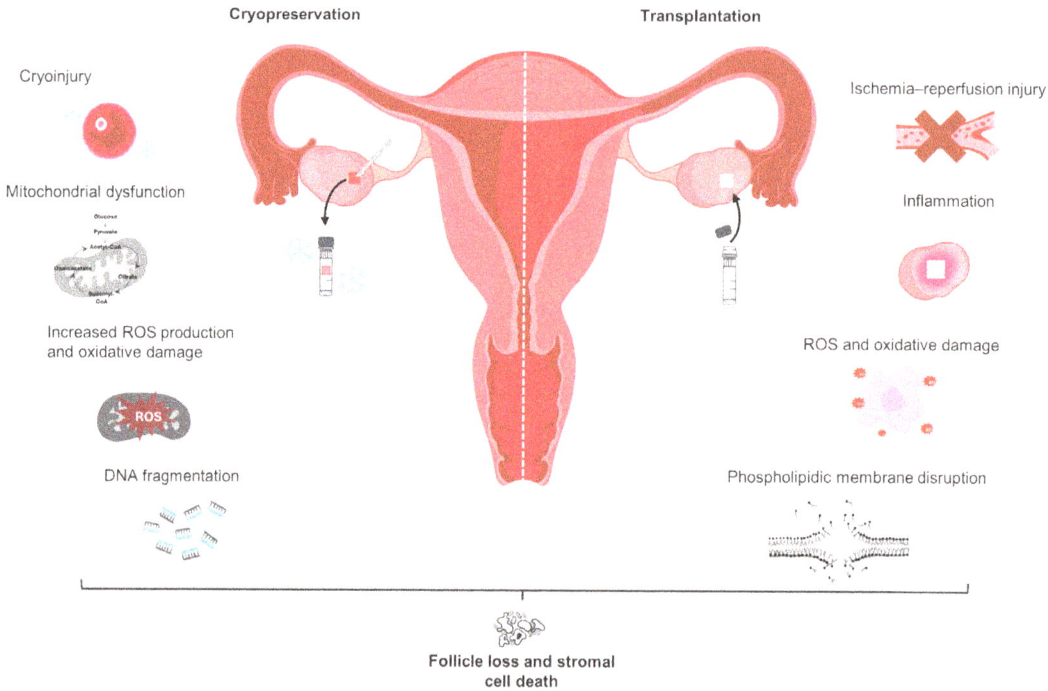

Figure 2. Cryopreservation and transplantation damage to ovarian tissue.

4. Prevention against Cryodamage

Multiple complementary approaches involve enhancing cryoprotectant solutions with supplements such as antioxidants, hormones, and anti-apoptotic agents. For instance, the combination of N-acetylcysteine (NAC) and pulsed electromagnetic fields (PEMFs) in vitrified mouse ovarian tissue demonstrated a synergistic effect in promoting angiogenesis and protecting the OT against oxidative stress and inflammation [94]. On the other hand, antioxidants such as vitamin E or selenium have been shown to mitigate oxidative stress during the freezing and thawing processes. In ducks, the administration of the antioxidant resveratrol, before cryopreservation, significantly upregulated the expressions of the VEGF, HIF-1α, Nrf2, CAT, and Bcl-2 mRNA genes, which are associated with increased antioxidant capacity (via SOD, CAT, and GSH peroxidase upregulation), decreased apoptosis, and enhanced angiogenesis post-transplantation [95].

Alternatively, pre-conditioning techniques such as ischemic preconditioning or hormonal priming can be applied to augment graft survival and function in the subsequent post-transplantation phase. The combined use of the hormone FSH and the anti-apoptotic agent S1P during vitrification has been shown to preserve the primordial follicle pool and suppress apoptosis [96]. The use of the anti-freezing protein during the warming procedure can also prevent OT damage and improve ovarian follicle morphology and apoptosis [97] (Table 3).

Table 3. Methods proposed to mitigate cryodamage to OT fragments.

Author, Date	Model	Treatment	Main Findings
Bedaiwy et al., 2006 [98]	Human	Slow-freezing; intact ovary with vascular pedicle; DMSO	75% and 78% primordial follicle viability
Westphal et al., 2017 [99]	Bovine, human	Slow-freezing; perfusion and submersion in DMSO	90–100% protection against cryodamage
Lee et al., 2021 [100]	Human	Slow-freezing; Z-VAD-FMK	Improved follicle preservation Improved follicular cell proliferation Prevention against DNA damage
Terren et al., 2021 [101]	Mouse	Slow-freezing; rapamycin and LY294002	Preservation of primordial follicle reserve
Kong et al., 2021 [97]	Bovine	Vitrification; anti-freezing protein (AFP)	↑ OT quality after xenotransplant Prevention against OT damage and apoptosis Improvement in follicle morphology
Rasaeifar et al., 2023 [94]	Mouse	Vitrification; NAC and PEMF	↑ angiogenesis Protection against oxidative stress Protection against inflammation
Wang et al., 2023 [96]	Mouse	Vitrification; FSH and S1P	Preservation of the primordial follicle pool ↓ follicular atresia Suppression of cell apoptosis
Qin et al., 2023 [95]	Duck	Vitrification; resveratrol	↑ VEGF, HIF-1α, Nrf2, CAT, and Bcl-2 mRNA expression ↓ TUNEL-positive cells

↑ Increase; ↓ Decrease.

With testicular tissue, most studies have addressed the need for optimizing CPA solutions and concentrations. DMSO is considered more effective for immature TT—which is more susceptible to CPA toxicity—whereas EG has been indicated for adult TT more [30]. Supplementation with trehalose has also been consistently reported to harbor positive results when it comes to reducing the number of apoptotic cells—via BAX downregulation and BCL-2 upregulation—and preserving testosterone production by cryopreserved Leydig cells [75,102–104]. This compound is known to promote the activity of SOD and CAT, antioxidant enzymes that protect cells against cryogenic-associated oxidative damage [75]. By contrast, vitamin A was reported to preserve SSC differentiation capacity and global cell division in TT while preventing spermatid DNA damage and nuclear alterations, ultimately promoting a higher spermatic yield [105] (Table 4; Figure 3).

Table 4. Methods proposed to mitigate cryodamage to TT fragments.

Author, Date	Model	Treatment	Main Findings
Zhang et al., 2015 [75]	Bovine	Slow-freezing; trehalose	↑ Viability ↑ Antioxidant enzyme activity (SOD and CAT) ↓ Oxidative damage
Dumont et al., 2016 [105]	Mouse	Vitrification; vitamin A	↑ Tissue development Improved differentiation of SSCs ↑ Cell division ↓ DNA damage ↓ Round spermatid nuclear alterations

Table 4. *Cont.*

Author, Date	Model	Treatment	Main Findings
Xi et al., 2019 [102]	Goat	Slow-freezing; trehalose	↓ Apoptosis Downregulation of BAX Upregulation of BCL-2, CREM, BOULE and HSP70-2 ↑ Testosterone production by Leydig cells
Jung et al., 2020 [103]	Monkey	Slow-freezing; trehalose, hypotaurine, necrostatin-1, melatonin	↑ Tissue viability ↓ Apoptosis
Zhu et al., 2021 [104]	Bovine	Slow-freezing; trehalose and KSR; uncontrolled slow-freezing	↓ Apoptosis ↑ Cell viability Preservation of structural integrity and seminiferous epithelial cohesion Maintenance of SSCs germline characteristics

↑ Increase; ↓ Decrease.

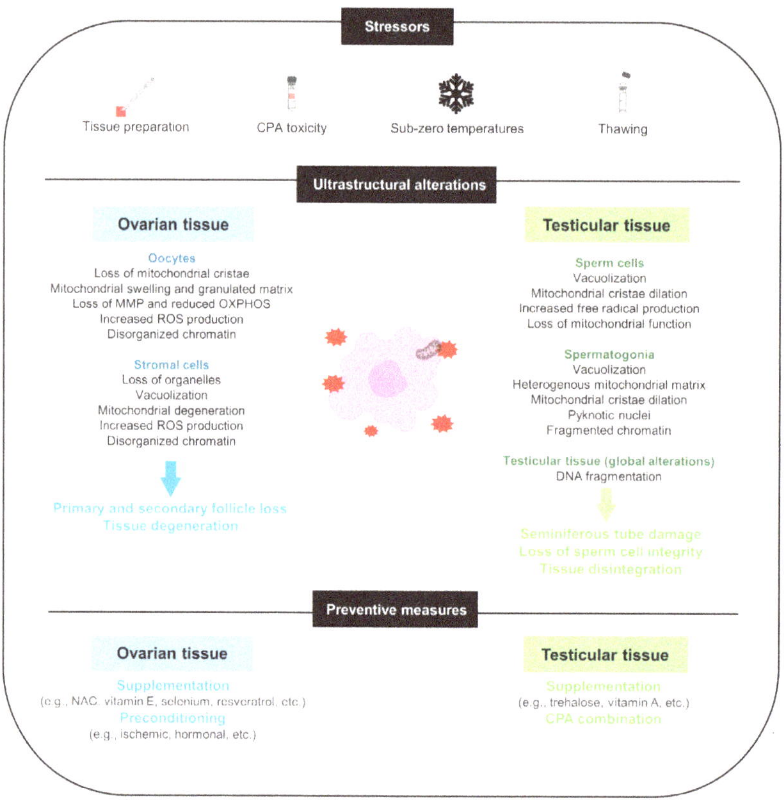

Figure 3. Gonadal tissue cryodamage and preventive measures.

5. Prevention against Ischemic Damage in Transplanted Gonadal Grafts

As previously discussed, the primary challenge encountered during gonadal tissue transplantation is ischemia and ischemia–reperfusion injury. Therefore, efforts have been primarily focused on reducing the damage caused by inadequate blood supply rather than on solely preventing cryoinjury.

In mice, the administration of hormones such as erythropoietin increased angiogenesis, reduced ischemic damage, decreased fibrosis, and maintained ovarian follicle proliferation after transplantation [106]. Taurine, on the other hand, was found to decrease oxidative stress and apoptosis and expedite angiogenesis by augmenting CD31 expression (Figure 4) [107]. In this context, the pro-angiogenic growth factor VEGF also has a prominent role in follicle growth as it promotes endothelial proliferation and triggers signaling pathways crucial for early follicle activation. These pathways include PI3K/Akt and the mammalian target of rapamycin (mTOR) [108]. Hence, as master regulators of primordial follicle recruitment, the pharmacological inhibition of PI3K—using LY294002—or the suppression of mTOR—using rapamycin or the NGF inhibitor K252a—was revealed to safeguard the tissue against follicle pool depletion and overexhaustion by effectively preventing the premature activation of primordial follicles from their dormant state [56,101,109–112]. This renders the tissue more suitable for clinical application. Moreover, treatments based on the recombinant anti-mullerian hormone (which acts as an inhibitor of primordial follicle activation) have also demonstrated efficacy in preserving the primordial follicle pool by suppressing their transition to primary follicles [56].

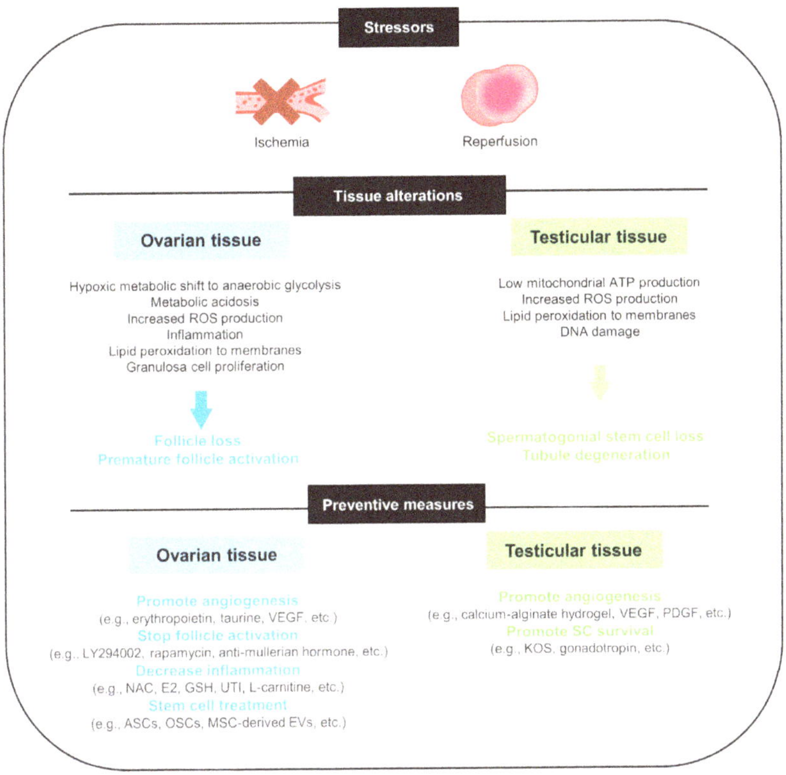

Figure 4. Prevention against ischemic damage in transplanted gonadal grafts.

As reoxygenation kinetics exacerbate oxidative damage, new strategies are also being developed with the goal of enhancing revascularization and limiting the prolonged exposure to ischemia. The daily administration of NAC (up to 7–12 days after transplantation) produced promising results by reducing IRI and promoting follicle survival in immunodeficient mice; these are effects that were attributed to the upregulation of the antioxidant defense system (increased SOD1, HMOX1, and CAT) and to a boost in anti-inflammatory and antiapoptotic mechanisms (via BCL2) [113]. The combination of NAC and estradiol

(E2) has produced similar outcomes [114]. The administration of glutathione (GSH) and ulinastatin (UTI), on the other hand, has helped block macrophage accumulation and increase the levels of VEGF, CD31, and SOD 1 and 2 in mice, who also presented lowered levels of IL6, TNF-α, and MDA [115]. Thus, various strategies aimed at mitigating inflammation and oxidative harm have been explored; these also include the use of L-carnitine and Etanercept, the latter of which is known to neutralize the activity of TNF-α and inhibit the release of cytokines, chemokines, and stress hormones [116,117].

Finally, adult stem cells exhibit suitable attributes when it comes to maintaining the follicle pool. They are considered promising tools for tissue regeneration and possess the ability to release paracrine factors that, in turn, modulate a wide variety of cellular mechanisms from apoptosis to inflammation [118,119]. Ergo, some authors have presented the usage of mesenchymal stem cells (MSCs) as a tool to protect against ischemic exposure [120–122]. Adipose stem cells (ASCs) were observed to encompass and penetrate OT grafts and increase vessel density and angiogenesis through the secretion of VEGF [123]. The resulting increase in angiogenesis is pivotal in elevating follicle survival rates and reducing apoptosis and follicular activation. One study demonstrates that oogonial stem cells (OSCs) can also be incorporated by the OT and partially restore normal ovarian function after chemotherapy; by maintaining the ability to differentiate into oocytes, these cells were successfully matured to produce a viable offspring through in vitro fertilization [124] (Table 5).

Table 5. Potential methods of mitigating IRI in OT fragments.

Author, Date	Model	Treatment	Main Findings
He et al., 2017 [109]	Mouse	K252a Rapamycin	↓ Primordial follicle activation
Eken et al., 2019 [116]	Rat	Etanercept	↑ GSH and SOD levels ↓ Inflammation and apoptosis
Manavella et al., 2019 [123]	Mouse	ASCs	↑ Vessel density
Celik et al., 2020 [56]	Rat	Rapamycin	↓ Primordial follicle activation
Liu et al., 2021 [111]	Mouse	Rapamycin	↓ Primordial follicle activation ↑ Ovarian survival rate ↓ Apoptosis
Olesen et al., 2021 [113]	Human	NAC	↑ Expressions of SOD1, HMOX1, and CAT ↓ IRI ↓ Follicle apoptosis ↑ Follicle density ↓ Expression of VEGFA
Li et al., 2021 [115]	Human	GSH, UTI, or GSH+UTI	↑ Follicle survival ↑ Antioxidant enzyme activity ↑ Angiogenesis ↓ Oxidative stress ↓ Inflammation
Ahmadi et al., 2021 [107]	Mouse	Taurine	Prevention against oxidative stress ↑ Angiogenesis ↓ Apoptosis ↑ Follicle survival and growth
Sanamiri et al., 2022 [117]	Mouse	L-carnitine	↑ Number of follicles ↑ Estradiol and progesterone production ↓IL-6, TNF-α and MDA levels

Table 5. *Cont.*

Author, Date	Model	Treatment	Main Findings
Rodrigues et al., 2023 [106]	Mouse	Erythropoietin	↑ Follicle viability ↓ Follicle degeneration ↑ Angiogenesis ↓ Fibrotic areas
Bindels et al., 2023 [112]	Mouse	Rapamycin or LY294002	↓ Follicle proliferation Maintenance of primordial follicle reserve
Celik et al., 2023 [125]	Mouse	Anti-Mullerian Hormone	↓ Primordial follicle loss
Ebrahimi & Nasiri, 2024 [114]	Mouse	Estradiol and NAC	↑ Primordial, preantral, and antral follicle numbers ↓ Levels of TNF-α and FGF-2 ↑ Levels of IL-1β and IL-6 ↑ Levels of VEGF

↑ Increase; ↓ Decrease.

Notably, MSCs also demonstrate a promising ability to produce large quantities of extracellular vesicles (EVs)—lipidic bilayer complexes capable of transporting cargo such as microRNAs (miRNA), small interfering RNA (siRNA), messenger RNA (mRNA), proteins, and lipids [126]. Due to their low immunogenicity, membrane integrity, and stability, EVs have been considered important cell-free therapeutic tools for translational applications [127]. Studies carried out in the context of organ and tissue transplantation have revealed that these EVs can be endocytosed and significantly reduce and attenuate inflammation and I/R damage [128–130]. Interestingly, recent reports demonstrate that these cells can also transfer viable mitochondria to damaged neighboring cells, thereby contributing to tissue regeneration [131,132]. Altogether, these reports provide the theoretical basis to support the idea that adult stem cells and EVs might be useful solutions to minimize IRI caused to gonadal grafted tissues, and that their usage and further research on them might be of relevant scientific and clinical interest.

While numerous other studies have demonstrated the efficacy of various compounds in enhancing ovarian cortex transplantation programs, there is still comparatively little research on testicular tissue transplantation. Nevertheless, some authors have ventured into similar strategies adapted to TTC. These include supplementation with diverse compounds, namely with gonadotropin (FSH/LH) and Knockout Serum Replacement (KSR) [133]. Concomitantly, Del Vento and colleagues were able to improve TT revascularization by encapsulating the grafts in calcium alginate hydrogels and delivering VEGF and platelet-derived growth factor (PDGF)-loaded polymeric nanoparticles [134].

In summary, strategies aimed at promoting early blood supply to the graft, mitigating germ cell burnout post-transplantation, and reinforcing the tissue's antioxidant, anti-apoptotic, and anti-inflammatory capacities have consistently been the primary focus of most studies. Although mitochondrial dysfunction can be seen at the basis of all these comorbidities, there is very little research targeting and prioritizing mitochondrial dysfunction and metabolic alterations in cryopreserved transplanted gonadal grafts.

6. Conclusions and Future Perspectives

With the rise in cancer survivors intrinsic to improved survival odds, there has been an accompanying demand for ART, and the cryopreservation of gonadal tissues has been increasingly carried out as a resort. There is still limited research focused on the impact that these protocols have on the energetic and biomolecular functions of reproductive structures and cells; ergo, to understand the shortfalls of fertility preservation techniques, scrutiny should go not only to the systemic, quantitative, and morphological alterations caused by cryostorage and transplantation, but also further into the ultrastructural, bioenergetic, and metabolic abnormalities caused by these techniques.

A lot of recent research has ventured into medium supplementation to mitigate cryodamage and IRI. Apropos of cryostorage, a combination of different permeating and non-permeating agents—namely DMSO and trehalose—stands out as a promising method to safeguard germ cell integrity. MSCs—with their low immunogenicity and ability to release protective EVs, healthy mitochondria, and anti-inflammatory, anti-apoptotic, and antioxidant factors—might also be a future tool for the prevention against mitochondrial dysfunction-associated tissue degeneration.

How these preventive measures safeguard mitochondrial function and oxidative and energetic balance remains to be confirmed and merits further research. We anticipate that by targeting the mitochondria, we might find an important solution for the protection of gonadal tissues against cryodamage and IRI.

Author Contributions: Conceptualization, I.M.; resources, J.R.-S. and A.P.S.; data curation, I.M., M.S. and A.B.; writing—original draft preparation, I.M., M.S. and A.B.; writing—review and editing, J.R.-S., A.P.S., M.S. and A.B.; supervision, J.R.-S., A.B. and A.P.S.; funding acquisition, J.R.-S. and A.P.S. All authors have read and agreed to the published version of the manuscript.

Funding: This work was financed by the European Regional Development Fund (ERDF) through the Centro 2020 Regional Operational Programme and through the COMPETE 2020—Operational Programme for Competitiveness and Internationalisation and Portuguese national funds via FCT—Fundação para a Ciência e a Tecnologia and Fundo Social Europeu (FSE) under projects UIDB/04539/2020, UIDP/04539/2020, and LA/P/0058/2020. I.M. and M.S. were funded by FCT Portugal under a PhD fellowship (2022.10535.BD and 2020.06180.BD, respectively). A.B was funded under a CEEC contract (CEECIND/00860/2018).

Institutional Review Board Statement: Not applicable.

Informed Consent Statement: Not applicable.

Data Availability Statement: Data sharing is not applicable.

Acknowledgments: We extend our sincere appreciation to the designer Rita Moniz for the illustrations provided.

Conflicts of Interest: The authors declare no conflicts of interest.

References

1. Sonigo, C.; Beau, I.; Binart, N.; Grynberg, M. The Impact of Chemotherapy on the Ovaries: Molecular Aspects and the Prevention of Ovarian Damage. *Int. J. Mol. Sci.* **2019**, *20*, 5342. [CrossRef] [PubMed]
2. Pai, H.D.; Baid, R.; Palshetkar, N.P.; Pai, A.; Pai, R.D.; Palshetkar, R. Oocyte Cryopreservation—Current Scenario and Future Perspectives: A Narrative Review. *J. Hum. Reprod. Sci.* **2021**, *14*, 340–349. [CrossRef] [PubMed]
3. Himpe, J.; Lammerant, S.; Van den Bergh, L.; Lapeire, L.; De Roo, C. The Impact of Systemic Oncological Treatments on the Fertility of Adolescents and Young Adults-A Systematic Review. *Life* **2023**, *13*, 1209. [CrossRef] [PubMed]
4. Howell, S.J.; Shalet, S.M. Testicular function following chemotherapy. *Hum. Reprod. Update* **2001**, *7*, 363–369. [CrossRef] [PubMed]
5. Keros, V.; Rosenlund, B.; Hultenby, K.; Aghajanova, L.; Levkov, L.; Hovatta, O. Optimizing cryopreservation of human testicular tissue: Comparison of protocols with glycerol, propanediol and dimethylsulphoxide as cryoprotectants. *Hum. Reprod.* **2005**, *20*, 1676–1687. [CrossRef] [PubMed]
6. Biedka, M.; Kuźba-Kryszak, T.; Nowikiewicz, T.; Żyromska, A. Fertility impairment in radiotherapy. *Contemp. Oncol.* **2016**, *20*, 199–204. [CrossRef] [PubMed]
7. Karavani, G.; Rottenstreich, A.; Schachter-Safrai, N.; Cohen, A.; Weintraub, M.; Imbar, T.; Revel, A. Chemotherapy-based gonadotoxicity risk evaluation as a predictor of reproductive outcomes in post-pubertal patients following ovarian tissue cryopreservation. *BMC Women's Health* **2021**, *21*, 201. [CrossRef] [PubMed]
8. Assi, J.; Santos, J.; Bonetti, T.; Serafini, P.C.; Motta, E.L.A.; Chehin, M.B. Psychosocial benefits of fertility preservation for young cancer patients. *J. Assist. Reprod. Genet.* **2018**, *35*, 601–606. [CrossRef] [PubMed]
9. Takae, S.; Iwahata, Y.; Sugishita, Y.; Iwahata, H.; Kanamori, R.; Shiraishi, E.; Ito, K.; Suzuki, Y.; Yamaya, Y.; Tanaka, K.; et al. Survey of understanding and awareness of fertility preservation in pediatric patients: Is conversation about fertility preservation unpleasant for pediatric patients? *Front. Endocrinol.* **2023**, *13*, 1074603. [CrossRef] [PubMed]
10. Oktay, K.; Harvey, B.E.; Partridge, A.H.; Quinn, G.P.; Reinecke, J.; Taylor, H.S.; Wallace, W.H.; Wang, E.T.; Loren, A.W. Fertility Preservation in Patients With Cancer: ASCO Clinical Practice Guideline Update. *J. Clin. Oncol. Off. J. Am. Soc. Clin. Oncol.* **2018**, *36*, 1994–2001. [CrossRef]

11. Valli-Pulaski, H.; Peters, K.A.; Gassei, K.; Steimer, S.R.; Sukhwani, M.; Hermann, B.P.; Dwomor, L.; David, S.; Fayomi, A.P.; Munyoki, S.K.; et al. Testicular tissue cryopreservation: 8 years of experience from a coordinated network of academic centers. *Hum. Reprod.* **2019**, *34*, 966–977. [CrossRef]
12. Goossens, E.; Jahnukainen, K.; Mitchell, R.T.; van Pelt, A.; Pennings, G.; Rives, N.; Poels, J.; Wyns, C.; Lane, S.; Rodriguez-Wallberg, K.A.; et al. Fertility preservation in boys: Recent developments and new insights. *Hum. Reprod. Open* **2020**, *2020*, hoaa016. [CrossRef]
13. Fayomi, A.P.; Peters, K.; Sukhwani, M.; Valli-Pulaski, H.; Shetty, G.; Meistrich, M.L.; Houser, L.; Robertson, N.; Roberts, V.; Ramsey, C.; et al. Autologous grafting of cryopreserved prepubertal rhesus testis produces sperm and offspring. *Science* **2019**, *363*, 1314–1319. [CrossRef]
14. European IVF Monitoring Consortium (EIM) for the European Society of Human Reproduction and Embryology (ESHRE); Smeenk, J.; Wyns, C.; De Geyter, C.; Kupka, M.; Bergh, C.; Cuevas Saiz, I.; De Neubourg, D.; Rezabek, K.; Tandler-Schneider, A.; et al. ART in Europe, 2019: Results generated from European registries by ESHRE. *Hum. Reprod.* **2023**, *38*, 2321–2338. [CrossRef]
15. Jahnukainen, K.; Ehmcke, J.; Nurmio, M.; Schlatt, S. Autologous ectopic grafting of cryopreserved testicular tissue preserves the fertility of prepubescent monkeys that receive sterilizing cytotoxic therapy. *Cancer Res.* **2012**, *72*, 5174–5178. [CrossRef]
16. Grynberg, M.; Poulain, M.; Sebag-Peyrelevade, S.; le Parco, S.; Fanchin, R.; Frydman, N. Ovarian tissue and follicle transplantation as an option for fertility preservation. *Fertil. Steril.* **2012**, *97*, 1260–1268. [CrossRef]
17. Practice Committee of the American Society for Reproductive Medicine. Electronic address: Asrm@asrm.org Fertility preservation in patients undergoing gonadotoxic therapy or gonadectomy: A committee opinion. *Fertil. Steril.* **2019**, *112*, 1022–1033. [CrossRef]
18. ESHRE Guideline Group on Female Fertility Preservation; Anderson, R.A.; Amant, F.; Braat, D.; D'Angelo, A.; Chuva de Sousa Lopes, S.M.; Demeestere, I.; Dwek, S.; Frith, L.; Lambertini, M.; et al. ESHRE guideline: Female fertility preservation. *Hum. Reprod. Open* **2020**, *2020*, hoaa052. [CrossRef]
19. Donnez, J.; Dolmans, M.M.; Demylle, D.; Jadoul, P.; Pirard, C.; Squifflet, J.; Martinez-Madrid, B.; van Langendonckt, A. Livebirth after orthotopic transplantation of cryopreserved ovarian tissue. *Lancet* **2004**, *364*, 1405–1410. [CrossRef]
20. Khattak, H.; Malhas, R.; Craciunas, L.; Afifi, Y.; Amorim, C.A.; Fishel, S.; Silber, S.; Gook, D.; Demeestere, I.; Bystrova, O.; et al. Fresh and cryopreserved ovarian tissue transplantation for preserving reproductive and endocrine function: A systematic review and individual patient data meta-analysis. *Hum. Reprod. Update* **2022**, *28*, 400–416. [CrossRef]
21. Fabbri, R.; Vicenti, R.; Macciocca, M.; Martino, N.A.; Dell'Aquila, M.E.; Pasquinelli, G.; Morselli-Labate, A.M.; Seracchioli, R.; Paradisi, R. Morphological, ultrastructural and functional imaging of frozen/thawed and vitrified/warmed human ovarian tissue retrieved from oncological patients. *Hum. Reprod.* **2016**, *31*, 1838–1849. [CrossRef]
22. Mazur, P. Cryobiology: The freezing of biological systems. *Science* **1970**, *168*, 939–949. [CrossRef] [PubMed]
23. Bakhach, J. The cryopreservation of composite tissues: Principles and recent advancement on cryopreservation of different type of tissues. *Organogenesis* **2009**, *5*, 119–126. [CrossRef] [PubMed]
24. Whaley, D.; Damyar, K.; Witek, R.P.; Mendoza, A.; Alexander, M.; Lakey, J.R. Cryopreservation: An Overview of Principles and Cell-Specific Considerations. *Cell Transplant.* **2021**, *30*, 963689721999617. [CrossRef]
25. Pegg, D.E. The relevance of ice crystal formation for the cryopreservation of tissues and organs. *Cryobiology* **2010**, *60* (Suppl. 3), S36–S44. [CrossRef] [PubMed]
26. Towey, J.J.; Dougan, L. Structural examination of the impact of glycerol on water structure. *J. Phys. Chem. B* **2012**, *116*, 1633–1641. [CrossRef] [PubMed]
27. Tan, Y.J.; Xiong, Y.; Ding, G.L.; Zhang, D.; Meng, Y.; Huang, H.F.; Sheng, J.Z. Cryoprotectants up-regulate expression of mouse oocyte AQP7, which facilitates water diffusion during cryopreservation. *Fertil. Steril.* **2013**, *99*, 1428–1435. [CrossRef] [PubMed]
28. Murray, K.A.; Gibson, M.I. Post-Thaw Culture and Measurement of Total Cell Recovery Is Crucial in the Evaluation of New Macromolecular Cryoprotectants. *Biomacromolecules* **2020**, *21*, 2864–2873. [CrossRef] [PubMed]
29. Lopes, É.P.F.; Tetaping, G.M.; Novaes, M.A.S.; Dos Santos, R.R.; Rodrigues, A.P.R. Systematic review and meta-analysis on patented and non-patented vitrification processes to ovarian tissue reported between 2000 and 2021. *Anim. Reprod.* **2023**, *20*, e20230065. [CrossRef] [PubMed]
30. Unni, S.; Kasiviswanathan, S.; D'Souza, S.; Khavale, S.; Mukherjee, S.; Patwardhan, S.; Bhartiya, D. Efficient cryopreservation of testicular tissue: Effect of age, sample state, and concentration of cryoprotectant. *Fertil. Steril.* **2012**, *97*, 200–208.e1. [CrossRef]
31. Chen, J.; Liu, X.; Hu, Y.; Chen, X.; Tan, S. Cryopreservation of tissues and organs: Present, bottlenecks, and future. *Front. Vet. Sci.* **2023**, *10*, 1201794. [CrossRef]
32. Newton, H.; Fisher, J.; Arnold, J.R.; Pegg, D.E.; Faddy, M.J.; Gosden, R.G. Permeation of human ovarian tissue with cryoprotective agents in preparation for cryopreservation. *Hum. Reprod.* **1998**, *13*, 376–380. [CrossRef] [PubMed]
33. Best, B.P. Cryoprotectant Toxicity: Facts, Issues, and Questions. *Rejuvenation Res.* **2015**, *18*, 422–436. [CrossRef] [PubMed]
34. Wu, K.; Laouar, L.; Dong, R.; Elliott, J.A.W.; Jomha, N.M. Evaluation of five additives to mitigate toxicity of cryoprotective agents on porcine chondrocytes. *Cryobiology* **2019**, *88*, 98–105. [CrossRef] [PubMed]
35. Crisol, M.; Yong, K.W.; Wu, K.; Laouar, L.; Elliott, J.A.W.; Jomha, N.M. Effectiveness of Clinical-Grade Chondroitin Sulfate and Ascorbic Acid in Mitigating Cryoprotectant Toxicity in Porcine Articular Cartilage. *Biopreservation Biobanking* **2022**, *20*, 401–408. [CrossRef] [PubMed]
36. Holmström, K.M.; Finkel, T. Cellular mechanisms and physiological consequences of redox-dependent signalling. *Nat. Rev. Mol. Cell Biol.* **2014**, *15*, 411–421. [CrossRef] [PubMed]

37. Shadel, G.S.; Horvath, T.L. Mitochondrial ROS signaling in organismal homeostasis. *Cell* **2015**, *163*, 560–569. [CrossRef] [PubMed]
38. Zhao, R.Z.; Jiang, S.; Zhang, L.; Yu, Z.B. Mitochondrial electron transport chain, ROS generation and uncoupling (Review). *Int. J. Mol. Med.* **2019**, *44*, 3–15. [CrossRef]
39. Valko, M.; Leibfritz, D.; Moncol, J.; Cronin, M.T.; Mazur, M.; Telser, J. Free radicals and antioxidants in normal physiological functions and human disease. *Int. J. Biochem. Cell Biol.* **2007**, *39*, 44–84. [CrossRef]
40. Juan, C.A.; Pérez de la Lastra, J.M.; Plou, F.J.; Pérez-Lebeña, E. The Chemistry of Reactive Oxygen Species (ROS) Revisited: Outlining Their Role in Biological Macromolecules (DNA, Lipids and Proteins) and Induced Pathologies. *Int. J. Mol. Sci.* **2021**, *22*, 4642. [CrossRef]
41. Salahudeen, A.K.; Huang, H.; Joshi, M.; Moore, N.A.; Jenkins, J.K. Involvement of the mitochondrial pathway in cold storage and rewarming-associated apoptosis of human renal proximal tubular cells. *Am. J. Transplant. Off. J. Am. Soc. Transplant. Am. Soc. Transpl. Surg.* **2003**, *3*, 273–280. [CrossRef]
42. Yard, B.; Beck, G.; Schnuelle, P.; Braun, C.; Schaub, M.; Bechtler, M.; Göttmann, U.; Xiao, Y.; Breedijk, A.; Wandschneider, S.; et al. Prevention of cold-preservation injury of cultured endothelial cells by catecholamines and related compounds. *Am. J. Transplant. Off. J. Am. Soc. Transplant. Am. Soc. Transpl. Surg.* **2004**, *4*, 22–30. [CrossRef] [PubMed]
43. Kanitkar, M.; Bhonde, R.R. Curcumin treatment enhances islet recovery by induction of heat shock response proteins, Hsp70 and heme oxygenase-1, during cryopreservation. *Life Sci.* **2008**, *82*, 182–189. [CrossRef] [PubMed]
44. Larsen, S.; Wright-Paradis, C.; Gnaiger, E.; Helge, J.W.; Boushel, R. Cryopreservation of human skeletal muscle impairs mitochondrial function. *Cryo Lett.* **2012**, *33*, 170–176.
45. Acin-Perez, R.; Benador, I.Y.; Petcherski, A.; Veliova, M.; Benavides, G.A.; Lagarrigue, S.; Caudal, A.; Vergnes, L.; Murphy, A.N.; Karamanlidis, G.; et al. A novel approach to measure mitochondrial respiration in frozen biological samples. *EMBO J.* **2020**, *39*, e104073. [CrossRef] [PubMed]
46. Xu, X.; Cowley, S.; Flaim, C.J.; James, W.; Seymour, L.; Cui, Z. The roles of apoptotic pathways in the low recovery rate after cryopreservation of dissociated human embryonic stem cells. *Biotechnol. Prog.* **2010**, *26*, 827–837. [CrossRef]
47. Bilodeau, J.F.; Chatterjee, S.; Sirard, M.A.; Gagnon, C. Levels of antioxidant defenses are decreased in bovine spermatozoa after a cycle of freezing and thawing. *Mol. Reprod. Dev.* **2000**, *55*, 282–288. [CrossRef]
48. Martín-Cano, F.E.; Gaitskell-Phillips, G.; Ortiz-Rodríguez, J.M.; Silva-Rodríguez, A.; Román, Á.; Rojo-Domínguez, P.; Alonso-Rodríguez, E.; Tapia, J.A.; Gil, M.C.; Ortega-Ferrusola, C.; et al. Proteomic profiling of stallion spermatozoa suggests changes in sperm metabolism and compromised redox regulation after cryopreservation. *J. Proteom.* **2020**, *221*, 103765. [CrossRef] [PubMed]
49. Roness, H.; Meirow, D. FERTILITY PRESERVATION: Follicle reserve loss in ovarian tissue transplantation. *Reproduction* **2019**, *158*, F35–F44. [CrossRef] [PubMed]
50. Nottola, S.A.; Camboni, A.; Van Langendonckt, A.; Demylle, D.; Macchiarelli, G.; Dolmans, M.M.; Martinez-Madrid, B.; Correr, S.; Donnez, J. Cryopreservation and xenotransplantation of human ovarian tissue: An ultrastructural study. *Fertil. Steril.* **2008**, *90*, 23–32. [CrossRef]
51. Ting, A.Y.; Yeoman, R.R.; Lawson, M.S.; Zelinski, M.B. In vitro development of secondary follicles from cryopreserved rhesus macaque ovarian tissue after slow-rate freeze or vitrification. *Hum. Reprod.* **2011**, *26*, 2461–2472. [CrossRef]
52. Newton, H.; Aubard, Y.; Rutherford, A.; Sharma, V.; Gosden, R. Low temperature storage and grafting of human ovarian tissue. *Hum. Reprod.* **1996**, *11*, 1487–1491. [CrossRef] [PubMed]
53. Donnez, J.; Silber, S.; Andersen, C.Y.; Demeestere, I.; Piver, P.; Meirow, D.; Pellicer, A.; Dolmans, M.M. Children born after autotransplantation of cryopreserved ovarian tissue. a review of 13 live births. *Ann. Med.* **2011**, *43*, 437–450. [CrossRef] [PubMed]
54. Silber, S.; Kagawa, N.; Kuwayama, M.; Gosden, R. Duration of fertility after fresh and frozen ovary transplantation. *Fertil. Steril.* **2010**, *94*, 2191–2196. [CrossRef] [PubMed]
55. Fabbri, R.; Pasquinelli, G.; Keane, D.; Magnani, V.; Paradisi, R.; Venturoli, S. Optimization of protocols for human ovarian tissue cryopreservation with sucrose, 1,2-propanediol and human serum. *Reprod. Biomed. Online* **2010**, *21*, 819–828. [CrossRef] [PubMed]
56. Celik, S.; Ozkavukcu, S.; Celik-Ozenci, C. Altered expression of activator proteins that control follicle reserve after ovarian tissue cryopreservation/transplantation and primordial follicle loss prevention by rapamycin. *J. Assist. Reprod. Genet.* **2020**, *37*, 2119–2136. [CrossRef] [PubMed]
57. Tian, T.; Zhao, G.; Han, D.; Zhu, K.; Chen, D.; Zhang, Z.; Wei, Z.; Cao, Y.; Zhou, P. Effects of vitrification cryopreservation on follicular morphology and stress relaxation behaviors of human ovarian tissues: Sucrose versus trehalose as the non-permeable protective agent. *Hum. Reprod.* **2015**, *30*, 877–883. [CrossRef] [PubMed]
58. Mathias, F.J.; D'Souza, F.; Uppangala, S.; Salian, S.R.; Kalthur, G.; Adiga, S.K. Ovarian tissue vitrification is more efficient than slow freezing in protecting oocyte and granulosa cell DNA integrity. *Syst. Biol. Reprod. Med.* **2014**, *60*, 317–322. [CrossRef] [PubMed]
59. Amorim, C.A.; David, A.; Van Langendonckt, A.; Dolmans, M.M.; Donnez, J. Vitrification of human ovarian tissue: Effect of different solutions and procedures. *Fertil. Steril.* **2011**, *95*, 1094–1097. [CrossRef] [PubMed]
60. Suzuki, N.; Yoshioka, N.; Takae, S.; Sugishita, Y.; Tamura, M.; Hashimoto, S.; Morimoto, Y.; Kawamura, K. Successful fertility preservation following ovarian tissue vitrification in patients with primary ovarian insufficiency. *Hum. Reprod.* **2015**, *30*, 608–615. [CrossRef]
61. Borges, E.N.; Silva, R.C.; Futino, D.O.; Rocha-Junior, C.M.; Amorim, C.A.; Báo, S.N.; Lucci, C.M. Cryopreservation of swine ovarian tissue: Effect of different cryoprotectants on the structural preservation of preantral follicle oocytes. *Cryobiology* **2009**, *59*, 195–200. [CrossRef]

62. Fabbri, R.; Vicenti, R.; Martino, N.A.; Dell'Aquila, M.E.; Pasquinelli, G.; Macciocca, M.; Magnani, V.; Paradisi, R.; Venturoli, S. Confocal laser scanning microscopy analysis of bioenergetic potential and oxidative stress in fresh and frozen-thawed human ovarian tissue from oncologic patients. *Fertil. Steril.* **2014**, *101*, 795–804. [CrossRef]
63. Leonel, E.C.R.; Corral, A.; Risco, R.; Camboni, A.; Taboga, S.R.; Kilbride, P.; Vazquez, M.; Morris, J.; Dolmans, M.M.; Amorim, C.A. Stepped vitrification technique for human ovarian tissue cryopreservation. *Sci. Rep.* **2019**, *9*, 20008. [CrossRef]
64. Wu, Q.; Ru, G.; Xiao, W.; Wang, Q.; Li, Z. Adverse effects of ovarian cryopreservation and auto-transplantation on ovarian grafts and quality of produced oocytes in a mouse model. *Clin. Sci.* **2023**, *137*, 1577–1591. [CrossRef]
65. Rodrigues, A.Q.; Picolo, V.L.; Goulart, J.T.; Silva, I.M.G.; Ribeiro, R.B.; Aguiar, B.A.; Ferreira, Y.B.; Oliveira, D.M.; Lucci, C.M.; de Bem, A.F.; et al. Metabolic activity in cryopreserved and grafted ovarian tissue using high-resolution respirometry. *Sci. Rep.* **2021**, *11*, 21517. [CrossRef]
66. Keros, V.; Hultenby, K.; Borgström, B.; Fridström, M.; Jahnukainen, K.; Hovatta, O. Methods of cryopreservation of testicular tissue with viable spermatogonia in pre-pubertal boys undergoing gonadotoxic cancer treatment. *Hum. Reprod.* **2007**, *22*, 1384–1395. [CrossRef]
67. Poels, J.; Van Langendonckt, A.; Many, M.C.; Wese, F.X.; Wyns, C. Vitrification preserves proliferation capacity in human spermatogonia. *Hum. Reprod.* **2013**, *28*, 578–589. [CrossRef]
68. Picton, H.M.; Wyns, C.; Anderson, R.A.; Goossens, E.; Jahnukainen, K.; Kliesch, S.; Mitchell, R.T.; Pennings, G.; Rives, N.; Tournaye, H.; et al. ESHRE Task Force on Fertility Preservation in Severe Diseases a European perspective on testicular tissue cryopreservation for fertility preservation in prepubertal and adolescent boys. *Hum. Reprod.* **2015**, *30*, 2463–2475. [CrossRef]
69. Kvist, K.; Thorup, J.; Byskov, A.G.; Høyer, P.E.; Møllgård, K.; Yding Andersen, C. Cryopreservation of intact testicular tissue from boys with cryptorchidism. *Hum. Reprod.* **2006**, *21*, 484–491. [CrossRef]
70. Curaba, M.; Poels, J.; van Langendonckt, A.; Donnez, J.; Wyns, C. Can prepubertal human testicular tissue be cryopreserved by vitrification? *Fertil. Steril.* **2011**, *95*, 2123-e9. [CrossRef]
71. Hajiaghalou, S.; Ebrahimi, B.; Shahverdi, A.; Sharbatoghli, M.; Beigi Boroujeni, N. Comparison of apoptosis pathway following the use of two protocols for vitrification of immature mouse testicular tissue. *Theriogenology* **2016**, *86*, 2073–2082. [CrossRef]
72. Lucio, C.F.; Regazzi, F.M.; Silva, L.C.G.; Angrimani, D.S.R.; Nichi, M.; Vannucchi, C.I. Oxidative stress at different stages of two-step semen cryopreservation procedures in dogs. *Theriogenology* **2016**, *85*, 1568–1575. [CrossRef]
73. Moubasher, A.E.; Taha, E.A.; Younis, A.; Fakhry, M.E.; Morsy, H. Testicular tissue oxidative stress in azoospermic patients: Effect of cryopreservation. *Andrologia* **2020**, *52*, e13817. [CrossRef]
74. Pukazhenthi, B.S.; Nagashima, J.; Travis, A.J.; Costa, G.M.; Escobar, E.N.; França, L.R.; Wildt, D.E. Slow freezing, but not vitrification supports complete spermatogenesis in cryopreserved, neonatal sheep testicular xenografts. *PLoS ONE* **2015**, *10*, e0123957. [CrossRef]
75. Zhang, X.G.; Wang, Y.H.; Han, C.; Hu, S.; Wang, L.Q.; Hu, J.H. Effects of trehalose supplementation on cell viability and oxidative stress variables in frozen-thawed bovine calf testicular tissue. *Cryobiology* **2015**, *70*, 246–252. [CrossRef]
76. Lima, D.B.C.; Silva, L.D.M.D.; Comizzoli, P. Influence of warming and reanimation conditions on seminiferous tubule morphology, mitochondrial activity, and cell composition of vitrified testicular tissues in the domestic cat model. *PLoS ONE* **2018**, *13*, e0207317. [CrossRef]
77. Farias, J.G.; Puebla, M.; Acevedo, A.; Tapia, P.J.; Gutierrez, E.; Zepeda, A.; Calaf, G.; Juantok, C.; Reyes, J.G. Oxidative stress in rat testis and epididymis under intermittent hypobaric hypoxia: Protective role of ascorbate supplementation. *J. Androl.* **2010**, *31*, 314–321. [CrossRef]
78. Lee, J.; Kong, H.S.; Kim, E.J.; Youm, H.W.; Lee, J.R.; Suh, C.S.; Kim, S.H. Ovarian injury during cryopreservation and transplantation in mice: A comparative study between cryoinjury and ischemic injury. *Hum. Reprod.* **2016**, *31*, 1827–1837. [CrossRef]
79. Prag, H.; Kula-Alwar, D.; Beach, T.; Gruszczyk, A.; Burger, N.; Murphy, P. Mitochondrial ROS production during ischemia-reperfusion injury. In *Oxidative Stress Eustress and Distress*; Sies, H., Ed.; Academic Press: Cambridge, MA, USA, 2020; pp. 513–538.
80. Kirmizi, D.A.; Baser, E.; Okan, A.; Kara, M.; Yalvac, E.S.; Doganyigit, Z. The effect of a natural molecule in ovary ischemia reperfusion damage: Does lycopene protect ovary? *Exp. Anim.* **2021**, *70*, 37–44. [CrossRef]
81. Kim, S.S.; Yang, H.W.; Kang, H.G.; Lee, H.H.; Lee, H.C.; Ko, D.S.; Gosden, R.G. Quantitative assessment of ischemic tissue damage in ovarian cortical tissue with or without antioxidant (ascorbic acid) treatment. *Fertil. Steril.* **2004**, *82*, 679–685. [CrossRef]
82. Della Rocca, Y.; Fonticoli, L.; Rajan, T.S.; Trubiani, O.; Caputi, S.; Diomede, F.; Pizzicannella, J.; Marconi, G.D. Hypoxia: Molecular pathophysiological mechanisms in human diseases. *J. Physiol. Biochem.* **2022**, *78*, 739–752. [CrossRef]
83. Akdemir, A.; Erbas, O.; Gode, F.; Ergenoglu, M.; Yeniel, O.; Oltulu, F.; Yavasoglu, A.; Taskiran, D. Protective effect of oxytocin on ovarian ischemia-reperfusion injury in rats. *Peptides* **2014**, *55*, 126–130. [CrossRef]
84. Aksak Karamese, S.; Toktay, E.; Unal, D.; Selli, J.; Karamese, M.; Malkoc, I. The protective effects of beta-carotene against ischemia/reperfusion injury in rat ovarian tissue. *Acta Histochem.* **2015**, *117*, 790–797. [CrossRef]
85. Murphy, M.P.; Hartley, R.C. Mitochondria as a therapeutic target for common pathologies. *Nat. Rev. Drug Discov.* **2018**, *17*, 865–886. [CrossRef]
86. Wu, M.Y.; Yiang, G.T.; Liao, W.T.; Tsai, A.P.; Cheng, Y.L.; Cheng, P.W.; Li, C.Y.; Li, C.J. Current Mechanistic Concepts in Ischemia and Reperfusion Injury. *Cell. Physiol. Biochem. Int. J. Exp. Cell. Physiol. Biochem. Pharmacol.* **2018**, *46*, 1650–1667. [CrossRef]

87. Tabet, F.; Touyz, R. Reactive Oxygen Species, Oxidative Stress, and Vascular Biology in Hypertension. In *Comprehensive Hypertension*; Lip, G.Y.H., Hall, J.E., Eds.; Mosby: London, UK, 2007; pp. 337–347. [CrossRef]
88. Ozkisacik, S.; Yazici, M.; Gursoy, H.; Culhaci, N. Does gradual detorsion protect the ovary against ischemia-reperfusion injury in rats? *Pediatr. Surg. Int.* **2014**, *30*, 437–440. [CrossRef]
89. Han, C.; Zeng, Q.; He, L.; Luan, Z.; Liu, R.; Zhang, G.; Liu, W. Advances in the mechanisms related to follicle loss after frozen-thawed ovarian tissue transplantation. *Transpl. Immunol.* **2023**, *81*, 101935. [CrossRef]
90. Gavish, Z.; Spector, I.; Peer, G.; Schlatt, S.; Wistuba, J.; Roness, H.; Meirow, D. Follicle activation is a significant and immediate cause of follicle loss after ovarian tissue transplantation. *J. Assist. Reprod. Genet.* **2018**, *35*, 61–69. [CrossRef]
91. Gavish, Z.; Peer, G.; Roness, H.; Cohen, Y.; Meirow, D. Follicle activation and 'burn-out' contribute to post-transplantation follicle loss in ovarian tissue grafts: The effect of graft thickness. *Hum. Reprod.* **2014**, *29*, 989–996. [CrossRef]
92. Arena, S.; Iacona, R.; Antonuccio, P.; Russo, T.; Salvo, V.; Gitto, E.; Impellizzeri, P.; Romeo, C. Medical perspective in testicular ischemia-reperfusion injury. *Exp. Ther. Med.* **2017**, *13*, 2115–2122. [CrossRef]
93. Li, J.T.; Zhang, L.; Liu, J.J.; Lu, X.L.; Wang, H.X.; Zhang, J.M. Testicular damage during cryopreservation and transplantation. *Andrologia* **2021**, *53*, e14191. [CrossRef]
94. Rasaeifar, K.; Zavareh, S.; Hajighasem-Kashani, M.; Nasiri, M. Effects of pulsed electromagnetic fields and N-acetylcysteine on transplantation of vitrified mouse ovarian tissue. *Electromagn. Biol. Med.* **2023**, *42*, 67–80. [CrossRef]
95. Qin, Q.; Li, Z.; Liu, R.; Liu, S.; Guo, M.; Zhang, M.; Wu, H.; Huang, L. Effects of resveratrol on HIF-1α/VEGF pathway and apoptosis in vitrified duck ovary transplantation. *Theriogenology* **2023**, *210*, 84–93. [CrossRef]
96. Wang, F.; Tian, Y.; Huang, L.; Qin, T.; Ma, W.; Pei, C.; Xu, B.; Han, H.; Liu, X.; Pan, P.; et al. Roles of follicle stimulating hormone and sphingosine 1-phosphate co-administered in the process in mouse ovarian vitrification and transplantation. *J. Ovarian Res.* **2023**, *16*, 173. [CrossRef]
97. Kong, H.S.; Hong, Y.H.; Lee, J.; Youm, H.W.; Lee, J.R.; Suh, C.S.; Kim, S.H. Antifreeze Protein Supplementation During the Warming of Vitrified Bovine Ovarian Tissue Can Improve the Ovarian Tissue Quality After Xenotransplantation. *Front. Endocrinol.* **2021**, *12*, 672619. [CrossRef]
98. Bedaiwy, M.A.; Hussein, M.R.; Biscotti, C.; Falcone, T. Cryopreservation of intact human ovary with its vascular pedicle. *Hum. Reprod.* **2006**, *21*, 3258–3269. [CrossRef]
99. Westphal, J.R.; Gerritse, R.; Braat, D.D.M.; Beerendonk, C.C.M.; Peek, R. Complete protection against cryodamage of cryopreserved whole bovine and human ovaries using DMSO as a cryoprotectant. *J. Assist. Reprod. Genet.* **2017**, *34*, 1217–1229. [CrossRef]
100. Lee, S.; Cho, H.W.; Kim, B.; Lee, J.K.; Kim, T. The Effectiveness of Anti-Apoptotic Agents to Preserve Primordial Follicles and Prevent Tissue Damage during Ovarian Tissue Cryopreservation and Xenotransplantation. *Int. J. Mol. Sci.* **2021**, *22*, 2534. [CrossRef]
101. Terren, C.; Nisolle, M.; Munaut, C. Pharmacological inhibition of the PI3K/PTEN/Akt and mTOR signalling pathways limits follicle activation induced by ovarian cryopreservation and in vitro culture. *J. Ovarian Res.* **2021**, *14*, 95. [CrossRef]
102. Xi, H.; Ren, F.; Zhang, X.; Li, Y.; Zhang, L.; Wen, F.; Feng, T.; Zhang, X.; Niu, T.; Hu, J.; et al. Trehalose protects testicular tissue of dairy goat upon cryopreservation. *Reprod. Domest. Anim. = Zuchthyg.* **2019**, *54*, 1552–1559. [CrossRef]
103. Jung, S.E.; Ahn, J.S.; Kim, Y.H.; Kim, B.J.; Won, J.H.; Ryu, B.Y. Effective cryopreservation protocol for preservation of male primate (*Macaca fascicularis*) prepubertal fertility. *Reprod. Biomed. Online* **2020**, *41*, 1070–1083. [CrossRef]
104. Zhu, W.Q.; Cai, N.N.; Jiang, Y.; Yang, R.; Shi, J.Z.; Zhu, C.L.; Zhang, B.Y.; Tang, B.; Zhang, X.M. Survivable potential of germ cells after trehalose cryopreservation of bovine testicular tissues. *Cryobiology* **2021**, *101*, 105–114. [CrossRef]
105. Dumont, L.; Oblette, A.; Rondanino, C.; Jumeau, F.; Bironneau, A.; Liot, D.; Duchesne, V.; Wils, J.; Rives, N. Vitamin A prevents round spermatid nuclear damage and promotes the production of motile sperm during in vitro maturation of vitrified pre-pubertal mouse testicular tissue. *Mol. Hum. Reprod.* **2016**, *22*, 819–832. [CrossRef]
106. Rodrigues, A.Q.; Silva, I.M.; Goulart, J.T.; Araújo, L.O.; Ribeiro, R.B.; Aguiar, B.A.; Ferreira, Y.B.; Silva, J.K.O.; Bezerra, J.L.S.; Lucci, C.M.; et al. Effects of erythropoietin on ischaemia-reperfusion when administered before and after ovarian tissue transplantation in mice. *Reprod. Biomed. Online* **2023**, *47*, 103234. [CrossRef]
107. Ahmadi, S.; Mehranjani, M.S. Taurine improves follicular survival and function of mice ovarian grafts through increasing CD31 and GDF9 expression and reducing oxidative stress and apoptosis. *Eur. J. Pharmacol.* **2021**, *903*, 174134. [CrossRef]
108. Shiratsuki, S.; Hara, T.; Munakata, Y.; Shirasuna, K.; Kuwayama, T.; Iwata, H. Low oxygen level increases proliferation and metabolic changes in bovine granulosa cells. *Mol. Cell. Endocrinol.* **2016**, *437*, 75–85. [CrossRef]
109. He, Y.; Peng, X.; Wu, T.; Yang, W.; Liu, W.; Zhang, J.; Su, Y.; Kong, F.; Dou, X.; Li, J. Restricting the induction of NGF in ovarian stroma engenders selective follicular activation through the mTOR signaling pathway. *Cell Death Dis.* **2017**, *8*, e2817. [CrossRef]
110. Celik, S.; Celikkan, F.T.; Ozkavukcu, S.; Can, A.; Celik-Ozenci, C. Expression of inhibitor proteins that control primordial follicle reserve decreases in cryopreserved ovaries after autotransplantation. *J. Assist. Reprod. Genet.* **2018**, *35*, 615–626. [CrossRef]
111. Liu, W.; Zhang, J.; Wang, L.; Liang, S.; Xu, B.; Ying, X.; Li, J. The protective effects of rapamycin pretreatment on ovarian damage during ovarian tissue cryopreservation and transplantation. *Biochem. Biophys. Res. Commun.* **2021**, *534*, 780–786. [CrossRef]
112. Bindels, J.; Squatrito, M.; Bernet, L.; Nisolle, M.; Henry, L.; Munaut, C. The mTOR Inhibitor Rapamycin Counteracts Follicle Activation Induced by Ovarian Cryopreservation in Murine Transplantation Models. *Medicina* **2023**, *59*, 1474. [CrossRef]

113. Olesen, H.Ø.; Pors, S.E.; Jensen, L.B.; Grønning, A.P.; Lemser, C.E.; Nguyen Heimbürger, M.T.H.; Mamsen, L.S.; Getreu, N.; Christensen, S.T.; Andersen, C.Y.; et al. N-acetylcysteine protects ovarian follicles from ischemia-reperfusion injury in xenotransplanted human ovarian tissue. *Hum. Reprod.* **2021**, *36*, 429–443. [CrossRef]
114. Ebrahimi, F.; Zavareh, S.; Nasiri, M. The Combination of Estradiol and N-Acetylcysteine Reduces Ischemia-Reperfusion Injuries of Mice Autografted Ovarian Tissue. *Biopreservation Biobanking* **2024**, *22*, 29–37. [CrossRef] [PubMed]
115. Li, Y.; Hu, Y.; Zhu, S.; Tuo, Y.; Cai, B.; Long, T.; Zhao, W.; Ye, X.; Lu, X.; Long, L. Protective Effects of Reduced Glutathione and Ulinastatin on Xeno-transplanted Human Ovarian Tissue Against Ischemia and Reperfusion Injury. *Cell Transplant.* **2021**, *30*, 963689721997151. [CrossRef] [PubMed]
116. Eken, M.K.; Ersoy, G.S.; Kaygusuz, E.I.; Devranoğlu, B.; Takır, M.; Çilingir, Ö.T.; Çevik, Ö. Etanercept protects ovarian reserve against ischemia/reperfusion injury in a rat model. *Arch. Med. Sci. AMS* **2019**, *15*, 1104–1112. [CrossRef] [PubMed]
117. Sanamiri, K.; Soleimani Mehranjani, M.; Shahhoseini, M.; Shariatzadeh, M.A. L-Carnitine improves follicular survival and function in ovarian grafts in the mouse. *Reprod. Fertil. Dev.* **2022**, *34*, 713–721. [CrossRef] [PubMed]
118. Moniz, I.; Ramalho-Santos, J.; Branco, A.F. Differential Oxygen Exposure Modulates Mesenchymal Stem Cell Metabolism and Proliferation through mTOR Signaling. *Int. J. Mol. Sci.* **2022**, *23*, 3749. [CrossRef] [PubMed]
119. Branco, A.; Moniz, I.; Ramalho-Santos, J. Mitochondria as biological targets for stem cell and organismal senescence. *Eur. J. Cell Biol.* **2023**, *102*, 151289. [CrossRef] [PubMed]
120. Christie, J.D.; Edwards, L.B.; Kucheryavaya, A.Y.; Aurora, P.; Dobbels, F.; Kirk, R.; Rahmel, A.O.; Stehlik, J.; Hertz, M.I. The Registry of the International Society for Heart and Lung Transplantation: Twenty-seventh official adult lung and heart-lung transplant report—2010. *J. Heart Lung Transplant.* **2010**, *29*, 1104–1118. [CrossRef]
121. Johnson, M.R.; Meyer, K.H.; Haft, J.; Kinder, D.; Webber, S.A.; Dyke, D.B. Heart Transplantation in the United States, 1999–2008. *Am. J. Transplant.* **2010**, *10*, 1035–1046. [CrossRef] [PubMed]
122. Young, J.B.; Hauptman, P.J.; Naftel, D.C.; Ewald, G.; Aaronson, K.; Dec, G.W.; Taylor, D.O.; Higgins, R.; Platt, L.; Kirklin, J. Determinants of early graft failure following cardiac transplantation, a 10-year, multi-institutional, multivariable analysis. *J. Heart Lung Transplant.* **2001**, *20*, 212. [CrossRef]
123. Manavella, D.D.; Cacciottola, L.; Payen, V.L.; Amorim, C.A.; Donnez, J.; Dolmans, M.M. Adipose tissue-derived stem cells boost vascularization in grafted ovarian tissue by growth factor secretion and differentiation into endothelial cell lineages. *Mol. Hum. Reprod.* **2019**, *25*, 184–193. [CrossRef]
124. White, Y.A.; Woods, D.C.; Takai, Y.; Ishihara, O.; Seki, H.; Tilly, J.L. Oocyte formation by mitotically active germ cells purified from ovaries of reproductive-age women. *Nat. Med.* **2012**, *18*, 413–421. [CrossRef] [PubMed]
125. Celik, S.; Ozkavukcu, S.; Celik-Ozenci, C. Recombinant anti-Mullerian hormone treatment attenuates primordial follicle loss after ovarian cryopreservation and transplantation. *J. Assist. Reprod. Genet.* **2023**, *40*, 1117–1134. [CrossRef] [PubMed]
126. Jia, Y.; Yu, L.; Ma, T.; Xu, W.; Qian, H.; Sun, Y.; Shi, H. Small extracellular vesicles isolation and separation: Current techniques, pending questions and clinical applications. *Theranostics* **2022**, *12*, 6548–6575. [CrossRef] [PubMed]
127. Baglio, S.R.; Pegtel, D.M.; Baldini, N. Mesenchymal stem cell secreted vesicles provide novel opportunities in (stem) cell-free therapy. *Front. Physiol.* **2012**, *3*, 359. [CrossRef] [PubMed]
128. Rampino, T.; Gregorini, M.; Germinario, G.; Pattonieri, E.F.; Erasmi, F.; Grignano, M.A.; Bruno, S.; Alomari, E.; Bettati, S.; Asti, A.; et al. Extracellular Vesicles Derived from Mesenchymal Stromal Cells Delivered during Hypothermic Oxygenated Machine Perfusion Repair Ischemic/Reperfusion Damage of Kidneys from Extended Criteria Donors. *Biology* **2022**, *11*, 350. [CrossRef] [PubMed]
129. Stone, M.L.; Zhao, Y.; Robert Smith, J.; Weiss, M.L.; Kron, I.L.; Laubach, V.E.; Sharma, A.K. Mesenchymal stromal cell-derived extracellular vesicles attenuate lung ischemia-reperfusion injury and enhance reconditioning of donor lungs after circulatory death. *Respir. Res.* **2017**, *18*, 212. [CrossRef] [PubMed]
130. Lonati, C.; Bassani, G.A.; Brambilla, D.; Leonardi, P.; Carlin, A.; Maggioni, M.; Zanella, A.; Dondossola, D.; Fonsato, V.; Grange, C.; et al. Mesenchymal stem cell-derived extracellular vesicles improve the molecular phenotype of isolated rat lungs during ischemia/reperfusion injury. *J. Heart Lung Transplant. Off. Publ. Int. Soc. Heart Transplant.* **2019**, *38*, 1306–1316. [CrossRef] [PubMed]
131. Vasanthan, J.; Gurusamy, N.; Rajasingh, S.; Sigamani, V.; Kirankumar, S.; Thomas, E.L.; Rajasingh, J. Role of Human Mesenchymal Stem Cells in Regenerative Therapy. *Cells* **2020**, *10*, 54. [CrossRef] [PubMed]
132. Li, C.; Cheung, M.K.H.; Han, S.; Zhang, Z.; Chen, L.; Chen, J.; Zeng, H.; Qiu, J. Mesenchymal stem cells and their mitochondrial transfer: A double-edged sword. *Biosci. Rep.* **2019**, *39*, BSR20182417. [CrossRef]
133. Medrano, J.V.; Vilanova-Pérez, T.; Fornés-Ferrer, V.; Navarro-Gomezlechon, A.; Martínez-Triguero, M.L.; García, S.; Gómez-Chacón, J.; Povo, I.; Pellicer, A.; Andrés, M.M.; et al. Influence of temperature, serum, and gonadotropin supplementation in short- and long-term organotypic culture of human immature testicular tissue. *Fertil. Steril.* **2018**, *110*, 1045–1057.e3. [CrossRef]
134. Del Vento, F.; Poels, J.; Vermeulen, M.; Ucakar, B.; Giudice, M.G.; Kanbar, M.; des Rieux, A.; Wyns, C. Accelerated and Improved Vascular Maturity after Transplantation of Testicular Tissue in Hydrogels Supplemented with VEGF- and PDGF-Loaded Nanoparticles. *Int. J. Mol. Sci.* **2021**, *22*, 5779. [CrossRef] [PubMed]

biology

MDPI

Article

The Cardiometabolic Impact of Rebaudioside A Exposure during the Reproductive Stage

Isabella Bracchi [1,2,3,†], Juliana Morais [2,3,4,†], João Almeida Coelho [4,5], Ana Filipa Ferreira [4,5], Inês Alves [4,5], Cláudia Mendes [4,5], Beatriz Correia [4,6], Alexandre Gonçalves [4,5], João Tiago Guimarães [1,7,8], Inês Falcão-Pires [4,5,*], Elisa Keating [1,9] and Rita Negrão [1,9,*]

1 Unit of Biochemistry, Department Biomedicine, Faculty of Medicine, University of Porto, 4200-319 Porto, Portugal; isabellabracchi@gmail.com (I.B.); keating@med.up.pt (E.K.)
2 CINTESIS, Center for Health Technology and Services Research, 4200-319 Porto, Portugal; ju_morais17@hotmail.com
3 Department of Functional Sciences, School of Health, Polytechnic Institute of Porto, 4200-072 Porto, Portugal
4 Department of Surgery and Physiology, Faculdade de Medicina, Universidade do Porto, 4200-319 Porto, Portugal; almeidacoelho.joao@gmail.com (J.A.C.); csmendes@med.up.pt (C.M.)
5 UniC@RISE, Unidade de Investigação e Desenvolvimento Cardiovascular, Faculdade de Medicina, Universidade do Porto, 4200-319 Porto, Portugal
6 Nutrition & Metabolism, NOVA Medical School | FCM, NOVA University Lisbon, 1169-056 Lisbon, Portugal
7 Clinical Pathology, São João University Hospital Center, 4200-319 Porto, Portugal
8 EPIUnit, Institute of Public Health, University of Porto, 4200-319 Porto, Portugal
9 CINTESIS@RISE, Faculty of Medicine, University of Porto, 4200-319 Porto, Portugal
* Correspondence: ipires@med.up.pt (I.F.-P.); ritabsn@med.up.pt (R.N.)
† These authors contributed equally to this work.

Simple Summary: Since foods rich in refined sugars promote obesity, the use of non-caloric sweeteners has gained popularity, and their consumption by pregnant women has increased. Stevia (a non-caloric sweetener) consumption was considered safe for humans by the European Food Safety Authority in a dose of up to 4 mg/kg body weight/day. However, the World Health Organization recommended in 2023 the restraint of these sweeteners at any life stage, highlighting the need for research on pregnant women and early stages of development. So, we aimed to study the effects of chronic consumption of the main sweetener compound of stevia (Rebaudioside A) during the reproductive stage. Female rats were treated with Rebaudioside A (4 mg steviol equivalents/kg body weight/day) in the drinking water from 4 weeks before mating until weaning. Food and water consumption, blood glucose and lipids, as well as heart structure, function and mitochondrial function, were assessed. Rebaudioside A decreased heart size, cardiomyocyte area and fibrosis without repercussions on cardiac or mitochondrial function. Both fasting blood glucose and cholesterol decreased. This work suggests that stevia consumption at this dose may be safe for females during the reproductive stage. However, more studies are mandatory to explore the effects of stevia consumption on offspring's health.

Abstract: The consumption of non-sugar sweeteners (NSS) has increased during pregnancy. The European Food Safety Agency suggested that steviol glycosides, such as Rebaudioside A (RebA), the major sweetener component of stevia, are safe for humans up to a dose of 4 mg/kg body weight/day. However, the World Health Organization recommended in 2023 the restraint of using NSS, including stevia, at any life stage, highlighting the need to study NSS safety in early periods of development. We aimed to study the mitochondrial and cardiometabolic effects of long-term RebA consumption during the reproductive stage of the life cycle. Female rats were exposed to RebA (4 mg steviol equivalents/kg body weight/day) in the drinking water from 4 weeks before mating until weaning. Morphometry, food and water consumption, glucose and lipid homeostasis, heart structure, function, and mitochondrial function were assessed. RebA showed an atrophic effect in the heart, decreasing cardiomyocyte cross-sectional area and myocardial fibrosis without repercussions on cardiac function. Mitochondrial and myofilamentary functions were not altered. Glucose tolerance and insulin sensitivity were not affected, but fasting glycemia and total plasma cholesterol decreased.

This work suggests that this RebA dose is safe for female consumption during the reproductive stage, from a cardiometabolic perspective. However, studies on the effects of RebA exposure on the offspring are mandatory.

Keywords: rebaudioside A; pregnancy; lactation; cardiometabolism

1. Introduction

Obesity is a multifactorial and complex disease and one of the most common risk factors for cardiovascular disease. Obesity prevalence is alarmingly high worldwide. The World Health Organization (WHO) European Regional Obesity Report states that obesity affected 23.3% of the adult population in the WHO European region in 2022 [1]. The report also estimates that more than 20% of European women have obesity before pregnancy [1].

Since excessive energy intake from foods rich in free sugars (such as sucrose, glucose, or fructose) promotes overweight and obesity [2], the use of non-sugar sweeteners (NSS) as low-calorie alternatives has gained popularity in recent decades as a means of preventing obesity. In fact, the USA authorities reported a 50% increase in the prevalence of low-calorie sweeteners consumption by pregnant women from 1999 to 2014 [3].

Stevia is a generic name attributed to the plant, leaves, and sweetener compounds of *Stevia rebaudiana* Bertoni [4]. It is a natural NSS, introduced in the market as a sweetener in the 1970s [4]. The sweet-tasting properties of stevia are due to steviol glycosides, of which rebaudioside A (RebA) is the major component with 200 to 400 times sweetening capacity compared with sucrose [4].

Paradoxically, the consumption of NSS has been associated with increased food intake, weight gain, and adiposity in animal and human studies, suggestive of increased cardiometabolic risk and altered gut microbiota [5,6].

Not surprisingly, this topic has raised controversy. The European Food Safety Authority (EFSA) Panel on Food Additive and Flavourings (FAF) concluded in 2021 that using steviol glycosides up to 4 mg steviol equivalents/kg body weight/day presented no safety concerns for humans [7]. On the other hand, the WHO released in May 2023 a guideline recommending the restraint of using NSS, including stevia, for weight gain control at any life stage [8]. Importantly, this guideline highlights the need for future research addressing the potential long-term effects of NSS use in children and in pregnant and lactating women.

Considering the above, this work aimed to study the cardiometabolic effects of a natural NSS long-term consumption during the reproductive stage of a rodent's life cycle, while searching for putative mitochondrial involvement. To address this objective, 8-week-old Sprague Dawley females were exposed to 4 mg steviol equivalents/kg body weight/day /kg body weight/day RebA, the human dose corresponding to the EFSA's acceptable daily intake (ADI) [9], in drinking water, for 13 weeks (from 4 weeks before mating, throughout pregnancy and lactation), until sacrifice at 21 weeks of age. Morphometry, food and water consumption, glucose and lipid homeostasis, and heart structure, function, and mitochondrial function were assessed.

2. Materials and Methods

2.1. Animals and Treatments

This project was approved by the Animal Welfare and Ethics Body (ORBEA) from the Faculty of Medicine of the University of Porto, Portugal, and by the Directorate General of Food and Veterinary of the Portuguese Government (0421/000/000/2022).

As depicted in Figure 1, 8-week-old female Sprague Dawley rats (Charles River Laboratories, Barcelona, Spain) were kept under controlled environmental conditions (22–24 °C and 12 h light/dark cycles) for 1 week before the beginning of the experimental treatment and thereafter. Beverage and food (were administered ad libitum during the entire experiment. Body weight, beverage, and food consumption were evaluated daily during this acclimation week and then weekly during the entire experiment. The naso-anal length was measured weekly. At 8 weeks, females were randomly distributed into two groups: (i) the RebA group (n = 8), which was consumed 4.71–5.61 mg steviol equivalents/kg body weight/day (according to the ADI set by the Scientific Committee on Food (SCF) and EFSA [9]) (Rebaudioside A 96% HPLC, 01432-0010, Sigma-Aldrich®, Lisbon, Portugal) in the drinking water starting 4 weeks before mating, throughout pregnancy, and until the end of lactation, for a total duration of 13 weeks of treatment; and (ii) the control group (Control, n = 8) receiving drinking water. Both groups received the same standard diet (Mmucedola$_{s.r.l.}$, 4RF21, Settimo Milanese, Italy). Animals' weight was measured weekly, and RebA concentration was adjusted twice a week according to beverage consumption. Upon mating, elicited according to estrous cycle staging, pregnancy was confirmed by vaginal plug detection and vaginal cytology, allowing for the estimation of the delivery date. Mating efficiency (the number of encounters with males until conception) was also evaluated, as well as the gestational age (in days) at birth, litter size (n pups), and female-to-male ratio of each litter.

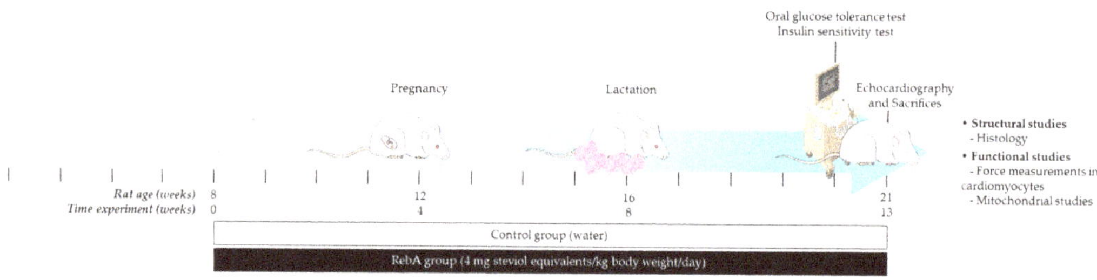

Figure 1. Experimental design. RebA, Rebaudioside A.

At 21 weeks of age, after weaning, female rats were sacrificed by exsanguination under anesthesia by intraperitoneal administration of 400 mg/mL sodium pentobarbital (Euthanimal, Nephar). Blood was obtained via cardiac puncture, and plasma and serum were separated and preserved at −80 °C for future analysis. Organs and tissues were dissected, weighed, and immediately frozen in liquid nitrogen and preserved at −80 °C or fixed in 10% formaldehyde (PanReac AppliChem, Castellar del Vallès, Spain) and processed until its inclusion in paraffin.

As considered equivalent to the body mass index in humans, the Lee index was determined using the following equation: Lee index = body weight$^{1/3}$ (g)/nasal–anal length (cm) × 1000.

Body surface area (BSA = 9.1 × body weight$^{.667}$(g)) was calculated and used to normalize echocardiographic dimensions, mass and organ weights.

2.2. Oral Glucose Tolerance Assessment and Insulin Sensitivity Assessment

Oral glucose tolerance test (OGTT) was performed in 7 h fasting animals after administering glucose (2 g/kg body weight, Fisher Scientific, London, UK) by gavage. Blood glucose concentration was measured with a FreeStyle Precision Neo system (Abbott, Amadora, Portugal) at 0, 15, 30, 60, 90, and 120 min of glucose oral gavage.

Insulin sensitivity test was performed in 7 h fasting animals after an intraperitoneal injection of insulin (0.75 U/Kg body weight, Actrapid®, Novo Nordisk®, Paço de Arcos, Portugal), and blood glucose concentration was measured as mentioned above.

2.3. Plasma Biochemical Markers Determination

Plasma biochemical markers were measured in the Central Laboratory, Department of Clinical Pathology, Centro Hospitalar Universitário São João, using conventional methods with an AU5400 automated clinical chemistry analyzer (Beckman-Coutler, Paço de Arcos, Portugal).

Hepatic function was evaluated by the determination of aspartate aminotransferase (AST), alanine aminotransferase (ALT), and alkaline phosphatase (ALP). Blood lipid parameters such as triglycerides, total cholesterol, and high-density lipoprotein cholesterol (HDL-c) were also measured, and low-density lipoprotein cholesterol (LDL-c) was calculated using the Friedwald equation.

2.4. Echocardiographic Evaluation

One day before euthanasia, each animal was anesthetized in a ventilated container (sevoflurane 5% for induction and 2.5–3% for maintaining anesthesia, Abbvie, Amadora, Portugal) to assess cardiac function. A linear 15 MHz probe (Sequoia 15L8W, UMI, Bellflower, CA, USA) and an echocardiograph Acuson Sequoia C512 (Siemens, Erlangen, Germany) were used to perform the transthoracic echocardiography. After 3 consecutive heartbeats, the recordings were averaged. M-mode was used to determine systolic and diastolic wall thickness, cavity dimensions, and transverse aortic root diameter via the parasternal short-axis view. The left ventricle (LV) mass, the ejection fraction, and the fractional shortening were calculated as previously described [10]. Mitral flow velocity tracings were obtained via pulsed-wave Doppler just above the mitral leaflets [10].

2.5. Mitochondrial Respiration Evaluation Using Permeabilized Cardiac Fibers

A portion of freshly isolated myocardium was immediately immersed in ice-cold BIOPS, a preservation solution composed of 10 mM Ca-EGTA buffer, 0.1 μM free calcium, 20 mM imidazole, 20 mM taurine, 50 mM K-MES, 0.5 mM DTT, 6.56 mM $MgCl_2$, 5.77 mM ATP, and 15 mM phosphocreatine with a pH of 7.1. Using two pairs of sharp forceps, the fiber bundles were mechanically separated in a small, ice-cold Petri dish and then placed into individual wells of a 12-well tissue culture plate with ice-cold BIOPS until all fibers were prepared. Subsequently, fiber bundles were submersed into a well with freshly prepared saponin solution (50 μg/mL of BIOPS) and incubated for 30 min with gentle agitation. Finally, the fibers were placed into 2 mL of ice-cold MiR06 [a mitochondrial respiration medium composed of MiR05 (0.5 mM EGTA, 3 mM $MgCl_2$, 60 mM lactobionic acid, 10 mM KH_2PO_4, 20 mM taurine, 20 mM HEPES, 110 mM D-sucrose, and 1 g/L essentially fatty acid-free bovine serum albumin (BSA) with a pH of 7.1) supplemented with 280 U/mL catalase] during 10 min on ice. Permeabilized fiber bundles were then carefully blotted on filter paper, weighed, and 1–2 mg wet weight was transferred into each chamber of the high-resolution respirometer (Oroboros Instruments, Innsbruck, Austria), containing 2 mL of MiR06 [11]. Using the high-resolution respirometer Oroboros Oxygraph-2k (Oroboros Instruments, Innsbruck, Austria), mitochondrial respiratory function was assessed. The Substrate-uncoupler-inhibitor titration (SUIT)-001 O2 pfi D002 protocol for permeabilized muscle fibers was followed at 37 °C (sequential addition of 5 mM pyruvate, 2 mM malate, 7.5 mM ADP, 10 μM cytochrome C, 0.5 μM CCCP, 10 mM glutamate, 10 mM succinate, 0.5 mM octanoylcarnitine, 0.5 μM rotenone, 10 mM glycerophosphate, 2.5 μM Antimicin A, 2 mM ascorbate, 0.5 mM TMPD, and 200 mM sodium azide). Oxygen flux rate and concentration were recorded and analyzed using DatLab software (Oroboros Datlab Version 7.0, Oroboros Instruments Innsbruck, Innsbruck, Austria). Oxygen flux was expressed in $pmol \cdot s^{-1} \cdot mg^{-1}$ normalized for the weight of the fiber bundle (mg). All reagents referred to in this section were the ones recommended by the Oroboros Instrument, Innsbruck, Austria (https://wiki.oroboros.at/index.php/OROBOROS_INSTRUMENTS).

2.6. Force Measurements in Isolated Permeabilized Cardiomyocytes

The specimen preparation protocol has been previously described [12]. In brief, LV myocardial tissue from each animal was cut into small pieces, mechanically disrupted, and incubated for 5 min in extraction solution (in mM: Na_2ATP, 5.97; MgCl, 6.28; $C_3H_6O_2$, 40.64; BES, 100; CaEGTA, 7; and Na_2PCr, 14.5) supplemented with 0.5% Triton X-100 (All from Merck Millipore, Burlington, MA, USA) at room temperature, to remove membrane structures. Cardiomyocytes were washed with extraction solution by consecutive centrifugations. An isolated cardiomyocyte was attached with glue between a force transducer and an electromagnetic motor length controller (Aurora Scientific Inc. (Aurora, ON, Canada) model 403A and model 315C-I, respectively). Passive tension (PT)-sarcomere length (SL) relationships ranging between 1.8 and 2.3 μm were acquired at 15 °C, with 0.1 μm step increases. Maximal activation at pCa 4.5 was used to calculate maximal calcium-activated isometric force (Total tension, Tt) and the slack test (the cell was shortened for 1 ms to 80% of its original length). A relaxing solution (in mM: Na_2ATP, 5.89; MgCl, 6.48; $C_3H_6O_2$, 40.76; BES, 100; CaEGTA, 6.97; and Na_2PCr, 14.5; all reagents were from Merck Millipore, Burlington, MA, USA), pCa 9.0, was used to determine passive tension (Tp). The cardiomyocyte cross-sectional area was used to normalize the force values to the cell's dimensions. Data acquisition was made by the ASI 600 A program with a sampling frequency of 2 KHz.

2.7. Histology

The heart (at the ventricular base) was sliced and fixed in 10% formaldehyde (PanReac AppliChem, Castellar del Vallès, Spain), dehydrated in ethanol (100%, 90% and 70% v/v), cleared in xylol (Fisher Scientific, London, UK), and impregnated in paraffin ("Epredia™ Paraffin Type 6", Epredia, Breda, The Netherlands). Five-micrometer slides were dewaxed, rehydrated, stained with Hematoxylin–Eosin (HE) (Hematoxylin H and Eosin Y 1% v/v alcoholic, Biognost, Zagreb, Croatia) to assess the cardiomyocyte area, or Picrosirius Red (Direct Red 80, Sigma-Aldrich, St. Louis, MO, USA), to assess myocardial fibrosis, and finally mounted with Entellan™ (rapid mounting medium for microscopy, Merck, Darmstadt, Germany). A photographic camera (Olympus XC30, Tokyo, Japan) coupled with an optic microscope (Leitz Wetzlar—Dialux 20, Wetzlar, Germany) was used to visualize and photograph the histological preparations. The area of 60 cardiomyocytes per animal was measured using Cell^B software serial number A5607500-74EBB51C (Olympus, Tokyo, Japan). To calculate the area of fibrosis and perivascular fibrosis, eight and five fields per animal, respectively, were photographed and analyzed using Image-Pro Pus 6 software (Media Cybernetics, Rockville, MD, USA).

2.8. Biomarker of Myocardial Fibrotic Assessment

Transforming growth factor-beta (TGF-β1), a powerful fibrogenic cytokine, was tested by ELISA following the standard protocol provided by Elabscience Corporation (Wuhan, China).

2.9. Statistical Analysis

Results are expressed as mean ± SEM. Statistical analysis was performed using GraphPad Prism software (Version 10.1.2). Shapiro–Wilk was used to assess parametric distribution. Comparison between the two groups was assessed by t-test. Comparisons between more than two groups were performed by one- or two-way ANOVA, and appropriate post hoc tests were used. The probability values < 0.05 were considered significant.

3. Results

3.1. Gestational and Morphometric Data

RebA did not affect mating efficiency, gestational age at birth, litter size, or female-to-male ratio of each litter (Table 1).

Figure 2 displays weight evolution as well as the daily amount of food and water intake. RebA did not affect weight gain or the Lee index until sacrifice (Figure 2A,B). Accordingly, RebA did not significantly change water or food consumption over time (Figure 2C,D), even though the RebA group drank more water at two time points after gestation.

Table 1. Gestational and morphometric data.

	Control				RebA				p-Value [b]
	Mean	±	SEM	(n)	Mean	±	SEM	(n)	
Mating efficiency (n mating attempts) [a]	1.9	±	0.4	(8)	2.5	±	0.5	(8)	0.300
Gestational age at birth (days)	21.5	±	0.3	(8)	21.9	±	0.1	(8)	0.224
Litter size (pups)	12.5	±	1.1	(8)	14.3	±	0.5	(8)	0.526
Female-to-male ratio	1.1	±	0.2	(6)	0.8	±	0.1	(8)	0.138
Body weight at euthanasia (g)	323.4	±	4.8	(8)	314.5	±	5.8	(8)	0.257

[a] Corresponds to the number of encounters with males until conception was confirmed. [b] t-test. RebA, rebaudioside A; SEM, standard error of the mean.

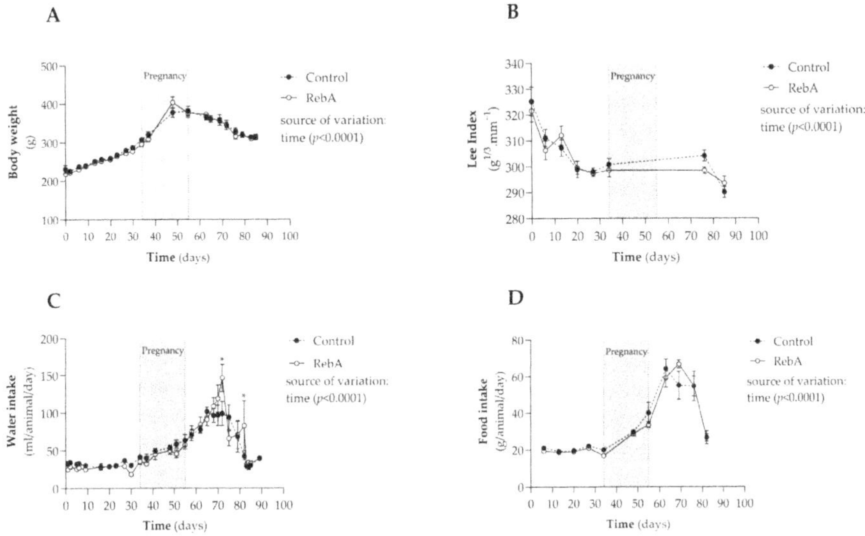

Figure 2. Body weight and feeding. Rebaudioside A in the drinking water (RebA) or drinking water alone (Control) was given from 4 weeks before mating (throughout pregnancy and lactation) until sacrifice at 21 weeks of age. During the study, (**A**) body weight, (**B**) Lee index, (**C**) water, and (**D**) food intake were measured. Results are presented as mean ± SEM (C or RebA, $n = 8$ each). Two-way ANOVA indicated a significant effect of time upon all measures ($p < 0.001$). * $p < 0.05$ versus Control (Bonferroni's multiple comparisons test).

Interestingly, RebA consumption reduced liver and heart weight, even after adjusting for BSA, as seen in Table 2.

Table 2. Organ weight adjusted for body surface area.

Organ Weight	Control				RebA				p-Value [b]
	Mean	±	SEM	(n)	Mean	±	SEM	(n)	
Liver/BSA (mg/cm^2)	23.3	±	0.38	(8)	21.6	±	0.31	(8)	0.005
Pancreas/BSA (mg/cm^2)	1.94	±	0.22	(7)	2.42	±	0.21	(8)	0.188
Heart/BSA (mg/cm^2)	26.8	±	0.05	(8)	25.0	±	0.04	(8)	0.031
Skeletal muscle/BSA (mg/cm^2)	4.73	±	0.17	(8)	4.87	±	0.06	(7)	0.505

[b] t-test; RebA, rebaudioside A; SEM, standard error of the mean.

3.2. Glycemic Control

At the end of the experiment (20 weeks of age), a significant reduction in fasting glycemia in the RebA group was observed when compared to the Control group

(72.8 ± 2.18 mg/dL versus 84.8 ± 3.04 mg/dL, Figure 3A). Nevertheless, RebA chronic consumption did not affect oral glucose tolerance (Figure 3B,C) or insulin sensitivity (Figure 3D).

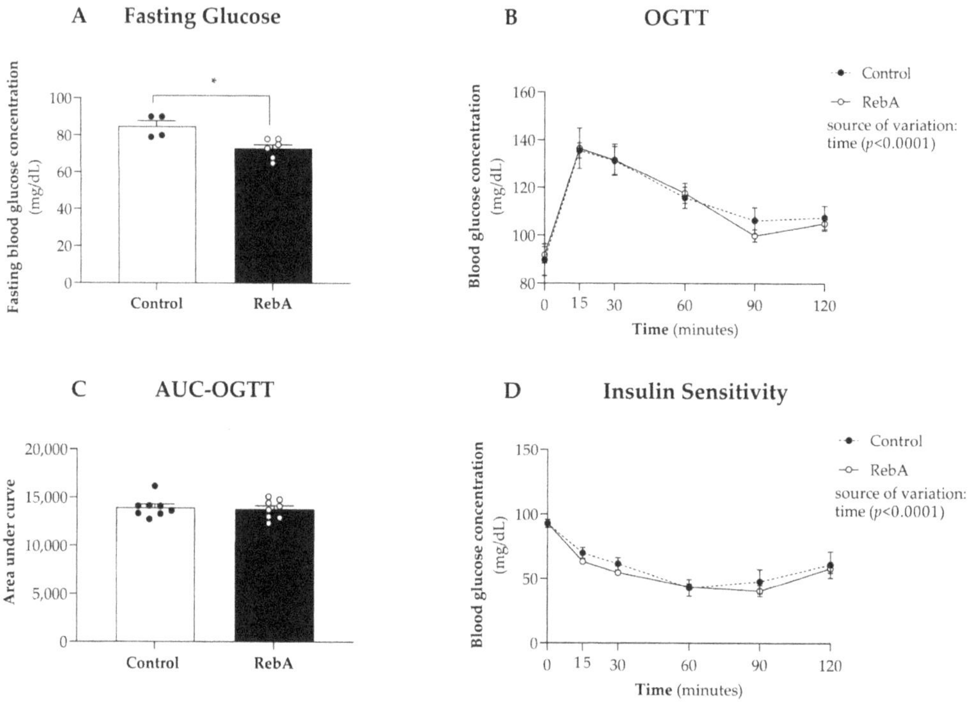

Figure 3. Glycemic control. Animals were treated with rebaudioside A in the drinking water (RebA) or with drinking water alone (Control) from 4 weeks before mating (throughout pregnancy and lactation) until sacrifice at 21 weeks of age. At 20 weeks of age, (**A**) fasting glycemia; (**B**) oral glucose tolerance test (OGTT); (**C**) the corresponding area under the curve (AUC); and (**D**) insulin sensitivity were measured. Data are represented as mean ± SEM (Control or RebA, $4 \leq n \leq 8$ each). Two-way ANOVA indicated a significant effect of time upon all measures ($p < 0.001$). * $p < 0.05$ versus Control (t-test).

Two-way ANOVA indicated a significant effect of time upon all measures ($p < 0.001$) (Figure 3B,D) but revealed no statistically significant effect of RebA treatment or interaction between treatment and time for any measured parameter.

3.3. *Plasma Biochemical Markers*

Figure 4 shows the plasma levels of triglycerides, total cholesterol, LDL-c, and HDL-c of all animals at 21 weeks of age. RebA group presented a significantly lower plasma concentration of total cholesterol (67.75 ± 2.46 mg/dL), LDL-c (27.88 ± 1.81 mg/dL) and HDL-c (43.63 ± 1.40 mg/dL) compared to control group (total cholesterol, 84.13 ± 6.04 mg/dL; LDL-c, 35.75 ± 3.11 mg/dL and HDL-c, 53.88 ± 4.09 mg/dL). Nevertheless, the ratio HDL-c/LDL-c was not different between the two groups (1.53 ± 0.05 mg/dL for Control and 1.60 ± 0.08 mg/dL for RebA, $p = 0.473$). Regarding triglyceride levels, no differences were found between groups.

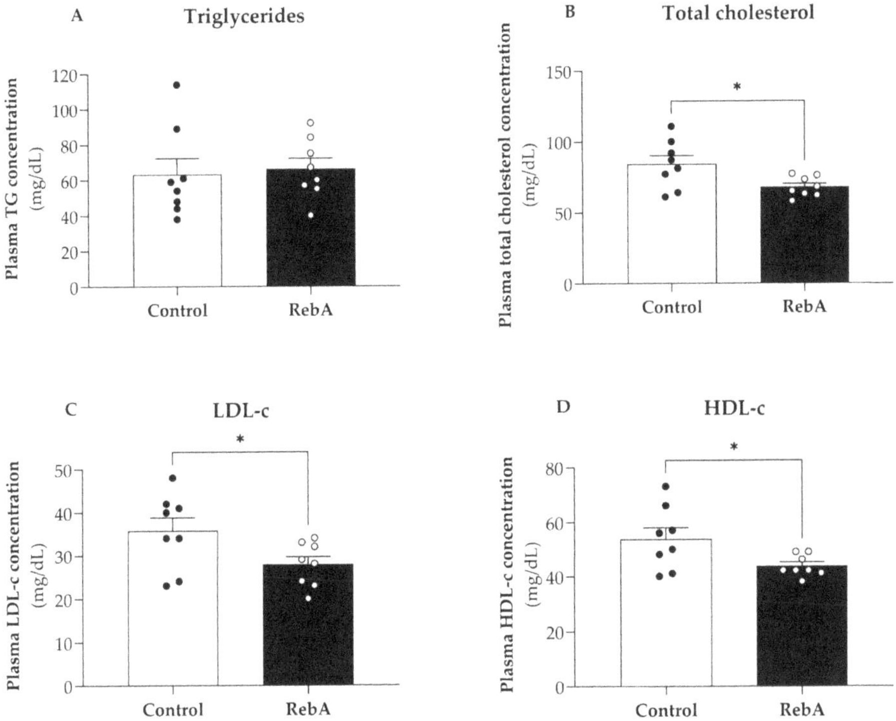

Figure 4. Lipid profile of animals at 21 weeks of age after treatment with rebaudioside A in the drinking water (RebA) or drinking water alone (Control) from 4 weeks before mating (throughout pregnancy and lactation) until sacrifice at 21 weeks of age. (**A**) Triglycerides, (**B**) total cholesterol, (**C**) low-density lipoprotein cholesterol (LDL-c), and (**D**) high-density lipoprotein cholesterol (HDL-c) were measured. Data are represented as mean ± SEM (Control or RebA, $n = 8$ each). T-test indicated a significant effect of RebA upon total cholesterol, LDL-c, and HDL-c. * $p < 0.05$ versus Control (t-test).

When evaluating the plasma activity of aspartate aminotransferase (AST), alanine aminotransferase (ALT), and alkaline phosphatase (ALP) at 21 weeks of age, no differences were found between groups.

3.4. Left Ventricle Cardiac Structure and Functional Characterization

The echocardiographic evaluation showed no differences in cardiac function between groups. Regarding structure, posterior LV wall thickness and relative wall thickness were significantly reduced in the RebA group (25% and 12% reductions compared to control, respectively, Table 3).

Subsequently, we aimed to explore if the slight cardiac atrophy assessed by decreased heart weight/BSA (Table 2) and by echocardiography (Table 3) had any cardiac functional impact. In vivo echocardiography further confirmed that this atrophic effect had no major impact on systolic or diastolic function (Table 3). Consistently, we showed that RebA reduced cardiomyocyte cross-sectional area (Control, 358.6 ± 7.486 vs. RebA, 288.5 ± 9.381 μm^2) (Figure 5A), cardiac interstitial fibrosis (Control, 3.99 ± 0.18 vs. RebA, 3.25 ± 0.13%) (Figure 5B), and perivascular fibrosis (Control, 18.29 ± 0.933 vs. RebA, 11.79 ± 0.583 μm^2) (Figure 5C).

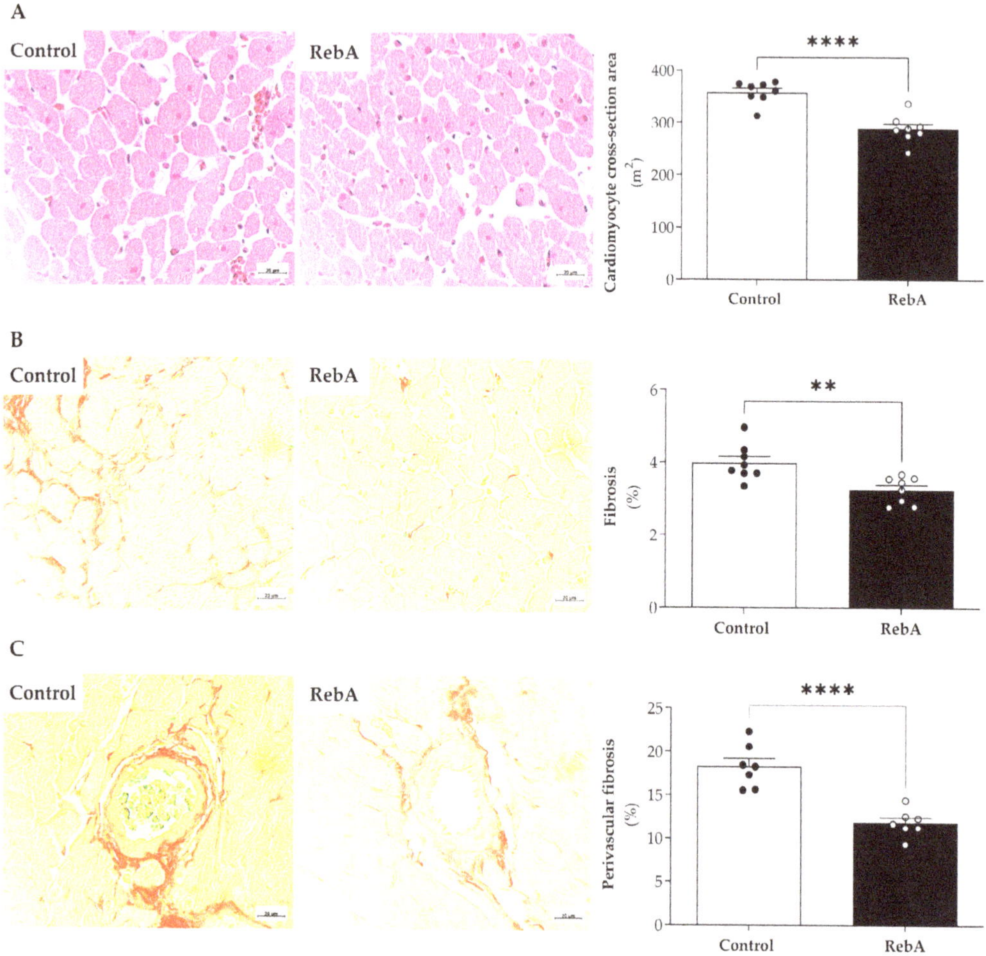

Figure 5. Cardiac morphological characterization at 21 weeks of age. Animals were treated from 4 weeks before mating (throughout pregnancy and lactation) until sacrifice (21 weeks of age) with rebaudioside A in the drinking water (RebA) or drinking water alone (Control). (**A**) Hematoxylin-eosin of left ventricular slices to assess cardiomyocyte cross-sectional area, (**B**) Picrosirius-red staining of left ventricular slices to assess fibrosis was measured, and (**C**) Picrosirius-red staining of left ventricular perivascular fibrosis. The representative sections of each group are represented at a magnification of ×40. Data are presented as mean ± SEM (Control or RebA, n = 8 each). T-test indicated a significant effect of RebA upon heart cardiomyocyte area, fibrosis, and perivascular fibrosis. ** $p < 0.05$ and **** $p < 0.0001$ versus Control (t-test).

In fact, despite the differences found in the values of cardiomyocyte fibrosis and perivascular fibrosis between groups, plasma levels of TGF-β1, a generally accepted promoter of myocardial fibrosis, was similar between groups (Figure 6).

The mechanical properties of single-skinned cardiomyocytes were measured to assess function at the cardiomyocyte level without interferences from the extracellular matrix (Figure 7A). Stiffness was similar between groups, as confirmed by similar passive tension–sarcomere length relationship curves and passive tension at 2.2 μm (Figure 7B,D).

Additionally, no changes were observed in the maximal developed tension or myofilament Ca^{2+} sensitivity (Figure 7C,E).

Table 3. In vivo echocardiographic evaluation of cardiac function and structure.

Parameter	Control Mean ± SEM	(*n*)	RebA Mean ± SEM	(*n*)	*p*-Value
Heart rate (bpm)	287.5 ± 6.9	(8)	269.2 ± 9.4	(8)	0.165
LV end-diastolic volume/BSA ($cm^3.cm^{-2}$)	1.260 ± 0.065	(8)	1.20 ± 0.054	(8)	0.604
LV end-systolic volume/BSA ($cm^3.cm^{-2}$)	0.049 ± 0.042	(8)	0.050 ± 0.040	(8)	0.969
Interventricular septum (mm)	1.48 ± 0.13	(8)	1.39 ± 0.13	(8)	0.171
Posterior LV wall (mm)	$0.004 \pm 85 \times 10^{-5}$	(8)	$0.003 \pm 12 \times 10^{-5}$	(8)	0.047
LV mass/BSA ($g{\cdot}cm^{-2}$)	1.614 ± 0.081	(8)	1.508 ± 0.060	(8)	0.329
Relative wall thickness	0.890 ± 0.025	(8)	0.780 ± 0.029	(8)	0.025
Ejection fraction (%)	75.38 ± 2.30	(8)	71.28 ± 1.43	(8)	0.176
Cardiac index $mL{\cdot}min{\cdot}cm^{-2}$	0.113 ± 0.005	(8)	0.102 ± 0.005	(8)	0.152
E/A	1.88 ± 0.54	(8)	2.15 ± 0.69	(8)	0.398
Tei index	0.44 ± 0.06	(8)	0.46 ± 0.10	(8)	0.748

RebA, rebaudioside A; SEM, standard error of the mean; BSA, body surface area; E/A: ratio between peak E and A waves of pulsed-wave Doppler mitral flow velocity; LV, left ventricle.

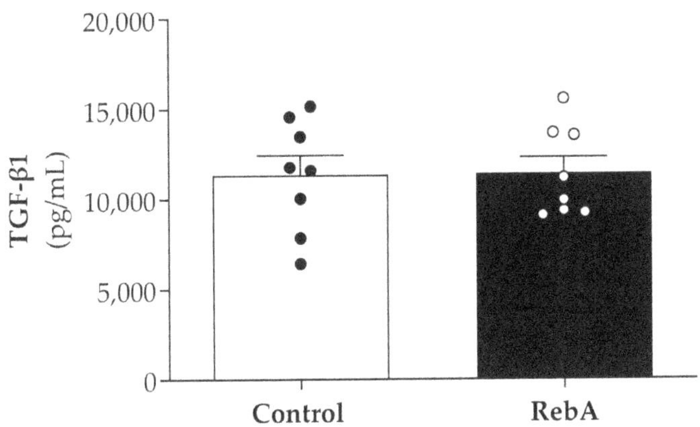

Figure 6. Plasma levels of TGF-β1 in animals treated from 4 weeks before mating (throughout pregnancy and lactation) until sacrifice (21 weeks of age) with rebaudioside A in the drinking water (RebA) or drinking water alone (Control).

The impact of RebA administration on cardiac mitochondrial respiratory function was evaluated by high-resolution respirometry of permeabilized cardiac fibers. RebA administration did not significantly affect mitochondrial respiratory function. Namely, no differences were observed in mitochondrial oxygen fluxes using Complex I and II substrates (Figure 8). Similarly, mitochondrial outer membrane integrity and the stimulation of respiration by fatty acid oxidation were unaffected (Cyt and Oct, Figure 8).

A trend towards increased Complex IV-associated respiration was observed with the administration of RebA (Δ20.4%) (Figure 8). Nevertheless, the values are very scattered, and there are no significant differences between groups.

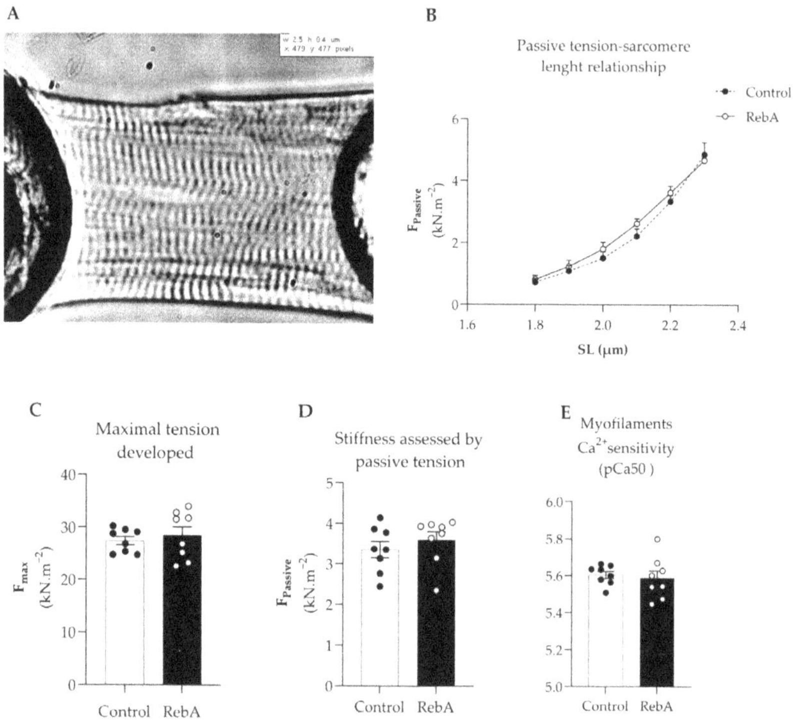

Figure 7. Force measurements in isolated permeabilized cardiomyocytes of the left ventricle (LV). Rebaudioside A in the drinking water (RebA) or drinking water alone (Control) was given from 4 weeks before mating (throughout pregnancy and lactation) until sacrifice at 21 weeks of age. (**A**) Representative image of a skinned cardiomyocyte stretched at 2.2 μm, (**B**) stiffness assessed by passive tension–sarcomere length relationship, (**C**) maximal tension developed, (**D**) stiffness assessed by passive tension, and (**E**) myofilament Ca^{2+}-sensitivity expressed by pCa50. Data are presented as mean ± SEM (Control or RebA, n = 8 each).

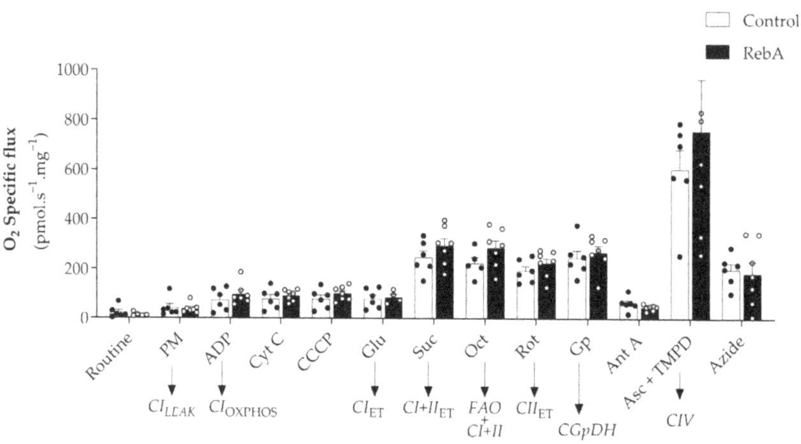

Figure 8. Heart mitochondrial function assessed by high-resolution respirometry, using the Oroboros Oxygraph-2k, of females treated with Rebaudioside A in the drinking water (RebA) or drinking water alone (Control) from 4 weeks before mating (throughout pregnancy and lactation) until sacrifice at

21 weeks of age. Results are presented as mean ± SEM (Control, $n = 6$ and RebA, $n = 7$). (T-test or Mann–Whitney test). PM: pyruvate + malate (Complex I, leak state); ADP: adenosine diphosphate (Complex I, OXPHOS state); Cyt C: cytochrome c (test for mitochondrial outer membrane integrity); CCCP (uncoupler); Glu: glutamate (Complex I, electron transfer (ET) state); Suc: succinate (Complex I+II, ET state); Oct: octanoylcarnitine (Fatty acid oxidation + Complex I+II, ET state); Rot: rotenone (Complex II, ET state); Gp: glycerophosphate (Complex II + glycerophosphate dehydrogenase, ET state); Ant A: antimycin A (residual oxygen consumption, ROX); Asc + TMPD: ascorbate + TMPD (Complex IV); Azide: sodium azide.

4. Discussion

This work showed that long-term (13 weeks) RebA consumption during the reproductive stage of female rats with the human ADI defined by EFSA did not majorly impact the cardiometabolic health of female rats.

Interestingly, RebA showed an atrophic effect in the heart without any repercussions on cardiac function. This result was further confirmed histologically, as demonstrated by a decreased cardiomyocyte cross-sectional area. Importantly, myocardial fibrosis was reduced in the RebA group, while mitochondrial and myofilamentary function was preserved.

Glucose homeostasis was also not majorly affected by RebA consumption, except for a reduction in fasting glycemia at the end of the study, for values close to the lowest value of the rat's euglycemic range (70–180 mg/dL) [13]. Sunanarunsawat and colleagues demonstrated increased insulin and decreased glucagon serum levels in diabetic rats, but not in the normoglycemic group, after receiving unspecified stevioside (0.25 g/kg body weight) or aqueous extract of *Stevia rebaudiana* (4.66 g/kg body weight) for 8 weeks [14]. These authors concluded that the beneficial impact of *Stevia rebaudiana* on glucagon and insulin levels could underlie its anti-hyperglycemic actions [14]. In our study, although the rats were normoglycemic, we detected a slight hypoglycemic trend induced by RebA as fasting glycemia decreased from 84.8 ± 3.04 mg/dL in the control group to 72.8 ± 2.18 mg/dL in the RebA group, in line with previous reports claiming that RebA reduces glycemia in humans [15–17] and in rats [18]. Moreover, the anti-hyperglycemic effects of stevia have been ascribed to the properties of stevioside and RebA as agonists of insulin receptors, causing an increase in glucose uptake by cardiac fibroblasts [19].

In our study, the observed decrease in liver weight could contribute to the observed hypoglycemic effect of RebA since the liver is the major source of glucose during fasting. Although other authors have shown no differences in liver weight, they report RebA (40 mg/Kg/day i.p.) to prevent liver injury, oxidative stress, and liver fibrosis caused by thioacetamide (200 mg/kg) [20]. In high-fat diet-induced nonalcoholic steatohepatitis obese mice, the administration of RebA decreased fasting glucose levels and hepatic stress enzymes, such as alanine aminotransferase (ALT) and plasma aspartate aminotransferase (AST) at 15 weeks post-intervention [21]. The authors suggest that hepatoprotection induced by RebA can be associated with, or even mediated by, improved pancreatic endocrine function that leads to anti-hyperglycemic effects [21]. Despite the observed decrease in in liver weight upon RebA treatment, we did not observe any changes in the hepatic ALT, AST, and ALP enzymes, suggesting that RebA at treatment dosage did not cause hepatic toxicity or hepatoprotection, probably because females were not submitted to a diet or metabolic challenge. Importantly, RebA doses used in the above-mentioned studies were higher than the dose used in the present study, which may also underlie variations in its biological effects. It is known that rat's liver increases during pregnancy because of the proliferation of hepatocytes, a process that is reverted during weaning by hepatocytes's death and liver remodeling [22]. As we could observe that RebA exposure decreased liver weight after 21 weeks, it would be interesting to evaluate liver changes during pregnancy and weaning to understand if this decrease in liver size observed only in dams exposed to RebA was already seen during pregnancy and weaning and to further understand the effects on offspring health.

RebA treatment also improved lipid homeostasis as it decreased total plasma cholesterol and LDL-c while maintaining the HDL-c/LDL-c ratio. Dyslipidemia is one of the major cardiovascular risk factors. In fact, total plasma cholesterol is directly associated with cardiovascular risk, as well as the decrease in HDL-c/LDL-c ratio. Although we could not observe an increase in the ratio HDL-c/LDL-c, the decrease in total plasma cholesterol upon RebA treatment already represents a better cardiovascular profile. Saravanan and Ramachandran also observed a decrease in total plasma cholesterol upon administration of a higher dose of RebA treatment (200 mg/kg/day for 45 days) on diabetic animals [23]. Ilias et al. suggested that RebA promotes the internalization of cholesterol by hepatocytes, modulating the expression of genes involved in cholesterol metabolism, such as *HMGCR*, *LDLR*, and *ACAT2* [24], which may, in part, explain our results.

Despite the anti-diabetic actions, stevia derivatives are also reported to have anti-fibrotic effects [25], corroborating our results. Our study was carried out in healthy female rats. Pregnancy is expected to physiologically induce cardiac hypertrophy and decreased fibrosis, which are expected to revert in rodents 14 days after delivery [26], a process called postpartum cardiac reverse remodeling. In our study, RebA-fed females showed cardiac atrophy and decreased cardiac fibrosis far beyond the period of reverse remodeling (40 days after delivery). These alterations may underlie the observed LV atrophy.

The anti-fibrotic properties observed for Reb A are of great therapeutic potential and deserve to be further explored. Indeed, our data agree with the study by Zhao et al., who have shown that a non-identified stevioside reduced cardiac fibrosis in Type 1 diabetic mice by modulating the expression of matrix metallopeptidases while increasing glucose tolerance [27]. Conversely to our observations, stevioside increased heart weight but in diabetic animals, which, in the case of Zhao's study, is beneficial as it counterbalances the type 1 diabetes-induced pathologic atrophy. It is important to note that, in that study, stevioside was used in a dose more than 10 times higher than the dose administered in our study.

To understand whether the morphological adaptations caused by RebA (reduced heart weight and decreased posterior and relative wall thicknesses) impacted cardiac function, we carried out in vivo echocardiographic and in vitro single-skinned cardiomyocyte evaluations. The observed structural changes did not affect cardiac myofilamentary function as assessed by preserved ejection fraction, cardiac output, and E/A between groups. Accordingly, in vitro, we did not find differences in cardiomyocyte contractile force, stiffness, or sensitivity for Ca^{2+} between groups. However, we cannot rule out that these results can be time- or dose-dependent.

Known as critical metabolic players, mitochondria have been recognized as essential for multiple functions beyond energy production, regulating cell apoptosis, inflammation, and immunological processes [28,29]. It is also known that they are dysfunctional in several pathological conditions, such as obesity and diabetes [30]. Hepatic lipid accumulation may result from mitochondrial dysfunction [31], and several diabetic complications can be, in part, attributed to excessive production of ROS by mitochondria in a chronic hyperglycemia environment, increasing oxidative stress and activating stress-response pathways. Interestingly, RebA extended the lifespan and health of C. elegans via the reduction in ROS, decreasing aging lipid accumulation [32]. In addition to this, the microbiome–mitochondrion axis is currently suggested as an important player in cardiometabolic fitness [33,34], and RebA consumption has been described as a modulator of gut microbiota in obese dams [35] and in male rats [36].

Studies assessing the effect of *Stevia rebaudiana* (or their components, stevioside and rebaudioside) on mitochondrial function are scarce. To the best of our knowledge, this is the first study to explore the effects of steviol glycosides (RebA) on mitochondrial respiration using high-resolution respirometry. In accordance with metabolic and cardiac function results, we reported no differences in the function of cardiac mitochondria of female rats after 13 weeks of RebA treatment (4.71–5.61 mg steviol equivalents/kg body weight/day) when compared to the control group. However, a non-significant 20% increase in oxygen flux was observed in complex IV. Mutations and deficiencies in complex IV have been associated with dilated, hypertrophic, and histiocytoid cardiomyopathies [37]. In addition, in a model of insulin resistance with metabolic syndrome, myocardial mitochondria were smaller but had an increased amount of mitochondrial complex IV proteins reflecting an adaptative mitochondrial activity [38]. As we observed, RebA promoted a reduced heart weight, and the effect in Complex IV could be an adaptative response. Nonetheless, the results obtained are very scattered and non-significant in the RebA group.

Despite this, unravelling whether RebA chronic consumption could interfere with the microbiome–mitochondrion axis would be interesting.

In human breast cancer cells (MCF-7), stevioside is a potent inducer of apoptosis via altering mitochondrial transmembrane potential [39]. In rats supplemented with whey protein sweetened with 0.2% S. rebaudiana extract, peroxisome proliferator-activated receptor γ coactivator 1-α (PGC-1α), an important mitochondrial biogenesis marker, was significantly higher when compared with control animals [40]. In line with our results, Han and colleagues also demonstrated that mitochondrial activity was enhanced in the skeletal muscle of diabetic mice treated with a high dose of stevia extract (500 mg/kg/day) but not in the stevioside group (40 mg/kg/day) [41].

The physiological actions of RebA are still unclear due to the high heterogeneity of studies, the huge differences in doses used, the times of intervention, and stevia derivatives. In a systematic review with meta-analysis including 756 participants, RebA did not improve blood pressure or cardiovascular risk in contrast to stevioside, which seems to decrease blood pressure and fasting glycemia, although the small effect and the robustness of the results are limited to the heterogeneity of the studies included [42].

The fact that we did not find major cardiometabolic effects may be explained by the dose administrated, the one recommended by EFSA as safe for humans (4 mg/kg body weight/day). The more marked effects obtained in other studies described above may reflect the use of higher doses or combined with reducing glucose ingested. Considering that steviol glycoside is currently the third most common NSS across all food groups [43], new studies regarding exposures during the reproductive stage with higher doses of RebA are needed to analyze the effects of overconsumption of glucosylated steviol glycosides in comparison to the effects of recommended doses [9]. Although the absence of significant cardiometabolic alterations may indicate that this RebA dose is safe regarding female consumption during the reproductive stage, we did not evaluate these cardiometabolic parameters during pregnancy and lactation, which is a limitation of this study. The fact that RebA did not affect mating efficiency, gestational age at birth, litter size, or female-to-male ratio of each litter is also important regarding safety during the reproductive stage of the life cycle as they are indicators of successful reproduction.

Nevertheless, concerns have been raised regarding the safety of RebA consumption during pregnancy as it may pass the placenta [44] and induce metabolic disease in the offspring in the long term [35]. This issue deserves future research.

5. Conclusions

In conclusion, our work shows that chronic RebA consumption during the reproductive stage in the human dose recommended as safe by EFSA (4 mg/kg/day) induced a hypoglycemic effect without altering glucose tolerance or insulin sensitivity and improved blood lipid profile. Additionally, RebA consumption reduced cardiac fibrosis, preserving cardiac, myofilamentary, and mitochondrial function.

Author Contributions: I.B.: Conceptualization, data curation, formal analysis, visualization, writing—original draft, review, and editing. J.M.: Data curation, formal analysis, visualization, writing—original draft, review, and editing. J.A.C.: Data curation, investigation, software, and writing—review and editing. A.F.F.: Data curation, investigation, and software. I.A.: Data curation, investigation, software, and writing—review and editing. C.M.: Data curation, investigation, and software. B.C.: Data curation and investigation. A.G.: Data curation, investigation, and software. J.T.G.: Formal analysis, resources, writing—original draft, review, and editing. I.F.-P.: Conceptualization, formal analysis, resources, writing—original draft, review and editing, supervision, and validation. E.K.: Conceptualization, methodology, formal analysis, investigation, writing—original draft, review and editing, supervision, project administration, funding acquisition, and validation. R.N.: Conceptualization, methodology, formal analysis, investigation, writing—original draft, review and editing, supervision, project administration, funding acquisition, and validation. All authors have read and agreed to the published version of the manuscript.

Funding: This work was financed by national funds via the Northern Regional Operational Program under the HEALTH-UNORTE project (NORTE-01-0145-FEDER-000039) and the FCT Fundação para a Ciência e a Tecnologia. I.P. within the scope of the projects "RISE—LA/P/0053/2020" and "CINTESIS—UIDB/4255/2020" and Cardiovascular R&D Center (UIDB/00051/2020 and UIDP/00051/2020). Isabella Bracchi was funded by the European Regional Development Fund (ERDF) via the Northern Regional Operational Program under the HEALTH-UNORTE project (NORTE-01-0145-FEDER-000039) and by FCT/MCTES (Foundation for Science and Technology and Ministry of Science, Technology and Higher Education) (2023.03003.BD). Juliana Morais was funded by FCT/MCTES (Foundation for Science and Technology and Ministry of Science, Technology and Higher Education) under CINTESIS by a Ph.D. scholarship (UI/BD/152306/2021).

Institutional Review Board Statement: The animal study protocol was approved by the Directorate General of Food and Veterinary of the Portuguese Government (protocol code 0421/000/000/2022) on 18 February 2022.

Informed Consent Statement: Not applicable.

Data Availability Statement: Data are contained within the article.

Conflicts of Interest: The authors declare no conflicts of interest.

References

1. *WHO European Regional Obesity Report 2022*; WHO Regional Office for Europe: Copenhagen, Denmark, 2022.
2. Johnson, R.K.; Appel, L.J.; Brands, M.; Howard, B.V.; Lefevre, M.; Lustig, R.H.; Sacks, F.; Steffen, L.M.; Wylie-Rosett, J. Dietary Sugars Intake and Cardiovascular Health. *Circulation* **2009**, *120*, 1011–1020. [CrossRef] [PubMed]
3. Sylvetsky, A.C.; Figueroa, J.; Rother, K.I.; Goran, M.I.; Welsh, J.A. Trends in Low-Calorie Sweetener Consumption Among Pregnant Women in the United States. *Curr. Dev. Nutr.* **2019**, *3*, nzz004. [CrossRef] [PubMed]
4. Ashwell, M. Stevia, Nature's Zero-Calorie Sustainable Sweetener: A New Player in the Fight Against Obesity. *Nutr. Today* **2015**, *50*, 129–134. [CrossRef]
5. Fowler, S.P.G. Low-calorie sweetener use and energy balance: Results from experimental studies in animals, and large-scale prospective studies in humans. *Physiol. Behav.* **2016**, *164*, 517–523. [CrossRef] [PubMed]
6. Azad, M.B.; Abou-Setta, A.M.; Chauhan, B.F.; Rabbani, R.; Lys, J.; Copstein, L.; Mann, A.; Jeyaraman, M.M.; Reid, A.E.; Fiander, M.; et al. Nonnutritive sweeteners and cardiometabolic health: A systematic review and meta-analysis of randomized controlled trials and prospective cohort studies. *Can. Med. Assoc. J.* **2017**, *189*, E929–E939. [CrossRef]
7. EFSA Panel on Food Additives and Flavourings (FAF); Younes, M.; Aquilina, G.; Engel, K.H.; Fowler, P.J.; Frutos Fernandez, M.J.; Fürst, P.; Gürtler, R.; Gundert-Remy, U.; Husøy, T.; et al. Safety evaluation of glucosylated steviol glycosides as a food additive in different food categories. *EFSA J.* **2022**, *20*, e07066. [CrossRef]
8. *Use of Non-Sugar Sweeteners: WHO Guideline*; World Health Organization: Geneva, Switzerland, 2023.
9. EFSA. Scientific Opinion on the safety of steviol glycosides for the proposed uses as a food additive. *EFSA J.* **2010**, *8*, 1537. [CrossRef]
10. Hamdani, N.; Franssen, C.; Lourenco, A.; Falcao-Pires, I.; Fontoura, D.; Leite, S.; Plettig, L.; Lopez, B.; Ottenheijm, C.A.; Becher, P.M.; et al. Myocardial titin hypophosphorylation importantly contributes to heart failure with preserved ejection fraction in a rat metabolic risk model. *Circ. Heart Fail.* **2013**, *6*, 1239–1249. [CrossRef]
11. Pesta, D.; Gnaiger, E. Preparation of permeabilized muscle fibers for diagnosis of mitochondrial respiratory function. *Mitochondr. Physiol. Netw.* **2015**, *14*, 1–5.
12. Gonçalves-Rodrigues, P.; Almeida-Coelho, J.; Gonçalves, A.; Amorim, F.; Leite-Moreira, A.F.; Stienen, G.J.M.; Falcão-Pires, I. In Vitro Assessment of Cardiac Function Using Skinned Cardiomyocytes. *J. Vis. Exp.* **2020**, e60427. [CrossRef]
13. Kirilmaz, O.B.; Salegaonkar, A.R.; Shiau, J.; Uzun, G.; Ko, H.S.; Lee, H.F.; Park, S.; Kwon, G. Study of blood glucose and insulin infusion rate in real-time in diabetic rats using an artificial pancreas system. *PLoS ONE* **2021**, *16*, e0254718. [CrossRef] [PubMed]
14. Suanarunsawat, T.; Klongpanichapak, S.; Rungseesantivanon, S.; Chaiyabutr, N. Glycemic effect of stevioside and Stevia rebaudiana in streptozotocin-induced diabetic rats. *East. J. Med.* **2004**, *9*, 51–56.
15. Maki, K.C.; Curry, L.L.; Reeves, M.S.; Toth, P.D.; McKenney, J.M.; Farmer, M.V.; Schwartz, S.L.; Lubin, B.C.; Boileau, A.C.; Dicklin, M.R.; et al. Chronic consumption of rebaudioside A, a steviol glycoside, in men and women with type 2 diabetes mellitus. *Food Chem. Toxicol.* **2008**, *46* (Suppl. S7), S47–S53. [CrossRef] [PubMed]

16. Shin, D.H.; Lee, J.H.; Kang, M.S.; Kim, T.H.; Jeong, S.J.; Kim, C.H.; Kim, S.S.; Kim, I.J. Glycemic Effects of Rebaudioside A and Erythritol in People with Glucose Intolerance. *Diabetes Metab. J.* **2016**, *40*, 283–289. [CrossRef]
17. Jan, S.A.; Habib, N.; Shinwari, Z.K.; Ali, M.; Ali, N. The anti-diabetic activities of natural sweetener plant Stevia: An updated review. *SN Appl. Sci.* **2021**, *3*, 517. [CrossRef]
18. Suanarunsawat, T.; Chaiyabutr, N. The effect of stevioside on glucose metabolism in rat. *Can. J. Physiol. Pharmacol.* **1997**, *75*, 976–982. [CrossRef]
19. Prata, C.; Zambonin, L.; Rizzo, B.; Maraldi, T.; Angeloni, C.; Vieceli Dalla Sega, F.; Fiorentini, D.; Hrelia, S. Glycosides from Stevia rebaudiana Bertoni Possess Insulin-Mimetic and Antioxidant Activities in Rat Cardiac Fibroblasts. *Oxid. Med. Cell Longev.* **2017**, *2017*, 3724545. [CrossRef]
20. Casas-Grajales, S.; Reyes-Gordillo, K.; Cerda-García-Rojas, C.M.; Tsutsumi, V.; Lakshman, M.R.; Muriel, P. Rebaudioside A administration prevents experimental liver fibrosis: An in vivo and in vitro study of the mechanisms of action involved. *J. Appl. Toxicol.* **2019**, *39*, 1118–1131. [CrossRef]
21. Xi, D.; Bhattacharjee, J.; Salazar-Gonzalez, R.-M.; Park, S.; Jang, A.; Warren, M.; Merritt, R.; Michail, S.; Bouret, S.; Kohli, R. Rebaudioside affords hepatoprotection ameliorating sugar sweetened beverage- induced nonalcoholic steatohepatitis. *Sci. Rep.* **2020**, *10*, 6689. [CrossRef]
22. Bartlett, A.Q.; Vesco, K.K.; Purnell, J.Q.; Francisco, M.; Goddard, E.; Guan, X.; DeBarber, A.; Leo, M.C.; Baetscher, E.; Rooney, W.; et al. Pregnancy and weaning regulate human maternal liver size and function. *Proc. Natl. Acad. Sci. USA* **2021**, *118*, e2107269118. [CrossRef]
23. Saravanan, R.; Ramachandran, V. Modulating efficacy of Rebaudioside A, a diterpenoid on antioxidant and circulatory lipids in experimental diabetic rats. *Environ. Toxicol. Pharmacol.* **2013**, *36*, 472–483. [CrossRef]
24. Ilias, A.N.; Ismail, I.S.; Hamzah, H.; Mohd Mohidin, T.B.; Idris, M.F.; Ajat, M. Rebaudioside A Enhances LDL Cholesterol Uptake in HepG2 Cells via Suppression of HMGCR Expression. *Rep. Biochem. Mol. Biol.* **2021**, *10*, 477–487. [CrossRef]
25. Wang, J.; Shen, W.; Zhang, J.-Y.; Jia, C.-H.; Xie, M.-L. Stevioside attenuates isoproterenol-induced mouse myocardial fibrosis through inhibition of the myocardial NF-κB/TGF-β1/Smad signaling pathway. *Food Funct.* **2019**, *10*, 1179–1190. [CrossRef] [PubMed]
26. Gonzalez, A.M.; Osorio, J.C.; Manlhiot, C.; Gruber, D.; Homma, S.; Mital, S. Hypertrophy signaling during peripartum cardiac remodeling. *Am. J. Physiol. Heart Circ. Physiol.* **2007**, *293*, H3008–H3013. [CrossRef]
27. Zhao, R.; Wang, J.; Qin, L.; Zhang, X.; Mei, Y. Stevioside improved hyperglycemia-induced cardiac dysfunction by attenuating the development of fibrosis and promoting the degradation of established fibrosis. *J. Funct. Foods* **2020**, *68*, 103895. [CrossRef]
28. Dela Cruz, C.S.; Kang, M.J. Mitochondrial dysfunction and damage associated molecular patterns (DAMPs) in chronic inflammatory diseases. *Mitochondrion* **2018**, *41*, 37–44. [CrossRef]
29. Weinberg, S.E.; Sena, L.A.; Chandel, N.S. Mitochondria in the regulation of innate and adaptive immunity. *Immunity* **2015**, *42*, 406–417. [CrossRef]
30. Wallace, D.C.; Fan, W.; Procaccio, V. Mitochondrial energetics and therapeutics. *Annu. Rev. Pathol.* **2010**, *5*, 297–348. [CrossRef] [PubMed]
31. Satapati, S.; He, T.; Inagaki, T.; Potthoff, M.; Merritt, M.E.; Esser, V.; Mangelsdorf, D.J.; Kliewer, S.A.; Browning, J.D.; Burgess, S.C. Partial resistance to peroxisome proliferator-activated receptor-alpha agonists in ZDF rats is associated with defective hepatic mitochondrial metabolism. *Diabetes* **2008**, *57*, 2012–2021. [CrossRef] [PubMed]
32. Li, P.; Wang, Z.; Lam, S.M.; Shui, G. Rebaudioside A Enhances Resistance to Oxidative Stress and Extends Lifespan and Healthspan in Caenorhabditis elegans. *Antioxidants* **2021**, *10*, 262. [CrossRef]
33. Franco-Obregón, A.; Gilbert, J.A. The Microbiome-Mitochondrion Connection: Common Ancestries, Common Mechanisms, Common Goals. *mSystems* **2017**, *2*, e00018-17. [CrossRef]
34. Gesper, M.; Nonnast, A.B.H.; Kumowski, N.; Stoehr, R.; Schuett, K.; Marx, N.; Kappel, B.A. Gut-Derived Metabolite Indole-3-Propionic Acid Modulates Mitochondrial Function in Cardiomyocytes and Alters Cardiac Function. *Front. Med.* **2021**, *8*, 648259. [CrossRef] [PubMed]
35. Nettleton, J.E.; Cho, N.A.; Klancic, T.; Nicolucci, A.C.; Shearer, J.; Borgland, S.L.; Johnston, L.A.; Ramay, H.R.; Noye Tuplin, E.; Chleilat, F.; et al. Maternal low-dose aspartame and stevia consumption with an obesogenic diet alters metabolism, gut microbiota and mesolimbic reward system in rat dams and their offspring. *Gut* **2020**, *69*, 1807–1817. [CrossRef] [PubMed]
36. Nettleton, J.E.; Klancic, T.; Schick, A.; Choo, A.C.; Shearer, J.; Borgland, S.L.; Chleilat, F.; Mayengbam, S.; Reimer, R.A. Low-Dose Stevia (Rebaudioside A) Consumption Perturbs Gut Microbiota and the Mesolimbic Dopamine Reward System. *Nutrients* **2019**, *11*, 1248. [CrossRef] [PubMed]
37. El-Hattab, A.W.; Scaglia, F. Mitochondrial Cardiomyopathies. *Front. Cardiovasc. Med.* **2016**, *3*, 25. [CrossRef] [PubMed]
38. Ren, J.; Pulakat, L.; Whaley-Connell, A.; Sowers, J.R. Mitochondrial biogenesis in the metabolic syndrome and cardiovascular disease. *J. Mol. Med.* **2010**, *88*, 993–1001. [CrossRef] [PubMed]
39. Paul, S.; Sengupta, S.; Bandyopadhyay, T.K.; Bhattacharyya, A. Stevioside induced ROS-mediated apoptosis through mitochondrial pathway in human breast cancer cell line MCF-7. *Nutr. Cancer* **2012**, *64*, 1087–1094. [CrossRef] [PubMed]
40. Lima, Y.C.; Kurauti, M.A.; da Fonseca Alves, G.; Ferezini, J.; Piovan, S.; Malta, A.; de Almeida, F.L.A.; Gomes, R.M.; de Freitas Mathias, P.C.; Milani, P.G.; et al. Whey protein sweetened with Stevia rebaudiana Bertoni (Bert.) increases mitochondrial biogenesis markers in the skeletal muscle of resistance-trained rats. *Nutr. Metab.* **2019**, *16*, 65. [CrossRef]

41. Han, J.-Y.; Park, M.; Lee, H.-J. Stevia (Stevia rebaudiana) extract ameliorates insulin resistance by regulating mitochondrial function and oxidative stress in the skeletal muscle of db/db mice. *BMC Complement. Med. Ther.* **2023**, *23*, 264. [CrossRef]
42. Onakpoya, I.J.; Heneghan, C.J. Effect of the natural sweetener, steviol glycoside, on cardiovascular risk factors: A systematic review and meta-analysis of randomised clinical trials. *Eur. J. Prev. Cardiol.* **2015**, *22*, 1575–1587. [CrossRef]
43. Redruello-Requejo, M.; González-Rodríguez, M.; Samaniego-Vaesken, M.D.L.; Montero-Bravo, A.; Partearroyo, T.; Varela-Moreiras, G. Low- and No-Calorie Sweetener (LNCS) Consumption Patterns Amongst the Spanish Adult Population. *Nutrients* **2021**, *13*, 1845. [CrossRef] [PubMed]
44. Halasa, B.C.; Sylvetsky, A.C.; Conway, E.M.; Shouppe, E.L.; Walter, M.F.; Walter, P.J.; Cai, H.; Hui, L.; Rother, K.I. Non-Nutritive Sweeteners in Human Amniotic Fluid and Cord Blood: Evidence of Transplacental Fetal Exposure. *Am. J. Perinatol.* **2023**, *40*, 1286–1291. [CrossRef] [PubMed]

biology

MDPI

Article

Maternal Obesity Programs the Premature Aging of Rat Offspring Liver Mitochondrial Electron Transport Chain Genes in a Sex-Dependent Manner

Consuelo Lomas-Soria [1,2], Guadalupe L. Rodríguez-González [1], Carlos A. Ibáñez [1], Luis A. Reyes-Castro [1], Peter W. Nathanielsz [3,4] and Elena Zambrano [1,5,*]

1 Departamento de Biología de la Reproducción, Instituto Nacional de Ciencias Médicas y Nutrición Salvador Zubirán, Mexico City 14080, Mexico; mconsuelo@conahcyt.mx (C.L.-S.); guadalupe.rodriguezg@incmnsz.mx (G.L.R.-G.); carlos_albertoibc@hotmail.com (C.A.I.); luis.reyesc@incmnsz.mx (L.A.R.-C.)
2 CONAHCyT-Cátedras, Investigador por México, Departamento de Biología de la Reproducción, Instituto Nacional de Ciencias Médicas y Nutrición Salvador Zubirán, Mexico City 14080, Mexico
3 Wyoming Center for Pregnancy and Life Course Health Research, Department of Animal Science, University of Wyoming, Laramie, WY 82071, USA; peter.nathanielsz@uwyo.edu
4 Department of Genetics, Texas Biomedical Research Institute, San Antonio, TX 78227, USA
5 Facultad de Química, Universidad Nacional Autónoma de México, Mexico City 04510, Mexico
* Correspondence: elena.zambranog@incmnsz.mx; Tel.: +52-55-5487-0900 (ext. 2417)

Simple Summary: Developmental programming is now an area of considerable interest throughout the biomedical research community as it is now well accepted that challenges during fetal and early neonatal life program the trajectory of the development and function of multiple systems across the life span. There is now also compelling evidence that developmental programming alters the trajectory of aging, beginning early in life. The present study links mitochondrial function to molecular signaling pathways that regulate life span and to the aging process; it demonstrates the role and importance of mitochondria in the predisposition to developing a fatty liver. The overall message we wish to emphasize is that hepatic aging in offspring caused by maternal obesity in rats involves changes in the mitochondrial function pathways that result in fatty livers. These processes show sexual dimorphism as they occur in males and females at different ages. These findings throw new light on the mechanisms that underlie the well-established sexual dimorphism in aging. We hope this paper will be a stimulus to similar studies on other tissues.

Abstract: We investigated whether maternal obesity affects the hepatic mitochondrial electron transport chain (ETC), sirtuins, and antioxidant enzymes in young (110 postnatal days (PND)) and old (650PND) male and female offspring in a sex- and age-related manner. Female Wistar rats ate a control (C) or high-fat (MO) diet from weaning, through pregnancy and lactation. After weaning, the offspring ate the C diet and were euthanized at 110 and 650PND. The livers were collected for RNA-seq and immunohistochemistry. Male offspring livers had more differentially expressed genes (DEGs) down-regulated by both MO and natural aging than females. C-650PND vs. C-110PND and MO-110PND vs. C-110PND comparisons revealed 1477 DEGs in common for males (premature aging by MO) and 35 DEGs for females. Analysis to identify KEGG pathways enriched from genes in common showed changes in 511 and 3 KEGG pathways in the male and female livers, respectively. Mitochondrial function pathways showed ETC-related gene down-regulation. All ETC complexes, *sirtuin2*, *sirtuin3*, *sod-1*, and *catalase*, exhibited gene down-regulation and decreased protein expression at young and old ages in MO males vs. C males; meanwhile, MO females down-regulated only at 650PND. Conclusions: MO accelerates the age-associated down-regulation of ETC pathway gene expression in male offspring livers, thereby causing sex-dependent oxidative stress, premature aging, and metabolic dysfunction.

Keywords: maternal obesity; aging; RNA-seq; liver; mitochondria; oxidative phosphorylation

1. Introduction

Obesity is considered a global pandemic and a worldwide public health issue [1]. In recent decades, the proportion of women of reproductive age who are overweight and obese has increased significantly, as has the incidence of obesity during pregnancy [2,3]. Human and controlled animal studies have shown that maternal obesity has detrimental lifelong consequences on offspring by programming their cells, tissues, and organs, as well as their structures and functions. Maternal obesity programs offspring metabolic disorders through several mechanisms, including metabolic, hormonal [4–7], and epigenetic changes [8,9], as well as through oxidative stress [10,11], a commonly proposed mechanism for liver injury and the progression of age-related diseases [10]. Non-alcoholic fatty liver disease (NAFLD) is the most prevalent form of liver disorder and is considered a global epidemic. Obese young children and adults are more likely to develop early liver diseases [12,13].

There is evidence that the onset of a fatty liver in offspring may occur early in development [14,15]. Moreover, maternal obesity accelerates the onset of offspring metabolic and liver dysfunction and shortens life span [10,16,17].

We have reported that maternal obesity programs premature metabolic aging in offspring in a sex-dependent manner, possibly due to increased oxidative stress, changes in steroid hormones, cardiovascular changes, and other functional alterations [10]. In most cases of programming by maternal obesity, such as NAFLD, we, and others, have observed a sexual dimorphism of outcomes as the male offspring of obese mothers exhibit more pronounced NAFLD characteristics (physiological, biochemical, histological, and gene changes) than the females [4,10].

Aging is a complex and dynamic biological process that, over time, causes a variety of structural, functional, molecular, and cellular damage, thereby increasing the risk of multiple diseases [18]. Cellular senescence, including telomere shortening and genomic and mitochondrial DNA damage, is a major cause of aging, and plays an important role in the progression of NAFLD and other liver diseases [19–21]. Mitochondrial dysfunction, such as a decreased oxidative capacity and increased reactive oxygen species (ROS) production, has been proposed as a cellular and molecular hallmark of aging [22,23].

Mitochondria are highly sensitive to their environmental conditions and undergo adaptations during the development of NAFLD diseases. Thus, mitochondrial alterations are implicated in liver aging and fatty liver diseases [24–30]. Mitochondrial dysfunction has been proposed as a central process in the development of liver disease programmed by maternal obesity [31]. Offspring of obese rodent mothers exhibit elevated oxidative stress and mitochondrial dysfunction in both fetal and young adult livers [32–35]. Some studies have evaluated the effects of maternal obesity programming on mitochondrial gene expression in offspring livers [15,36–38]. However, few studies have examined the extent to which these changes persist until old age. There is a need to determine whether adverse outcomes can be caused by aging and/or by maternal diet.

In the current study, RNA-seq was used to determine the difference in transcriptome changes between the male and female offspring of obese mothers at the young age of 110 and the old age of 650PND. We also measured protein products for key genes with altered expressions. We focused on the liver mitochondrial oxidative phosphorylation pathway in the young and old male and female offspring of control and obese mothers. Importantly, in our rat colony, the offspring of the control mothers (normally fed and normal weight) lived for ~850 days; whereas, the offspring of the obese mothers did not live for much longer than 650PND.

We hypothesized that maternal obesity: (1) produces sex-specific age-related liver transcriptome changes in offspring; (2) leads to offspring liver dysfunction by impairing antioxidant defenses and mitochondrial function; and (3) causes offspring hepatic mitochondrial electron transport chain (ETC) gene down-regulation, leading to an increase in reactive oxygen species (ROS) concentrations and liver damage.

2. Materials and Methods

2.1. Animals

The Animal Experimentation Ethics Committee of the Instituto Nacional de Ciencias Médicas y Nutrición Salvador Zubirán (INCMNSZ), Mexico City, Mexico (ethical approval code, CINVA 271 and 1868) approved all procedures, which are in accordance with the ARRIVE criteria for reporting animal studies [39,40]. Female albino Wistar rats were born and raised in the INCMNSZ animal facility, which is accredited by the Association for Assessment and Accreditation of Laboratory Animal Care International (AAALAC) and follows its standards. The rats were kept at 22–23 °C under controlled lighting (lights on from 07.00 to 19.00 h) with free access to food and water.

2.2. Experimental Design

First, 120-day-old female Wistar rats were randomly mated with proven fertile non-littermates to produce the founder generation (F0) of mothers. The F0 litters were adjusted to ten pups at birth (day 0), with at least four females [41]. At weaning (21 days old) F0 females were randomly assigned to one of the two experimental groups: control (F0C) or maternal obesity (F0MO) groups to be fed either a standard laboratory chow diet or a high-fat diet (HFD). The C diet consisted of standard laboratory chow (Zeigler Rodent RQ22-5, Gardners, PA, USA) containing 22.0% protein, 5.0% soy oil fat, 31.0% polysaccharide, 31.0% simple sugars, 4.0% fiber, 6.0% minerals, and 1.0% vitamins (*w*/*w*) (physiological fuel 3.4 kcal/g). The HFD was produced in the INCMNSZ's specialized dietary facility, with 23.5% protein, 20.0% lard, 5.0% soy oil fat, 20.2% polysaccharide, 20.2% simple sugars, 5.0% fiber, 5.0% mineral mix, 1.0% vitamin mix (*w*/*w*), and physiological fuel 4.8 kcal/g.

At 120 days, 10 female rats from the F0C group and 20 from the F0MO group were mated overnight (up to 5 days) with non-experimental males to produce offspring. Daily vaginal smears were obtained and the day a sperm plug was found was designated as day 0 of conception. To ensure similar pregnancy conditions, this study excluded litters with fewer than 9 or more than 14 pups. In addition, to achieve offspring homogeneity, on the second PND, all offspring litters studied were adjusted to 10 pups, with equal numbers of males and females whenever possible (C and MO). This adjustment to litter size had no effect on the metabolic variables as the litter size was considered normal.

2.3. Care and Maintenance of Offspring to Study for Developmental Programming and Aging Interactions

Our studies have routinely been conducted at 110PND, to obtain data at a young adult life stage, and at 650PND, to obtain data at a mature aged adult life stage. The litters were weaned at 21PND and males and females were divided into separate cages at weaning. After weaning, all offspring ate a control diet until the end of the experiment (110 and 650PND). There was no mixing of litters or sexes from different age groups. The offspring were maintained in this situation until PND50, after which, no more than 4 rats were placed in one cage. After 110PND the number was reduced to a minimum of 2 or a maximum of 3 per cage, as previously reported. All females at 110PND were evaluated during the diestrus phase of the ovarian cycle.

2.4. Offspring Tissue Collection

One male and one female from different litters were euthanized at 110 and 650PND by exsanguination through aortic punctures under isoflurane general anesthesia; this was conducted by the same experienced person under identical conditions at each timepoint (light period (12:00 to 14:00 h) and 6 h of fasting). Thus, the males and females evaluated at the two ages were groups of siblings. For each age group, the livers were dissected, cleaned, and weighed. The right inferior lobes were fixed in 4% paraformaldehyde and embedded in paraffin for immunohistochemical analysis. The left lobes were stored at −70 °C for RNA-seq analysis. We report data with the following number of animals per group and sex:

110PND—males: C $n = 6$, MO $n = 5$; females: C $n = 6$, MO $n = 5$; 650PND—males: C $n = 6$; MO $n = 6$; females: C $n = 6$ and MO $n = 6$.

2.5. RNA Extraction and cDNA Library Preparation and Sequencing

Liver tissue samples (10–20 mg) were homogenized with the BioSpec BeadBeater (BioSpec products, Bartlesville, OK, USA) and RNA was extracted using the Qiagen miRNeasy mini kit (Qiagen, Hilden, Germany), according to the manufacturer's instructions. RNA quantity and quality were determined using a Nanodrop spectrophotometer (Nanodrop Technologies, Wilmington, DE, USA). RNA was stored at −80 °C until it was used. cDNA libraries were generated from 1 μg of total RNA using an Illumina TruSeq RNA LS Sample Preparation kit v2, according to the manufacturer's instructions (Illumina, San Diego, CA, USA). The Agilent DNA 1000 was used to evaluate the quality and fragment size of the final individual cDNA libraries. The sequencing libraries were quantified using the KAPA Library Quantification kits for Illumina platforms. The libraries were normalized to 10 nM and diluted to 20 pM before loading on the cBot 2X100; the Illumina HiSeq 2500 sequencer was used for paired-end sequencing.

2.6. Bioinformatic Analysis

Output demultiplexed reads were exported to Partek Flow for analysis. Read FASTQ files were trimmed for quality to Phred 30 at each end. STAR aligner v2.3.1j was used to align trimmed reads to the *Rattus norvegicus* genomic reference (RGSC 5.0/rn5). Gene and transcript abundance were quantified against the rn5 RefSeq annotation and transcript abundance was normalized for all samples as a dataset using the Reads Per Kilobase per Million mapped reads (RPKM) values of all Refseq genes. To identify the functional pathways related to maternal obesity programming–aging interactions, we evaluated the differentially expressed genes (DEGs) between 650PND and 110PND in the male and female livers of the C and MO groups using pairwise comparisons with Partek Flow (Partek®, St. Louis, MO, USA). Genes were filtered based on >1 fold change (FC) and a nominal p-value of <0.05 (Student's t-test). All DEGs were mapped to the KEGG database (Kyoto Encyclopedia of Genes and Genomes) and searched for principal mitochondrial function-related pathways.

2.7. KEGG Pathway Analysis

The Web Gestalt application (WEB-based Gene SeT AnaLysis Toolkit) was used to perform analyses for enrichment KEGG pathways; the statistical significance p-value cutoff was set at 0.05 [42]. The KEGG is an online bioinformatics analysis system for over-represented pathways [43].

2.8. Liver Immunohistochemical (IHC) Analysis

Each liver's right inferior lobe was dissected, sectioned longitudinally, and immediately fixed in 4% paraformaldehyde in a neutral phosphate saline buffer. Following a 24 h fixation period, liver sections were dehydrated with ethanol at increasing concentrations from 75 to 95% and were then embedded in paraffin.

IHC analysis was carried out using the avidin–biotin complex (ABC) IHC method. Liver sections (4 μm) were deparaffinized, hydrated, and quenched for endogenous peroxidase with 0.3% hydrogen peroxide in PBS at room temperature for 30 min. To perform antigen retrieval, slides were placed in citrate buffer at pH 6.0 (ImmunoDNA Retriever Citrate, BioSB, Inc., Santa Barbara, CA, USA) and heated in a pressure cooker for 5 min. The sections were then incubated overnight at room temperature. The following primary antibodies were used for IHC analysis: anti Atp5f1, 1:500 (goat polyclonal SC-162552, Santa Cruz Biotechnology, Dallas, TX, USA); anti Ndufa10, 1:500 (mouse monoclonal SC-376357, Santa Cruz); anti Cox5a, 1:100 (mouse monoclonal SC-376907, Santa Cruz Biotechnology); anti Sdhc, 1:1000 (rabbit polyclonal SC-67256, Santa Cruz Biotechnology); anti Sirt-2, 1:1000 (mouse monoclonal SC-28292, Santa Cruz Biotechnology); anti Sirt-3, 1:300 (rabbit polyclonal SC-99143, Santa Cruz Biotechnology); anti Sod-1, 1:1000 (rabbit polyclonal SC-11407, Santa Cruz Biotechnology); Catalase, 1:600 (rabbit polyclonal SC-50508, Santa Cruz Biotechnology). Antibody binding was detected with a Vectastain Elite ABC kit (Vector Laboratories, Burlingame, CA, USA) and 3, 3′-diaminobenzidine as a chromogen. After tissue sections were stained, hematoxylin was used as a counterstain. Negative controls were performed without the primary antibody. Due to space limitations, the negative staining controls are presented as Supplementary Material. Twenty random digital images were taken of each rat using an Olympus BX51 microscope (Olympus Co. Model BX51RF, Tokyo, Japan). The staining areas of the images were analyzed using digital image analyzing software (ImageJ, U.S. National Institute of Health, Bethesda, MD, USA) and a color deconvolution plug-in.

2.9. Statistical Analysis

Gene expression is expressed as mean Log2 RPKM$\pm$ standard error of the mean (SEM). Immunohistochemical analyses are presented as mean $\pm$ SEM. A p-value < 0.05 was considered statistically significant. To analyze differences between the groups, we used the Tukey test (one-way ANOVA) for males and females separately. Analysis was performed with the Sigma Stat 3.5 statistical program (2005). Gene expression from RNA-seq data is shown as the mean of Log2FC and SEM based on normalized data. There was no overlap in DEGs between the sexes in the pathways examined, indicating that it was not necessary to compare males and females to determine sexual dimorphism.

3. Results

3.1. Liver Differentially Expressed Genes (DEGs)

We performed four different comparisons to evaluate the effects of maternal obesity at two different ages (young and old) and the effect of aging in the control group's and obese mothers group's offspring. The comparisons were as follows: (1) the effect of maternal diet on the young (MO-110PND vs. C-110PND); (2) the effect of maternal diet on the old (MO-650PND vs. C-650PND); (3) the effect of aging on the control groups (C-650PND vs. C-110PND); and 4) the effect of maternal obesity on aging (MO-650PND vs. MO-110PND). Males and females were analyzed separately.

The number of DEGs for male comparisons: (1) MO-110PND vs. C-110PND showed that 3030 genes were down- and 118 genes were up-regulated; (2) MO-650PND vs. C-650PND revealed that 35 genes were down- and 604 were up-regulated; (3) C-650PND vs. C-110PND indicated that 4218 genes were down- and 127 were up-regulated; (4) MO-650PND vs. MO-110PND showed that 480 genes were down- and 1285 were up-regulated.

The number of DEGs for female comparisons: (1) MO-110PND vs. C-110PND exhibited that 51 genes were down- and 127 genes were up-regulated; (2) MO-650PND vs. C-650PND revealed 9244 down- and 3 up-regulated genes; (3) C-650PND vs. C-110PND showed that 57 genes were down- and 415 were up-regulated; (4) MO-650PND vs. MO-110PND exhibited 3346 down- and 44 up-regulated genes.

Based on the DEG analysis for the effects of maternal obesity, we observed that 96% of the genes were down-regulated in male comparisons in both maternal obesity (MO-110PND vs. C-110PND) and age (C-650PND vs. C-110PND). We performed a Venn analysis to determine if the DEGs in both conditions shared common genes; then, we evaluated whether these genes are associated with premature aging (Figure 1).

The Venn diagram shows the distribution of DEGs by maternal diet in the young and by age in the control groups for males (Figure 1A) and for females (Figure 1B). Male Venn diagram with DEG comparisons: C-650PND vs. C-110PND and MO-110PND vs. C-110PND reveal that there are 1477 genes in common for both comparisons; we refer to these genes as genes involved in premature aging due to MO. In the same comparison, females only shared 35 genes. Clearly, maternal diet affects more genes involved in premature aging in males compared to females.

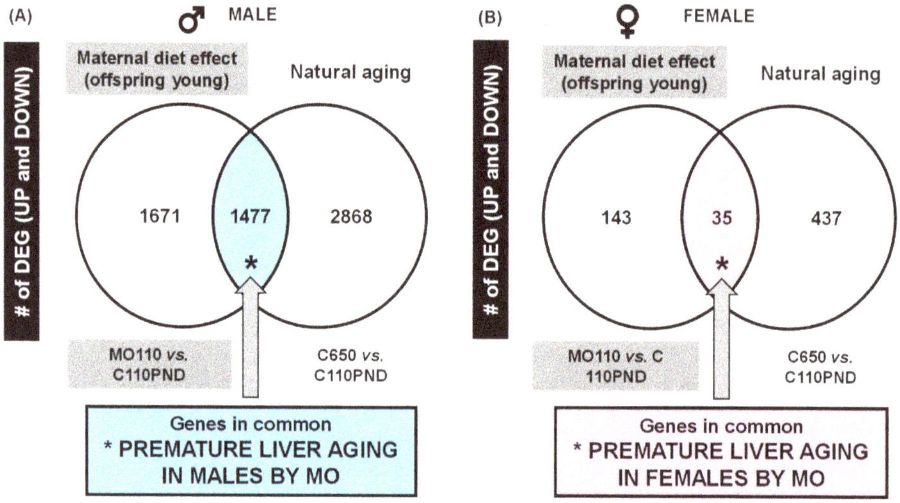

Figure 1. Venn diagram of up- and down-regulated liver genes, (**A**) males and (**B**) females.

3.2. KEGG Pathway Analysis for Prematurely Aging Genes in Males and Females

Using the lists of 1477 and 35 common genes (premature aging) in males and females, respectively, we performed an over-represented analysis to identify the KEGG pathways enriched from these two DEG lists (Supplementary Tables S1 and S2). The two lists were mapped to KEGG pathways separately; we found that fifty-one KEGG pathways showed significant changes in the male livers but just three did so in the livers of the females. Table 1 shows the most significant KEGG pathways (by *p*-value). In males (Table 1A), the pathways related to liver metabolism and aging, oxidative phosphorylation, and NAFLD are at the top of the KEGG pathway analysis; however, in females (Table 1B), there were only three pathways that changed significantly.

Table 1. List of the most significant KEGG pathways enriched with DEGs by *p*-value (up- and down-regulated), showing premature aging for males (**A**) and females (**B**).

(A). MALE. Id Pathway	Name	Size	*p*-Value
rno01100	Metabolic pathways	1380	$<2.2 \times 10^{-16}$
rno00280	Valine, leucine, and isoleucine degradation	56	1.7×10^{-6}
rno00640	Propanoate metabolism	32	1.0×10^{-5}
rno00190	Oxidative phosphorylation	143	4.1×10^{-5}
rno04932	Non-alcoholic fatty liver disease (NAFLD)	159	9.4×10^{-5}
rno04714	Thermogenesis	243	9.5×10^{-5}
rno00260	Glycine, serine, and threonine metabolism	40	1.0×10^{-4}
rno00310	Lysine degradation	61	1.1×10^{-4}
rno00140	Steroid hormone biosynthesis	84	1.1×10^{-4}
rno01200	Carbon metabolism	127	1.4×10^{-4}
rno00270	Cysteine and methionine metabolism	49	1.7×10^{-4}
rno00630	Glyoxylate and dicarboxylate metabolism	30	2.2×10^{-4}
rno03022	Basal transcription factors	45	1.3×10^{-3}
rno00760	Nicotinate and nicotinamide metabolism	32	1.8×10^{-3}
rno00380	Tryptophan metabolism	47	1.9×10^{-3}

Table 1. *Cont.*

(A). MALE. Id Pathway	Name	Size	*p*-Value
rno04122	Sulfur relay system	9	2.8×10^{-3}
rno04142	Lysosome	129	2.8×10^{-3}
rno00510	*N*-Glycan biosynthesis	51	3.6×10^{-3}
rno03420	Nucleotide excision repair	47	6.6×10^{-3}
rno04144	Endocytosis	275	6.6×10^{-3}
rno04217	Necroptosis	161	7.5×10^{-3}
rno04120	Ubiquitin mediated proteolysis	141	7.6×10^{-3}
rno00670	One carbon pool by folate	18	8.3×10^{-3}
rno00830	Retinol metabolism	85	9.1×10^{-3}
rno03060	Protein export	26	1.0×10^{-2}
rno00053	Ascorbate and aldarate metabolism	27	1.2×10^{-2}
rno00563	Glycosylphosphatidylinositol (GPI)-anchor biosynthesis	27	1.2×10^{-2}
rno00650	Butanoate metabolism	28	1.5×10^{-2}
rno04141	Protein processing in the endoplasmic reticulum	164	1.8×10^{-2}
rno00071	Fatty acid degradation	47	2.0×10^{-2}
rno00350	Tyrosine metabolism	40	2.5×10^{-2}
rno04146	Peroxisome	88	2.8×10^{-2}
rno00410	Beta-Alanine metabolism	33	3.2×10^{-2}
rno00730	Thiamine metabolism	17	3.2×10^{-2}
rno00920	Sulfur metabolism	10	3.3×10^{-2}
rno00330	Arginine and proline metabolism	52	3.5×10^{-2}
rno00010	Glycolysis/Gluconeogenesis	72	3.8×10^{-2}
rno00980	Metabolism of xenobiotics by cytochrome P450	74	4.5×10^{-2}
rno03040	Spliceosome	138	4.7×10^{-2}
(B). FEMALE Id pathway	**Name**	**Size**	***p*-Value**
rno04064	NF-kappa B signaling pathway	97	5.4×10^{-3}
rno00230	Purine metabolism	182	1.8×10^{-2}
rno04060	Cytokine–cytokine receptor interaction	269	3.8×10^{-2}

3.3. *Pathway Analysis Related to Mitochondria*

To determine that the pathways implicated in the MO-110PND vs. C-110PND and C-650PND vs. C-110PND comparisons were enriched and significant separately, we evaluated the over-represented analysis of the pathways of DEGs in each comparison using three different databases: KEGG, Wikipathway, and Reactome. In Table 2A–C, the results of the male DEGs in each database are displayed. For the analysis, we focused on mitochondrial function-related pathways; for each comparison, oxidative phosphorylation was significantly enriched and all DEGs in the pathways were down-regulated.

Table 2. List of (**A**) KEGG, (**B**) Wikipathway, and (**C**) Reactome enrichment pathways from DEGs (up- and down-regulated) in male livers from the MO-110PND vs. C-110PND and C-650PND vs. C-110PND comparisons.

(A). KEGG Pathway Comparison		*p*-Value	Genes Down	Genes Up
MO-110PND vs. C-110PND Maternal diet effect (young)	Oxidative phosphorylation	7.8×10^{-5}	39	0
	Lysosome	1.7×10^{-4}	37	0
	Ribosome	3.0×10^{-3}	41	0
	Peroxisome	9.5×10^{-3}	23	0
	Citrate cycle (TCA cycle)	1.1×10^{-2}	11	0
C-650PND vs. C-110PND Aging effect in controls	Peroxisome	$<2.2 \times 10^{-16}$	55	0
	Oxidative phosphorylation	2.9×10^{-14}	68	0
	Mitophagy	1.6×10^{-4}	27	0
	Lysosome	8.6×10^{-4}	43	0
	Citrate cycle (TCA cycle)	7.2×10^{-2}	11	0

Table 2. *Cont.*

(B). Wikipathway				
Comparison		***p*-Value**	**Genes Down**	**Genes Up**
MO-110PND vs. C-110PND Maternal diet effect (young)	Oxidative phosphorylation	1.0×10^{-3}	22	0
	Electron Transport Chain	1.5×10^{-3}	30	0
	TCA Cycle	1.7×10^{-2}	10	0
	Oxidative Stress	1.9×10^{-2}	12	0
C-650PND vs. C-110PND Aging effect in controls	Electron Transport Chain	1.0×10^{-10}	51	0
	Mitochondrial LC-Fatty Acid Beta-Oxidation	1.5×10^{-7}	14	0
	Oxidative phosphorylation	8.1×10^{-7}	32	0
	Oxidative stress	1.4×10^{-5}	20	0
	TCA Cycle	7.3×10^{-2}	10	0
(C). Reactome				
Comparison		***p*-Value**	**Genes Down**	**Genes Up**
MO-110PND vs. C-110PND Maternal diet effect (young)	Mitochondrial translation termination	5.2×10^{-14}	46	0
	Mitochondrial translation	9.5×10^{-14}	46	0
	The citric acid (TCA) cycle and respiratory electron transport	1.3×10^{-6}	46	0
	Respiratory electron transport	7.1×10^{-5}	25	0
	Citric acid cycle (TCA cycle)	9.8×10^{-4}	10	0
	Pyruvate metabolism and Citric Acid (TCA) cycle	1.3×10^{-3}	17	0
	Peroxisomal protein import	1.9×10^{-3}	18	0
C-650PND vs. C-110PND Aging effect in controls	Mitochondrial translation	$<2.2 \times 10^{-16}$	66	0
	Mitochondrial translation termination	$<2.2 \times 10^{-16}$	66	0
	Mitochondrial translation elongation	$<2.2 \times 10^{-16}$	65	0
	Peroxisomal protein import	2.5×10^{-10}	47	0
	Respiratory electron transport	3.4×10^{-10}	39	0

3.4. Oxidative Phosphorylation KEGG Pathway

In accordance with the aims of this study, we restricted our detailed analysis to changes in genes related to the oxidative phosphorylation KEGG pathway (Table 3). This pathway showed no overlap in DEGs between sexes or diet comparisons, clearly demonstrating a sex-dependent aging and maternal diet effect on the liver transcriptome.

Table 3. List of DEGs for males and females in each comparison of the oxidative phosphorylation KEGG pathway.

Comparison	Genes, Male	*p*-Value	Genes, Female	*p*-Value
(1) MO-110PND vs. C-110PND Maternal diet effect (young)	*atp5d, atp5g2, atp5i, atp5o, atp6v0a1, atp6v1f, cox15, cox5b, cox7a2l, cyc1, lhpp, ndufa10l1, ndufa11, ndufa12, ndufa9, ndufb10, ndufb11, ndufb2, ndufb3, ndufb6, ndufb8, ndufc2, ndufs1, ndufs2, ndufs7, ndufs8, ndufv1, ndufv2, ndufv3, ppa2, sdha, sdhb, tcirg1, uqcr11, uqcrc1, uqcrc2,*	7.8×10^{-5}	*cox6a*	---

Table 3. *Cont.*

Comparison	Genes, Male	*p*-Value	Genes, Female	*p*-Value
(2) MO-650PND vs. C-650PND Maternal diet effect (old)	*atp6v0a4*, ***atp6v0a2***	----	*atp5f1a, atp5f1b, atp5f1c, atp5f1c, atp5f1d, atp5f1e, atp5mc1, atp5mc2, atp5me, atp5mf, atp5mg, atp5pb, atp5pd, atp5pf, atp5po, atp6ap1, atp6v0a1, atp6v0a2, atp6v0a2, atp6v0c, atp6v0d1, atp6v0d2, atp6v0e1, atp6v1a, atp6v1b2, atp6v1c1, atp6v1c2, atp6v1d, atp6v1e1, atp6v1f, atp6v1g1, atp6v1h, cox15, cox17, cox4i1, cox5a, cox5b, cox6a1, cox6b1, cox6c, cox7a2, cox7a2l, cox7a2l2, cox7b, cox7c, cox8a, cox8b, cyc1, lhpp, ndufa1, ndufa10, ndufa10l1, ndufa11, ndufa12, ndufa13, ndufa2, ndufa4, ndufa5, ndufa6, ndufa7, ndufa8, ndufa9, ndufab1, ndufb10, ndufb11, ndufb2, ndufb3, ndufb4, ndufb5, ndufb6, ndufb7, ndufb8, ndufb9, ndufc2, ndufs1, ndufs2, ndufs3, ndufs4, ndufs5, ndufs6, ndufs7, ndufs8, ndufv1, ndufv2, ndufv3, ppa1, ppa2, sdha, sdhb, sdhc, sdhd, tcirg1, uqcr10, uqcr11, uqcrb, uqcrc2, uqcrfs1, uqcrh, uqcrq*	1.3×10^{-8}
(3) C-650PND vs. C-110 PND Aging effect in controls	*atp5f1c, atp5mc1, atp5me, atp5mf, atp5mg, atp5pb, atp5pd, atp5pf, atp5po, atp6v0a2, atp6v0c, atp6v0d1, atp6v0e1, atp6v1a, atp6v1f, atp6v1g1, atp6v1h, cox15, cox17, cox4i1, cox5a, cox5b, cox6a1, cox6b1, cox6c, cox7a2, cox7a2l, cox7a2l2, cox7b, cox7c, cox8a, ndufa1, ndufa10l1, ndufa11, ndufa12, ndufa13, ndufa2, ndufa4, ndufa5, ndufa6, ndufa7, ndufa8, ndufa9, ndufb10, ndufb11, ndufb2, ndufb3, ndufb4, ndufb5, ndufb6, ndufb7, ndufb9, ndufs3, ndufs5, ndufs6, ndufs8, ndufv1, ndufv2, ndufv3, ppa1, ppa2, sdhb, sdhc, sdhd, tcirg1, uqcr10, uqcrb, uqcrfs1, uqcrh, uqcrq*	2.42×10^{-14}	***cox6a, cox8, atpev1c***	---
(4) MO-650PND vs. MO-110PND Aging effect in MO	*Cox8*	---	*ap2s1, apaf1, atp5f1c, atp5f1d, atp5f1e, atp5mc1, atp5mc2, atp5pb, atp5pd, atp5pf, atp5po, bax, casp3, cox4i1, cox5a, cox5b, cox6a1, cox6b1, cox6c, cox7a2, cox7a2l, cox7a2l2, cox7b, cox7c, cox8a, cox8b, crebbp, creb3l1, cycs, cyct, cyct, dlg4, dnah1, gpx1, hdac2, ndufa1, ndufa10, ndufa11, ndufa12, ndufa13, ndufa2, ndufa4, ndufa5, ndufa6, ndufa7, ndufa9, ndufab1, ndufb10, ndufb11, ndufb2, ndufb3, ndufb4, ndufb5, ndufb6, ndufb7, ndufb9, ndufc2, ndufs3, ndufs4, ndufs5, ndufs6, ndufs7, ndufs8, ndufv2, ndufv3, plcb1, polr2f, polr2g, polr2h, polr2i, polr2j, polr2k, pparg, sdhd, slc25a5, sod1, sod2, uqcr10, uqcr11, uqcr11, uqcrb, uqcrfs1, uqcrh, uqcrq, vdac3*	$<2.2 \times 10^{-16}$

The genes in bold were up-regulated between comparisons in each sex.

Figure 2 shows the overlapping genes between the comparisons for aging (1) C-650PND vs. C-110PND and for programming by obesity (2) MO-110PND vs. C-110PND. Genes that were in common in these two comparisons were involved in premature liver aging, specifically in the oxidative phosphorylation KEGG pathway (Figure 2A) and on the ETC Wikipathway (Figure 2B).

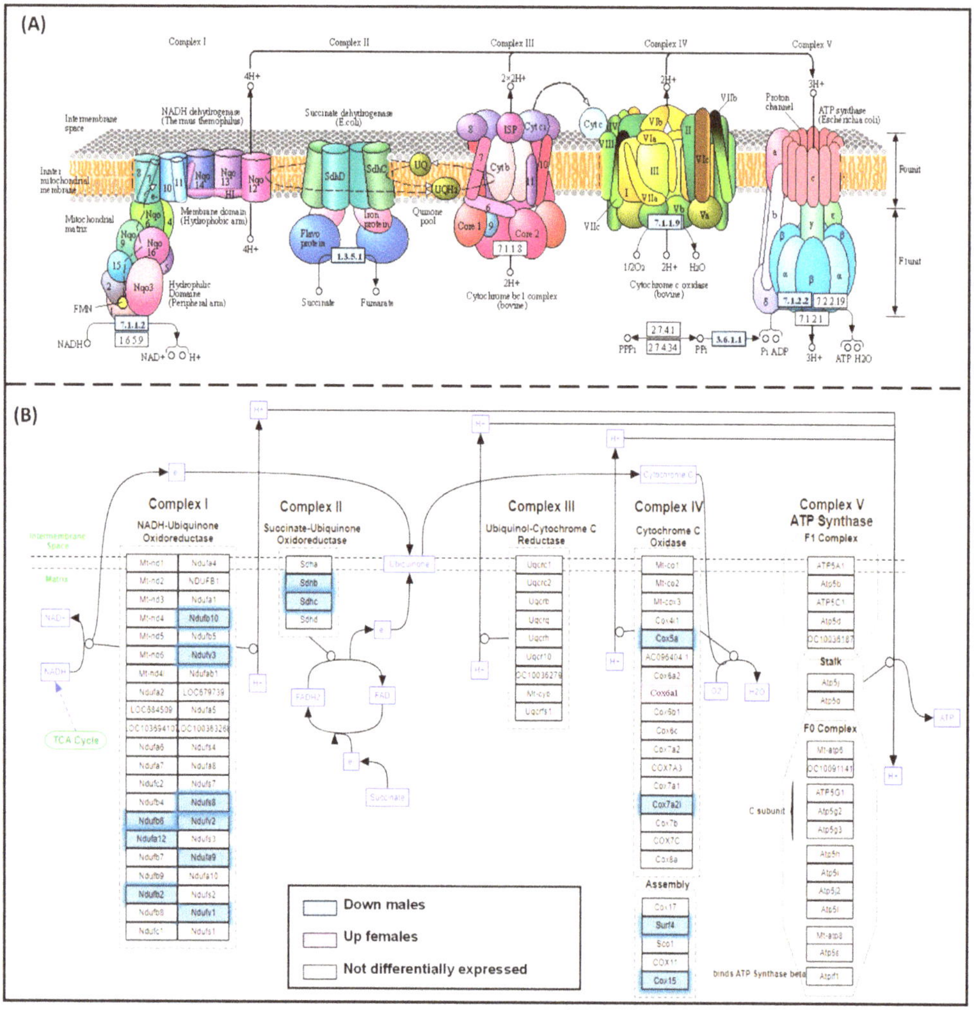

Figure 2. Overlapping genes for (**A**) the oxidative phosphorylation KEGG pathway and (**B**) the electron transport chain (Wikipathway) between the comparisons C-650PND vs. C-110PND and MO-110PND vs. C-110PND, enriched with common DEGs of male premature aging. Genes that were down-regulated in both comparisons are indicated in blue.

3.5. Male and Female Liver Oxidative Phosphorylation Complexes

We selected one representative gene from each oxidative phosphorylation complex. In males, the genes *ndufa10* (Complex I), *sdhc* (Complex II), *cox5a* (Complex IV), and *atp5f1* (Complex V) were down-regulated in the groups MO-110PND, C-650PND, and MO-650PND in comparison to the C-110PND group (Figure 3A–D). In contrast, the gene expression of *ndufa10*, *sdhc*, *cox5a*, and *atp5f1* was down-regulated only in MO-650PND females (Figure 4A–D).

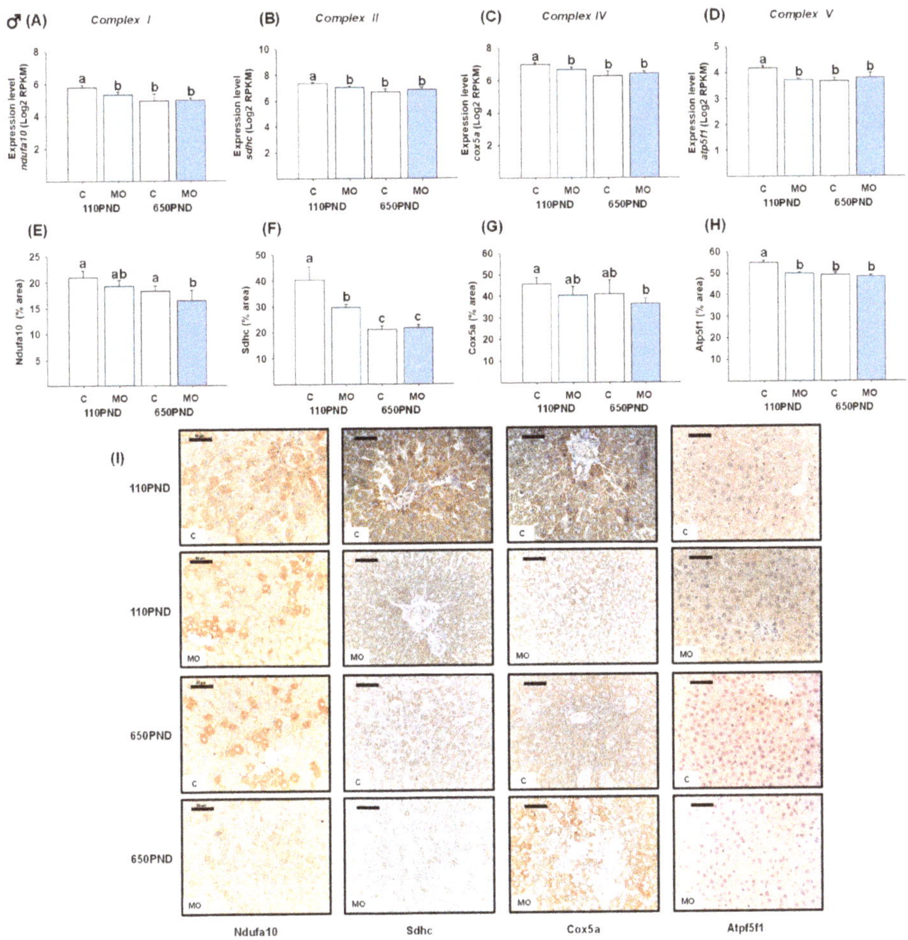

Figure 3. Male hepatic gene expression and protein abundance of four proteins in oxidative phosphorylation complexes in the control (C) and maternal obesity (MO) groups. Gene expression level (Log2 RPKM) of (**A**) *ndufa10;* (**B**) *sdhc*; (**C**) *cox5a*; (**D**) *atp5f1*; the immunostained area (%) of (**E**) Ndufa10; (**F**) Sdhc; (**G**) Cox5a; (**H**) Atp5f1; and (**I**) representative IHC micrograph (40×). Data for RNA-seq, mean Log2 RPKM ± SEM. Protein values are mean ± SEM. $p < 0.05$ for data not sharing a lowe case letter between groups. N = 5–6 rats/group/litter. PND = Postnatal days. Scale bar: 50 μm.

To determine whether changes in gene expression are associated with changes in gene protein products, proteins encoded by the *ndufa10*, *sdhc*, *cox5a, and atp5f1* genes were quantified by an IHC analysis. Males in the MO-110PND, C-650PND, and MO-650PND groups exhibited a lower liver fractional area being stained for Sdhc and Atp5f1 proteins than those in the C110-PND group; for the Ndufa10 and Cox5b proteins, only the MO-650PND group differed from the C-110PND group (Figure 3E–H). In contrast, the results for females varied across all proteins evaluated. The percentage of the Ndufa10 protein's stained area was higher in MO-650PND compared to C-110PND, with no differences between the MO-110PND and C-650PND groups. In terms of the Sdhc protein, C650-PND and MO-650PND had higher percentages of stained areas compared to the C and MO groups at younger ages. The Cox5a protein was similar in all groups; whereas, the groups from obese mothers, regardless of age, exhibited lower percentages of stained areas for the Atp5f1 protein (Figure 4E–H). Figures 3I and 4I show representative sections stained by IHC analysis for all of the oxidative phosphorylation proteins for males and females, respectively.

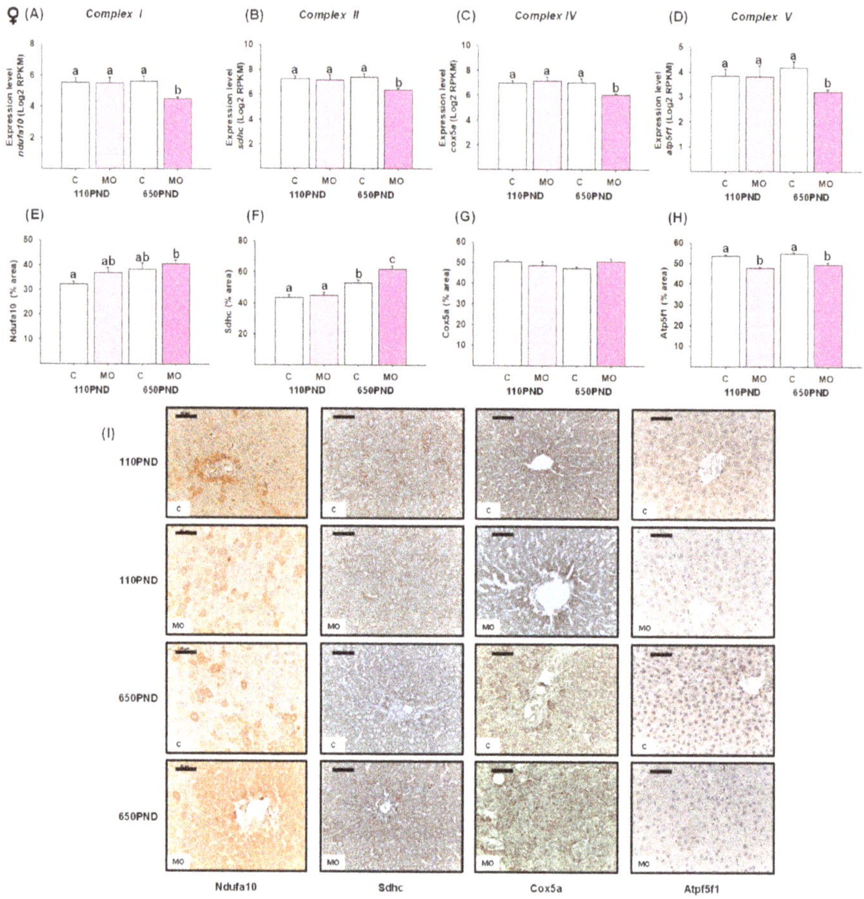

Figure 4. Female hepatic changes in gene expression and abundance of proteins in four oxidative phosphorylation complexes in the control (C) and maternal obesity (MO) groups. Gene expression (Log2 RPKM) of (**A**) *ndufa10;* (**B**) *sdhc;* (**C**) *cox5a;* (**D**) *atp5f1;* the immunostained area (%) of (**E**) Ndufa10; (**F**) Sdhc; (**G**) Cox5a; (**H**) Atp5f1; and (**I**) representative IHC micrograph (40×). Data for RNA-seq, mean Log2 RPKM ± SEM. Protein values are mean ± SEM. $p < 0.05$ for data not sharing a lower case letter between groups. n = 5–6 rats/group/litter. PND = Postnatal days. Scale bar: 50 μm.

3.6. Male and Female Liver Sirtuins

The *sirt-2* mRNA expression and protein content were both decreased in all groups in comparison to the C-110PND group (Figure 5A,B). Despite C-650PND exhibiting the lowest level of *sirt-3* gene expression, the protein abundance did not differ from C110PND; for the groups representing maternal obesity (MO-110PND and MO-650PND), both gene and protein contents were lower compared to C-110PND (Figure 5D,E). Figure 5C,F show representative sections stained by IHC analysis for the Sirt-2 and Sirt-3 proteins, respectively.

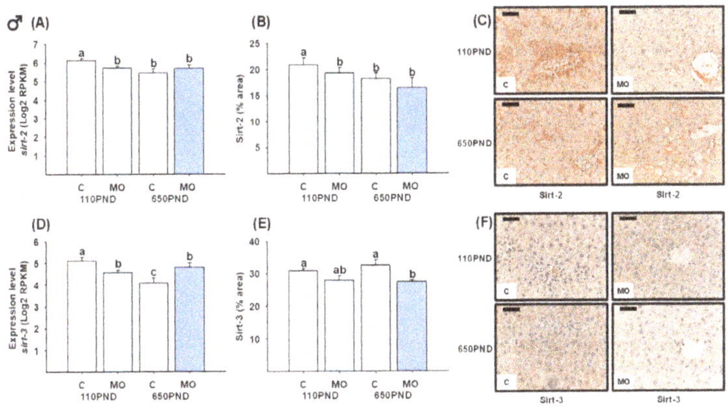

Figure 5. Male hepatic gene expression and protein abundance of Sirt-2 and Sirt-3 in the control (C) and maternal obesity (MO) groups. (**A**) Expression level of *sirt-2* (Log2 RPKM); (**B**) Sirt-2 immunostained area (%); (**C**) representative IHC micrograph of Sirt-2 (40×); (**D**) expression level of *sirt-3* (Log2 RPKM); (**E**) Sirt-3 immunostained area (%); and (**F**) representative IHC micrograph of Sirt-3 (40×). Data for RNA-seq, mean Log2 RPKM ± SEM. Protein values are mean ± SEM. $p < 0.05$ for data not sharing a lower case letter between groups. n = 5–6 rats/group/litter. PND = Postnatal days. Scale bar: 50 µm.

In terms of sirtuin gene expression in female livers, only the MO-650PND group showed a decrease in *sirt-2* and *sirt-3* (Figure 6A and D, respectively). However, unexpectedly Sirt-2 and Sirt-3 protein content was higher in C-650PND, and even higher in MO-650PND, compared to MO-110PND and C-110PND (Figure 6B,E). Figure 6C,F show the representative sections stained by IHC analysis for the Sirt-2 and Sirt-3 proteins, respectively.

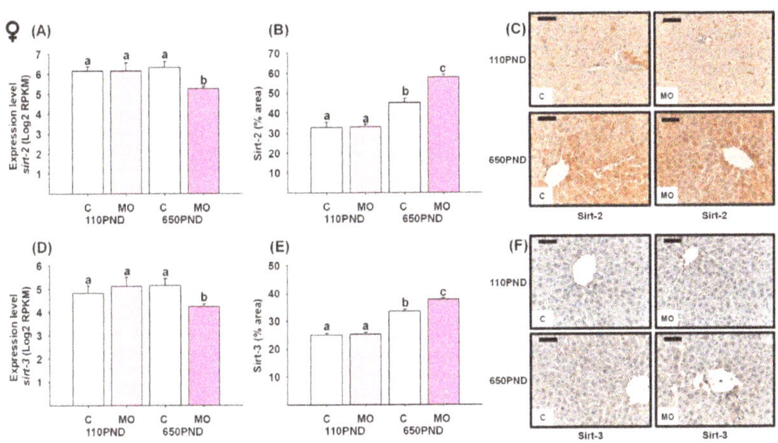

Figure 6. Female hepatic gene expression and protein abundance of Sirt-2 and Sirt-3 in the control (C) and maternal obesity (MO) groups. (**A**) Expression level of *sirt-2* (Log2 RPKM); (**B**) Sirt-2 immunostained area (%); (**C**) representative IHC micrograph of Sirt-2 (40×); (**D**) expression level of *sirt-3* (Log2 RPKM); (**E**) Sirt-3 immunostained area (%); and (**F**) representative IHC micrograph of Sirt-3 (40×). Data for RNA-seq, mean Log2 RPKM ± SEM. Protein values are mean ± SEM. $p < 0.05$ for data not sharing a lower case letter between groups. n = 5–6 rats/group/litter. PND = Postnatal days. Scale bar: 50 µm.

3.7. Male and Female Liver Sod-1 and Catalase

For males, the groups C-650PND and MO-650PND presented less gene expression and a lower protein percentage of the area stained for Sod-1 and Cat compared to C-110PND (Figure 7A,B,D,E). Figure 7C,F show representative sections stained by IHC analysis for *Sod-1* and *catalase* proteins, respectively.

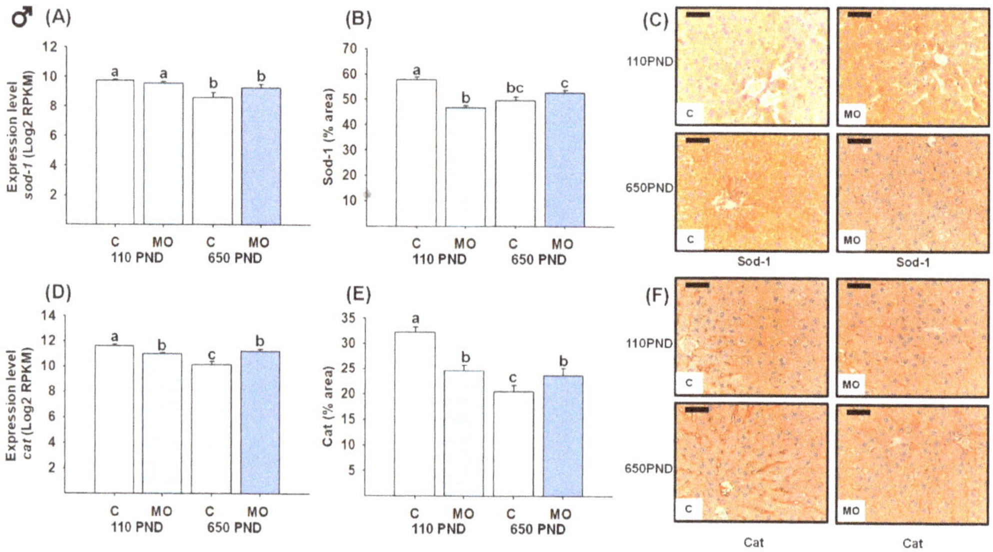

Figure 7. Male hepatic gene expression and protein abundance of Sod-1 and Catalase in the control (C) and maternal obesity (MO) groups. (**A**) Expression level of *sod-1* (Log2 RPKM); (**B**) Sod-1 immunostained area (%); (**C**) representative IHC micrograph of Sod-1 (40×); (**D**) expression level of *catalase* (Log2 RPKM); (**E**) Cat immunostained area (%); and (**F**) representative IHC micrograph of Cat (40×). Data for RNA-seq, mean Log2 RPKM ± SEM. Protein values are mean ± SEM. $p < 0.05$ for data not sharing a lower case letter between groups. n = 5–6 rats/group/litter. PND = Postnatal days. Scale bar: 50 μm.

In females, *sod-1* and *catalase* gene expression were only down-regulated in the MO-650PND group in comparison to all groups (Figure 8A and D, respectively). However, when it came to the Sod-1 protein, MO-650PND had a higher protein percentage of area stained than C-110PND and C-650PND (Figure 8B). Regarding the catalase protein, C-650PND and MO-650PND exhibited higher protein concentrations than C-110PND and MO-110PND (Figure 8E). Figure 8C,F show representative sections stained by IHC analysis for the Sod-1 and catalase proteins, respectively.

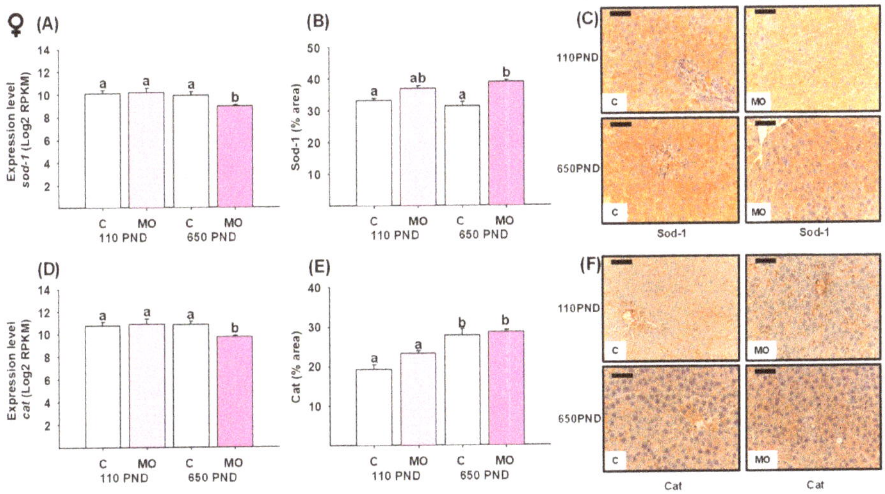

Figure 8. Female hepatic gene expression and protein abundance of Sod-1 and catalase in the control (C) and maternal obesity (MO) groups. (**A**) Expression level of *sod-1* (Log2 RPKM); (**B**) Sod-1 immunostained area (%); (**C**) representative micrograph of Sod-1 (40×); (**D**) expression level of *cat* (Log2 RPKM); (**E**) Cat immunostained area (%); and (**F**) representative micrograph of Cat (40×). Data for RNA-seq, mean Log2 RPKM ± SEM. Protein values are mean ± SEM. $p < 0.05$ for data not sharing a lower case letter between groups. n = 5–6 rats/group/litter. PND = Postnatal days. Scale bar: 50 µm.

4. Discussion

Exposure to a high-fat diet prior to and/or during pregnancy and lactation has long-term consequences for both mothers and their offspring. Maternal obesity increases offspring liver fat accumulation, which negatively affects offspring metabolism and predisposes neonates and children to obesity and NAFLD, increasing oxidative damage, inflammation, insulin resistance, lipid metabolism, and mitochondrial function [31]. The fetal liver function is immature and vulnerable to dysregulated maternal metabolism. Exposing the fetus to an excess of metabolic fuels from an obese mother during gestation contributes to the programming of NAFLD in childhood [36,38,44]. Studies in rodents [4,10,45], ewes [15], and non-human primates [46] have shown that maternal obesity programs offspring to develop hepatic metabolic disorders later in life and correlates with the severity of childhood NAFLD [47].

There is also considerable interest in the potential that developmental programming can alter the trajectory of aging [48–50]. Aging is a multifactorial degenerative process in which physiological and metabolic processes decline and is a risk factor for the development of metabolic diseases [51]. The natural biological changes that occur during aging differ among major organs and are sexually dimorphic [52]. In this regard, males aged earlier than females [53]. In humans, fatty liver disease is more severe and has a worse prognosis in the elderly than in young adults [54].

In addition to alterations in genes, proteins, and metabolites, liver aging is accompanied by a redox imbalance and a decline in hepatic metabolism. Among the alterations associated with liver aging, several signaling pathways are implicated, such as those related to xenobiotic metabolism, lipid metabolism, oxidative stress [55], cell growth [56], immune cell responses [53,57], metabolic processes, cell activation [57], and inflammatory processes [58,59].

In our animal model, the male and female offspring of obese mothers have higher adiposity indexes, triglycerides, and insulin resistance compared to those of control mothers. Males from the MO group exhibit greater physiological and histological NAFLD characteristics than females at 110 days [4]. Also, human studies indicate that the prevalence of NAFLD is higher in men [60]. However, little is known about developmental programming–aging interactions and the molecular mechanisms of NAFLD programmed by MO.

Our observations showed that where genes that were down-regulated in C-650PND vs. C-110PND (natural aging) were also down-regulated in the MO-110PND vs. C-110PND comparison (effect of maternal diet at a young age) they were considered to be genes programmed by maternal obesity to age prematurely. Furthermore, at a young age, we observed sex differences in the gene expression profiles between the offspring of obese mothers and offspring born to the control mothers, as well as in the natural liver aging course in our animal model at old age (650PND) vs. young age (110PND), with males again having more pronounced changes. Clearly, in all studies, the sexual dimorphism of the outcomes must be addressed in determining the underlying mechanisms involved.

In the MO-programmed NAFLD phenotype, we have also previously observed important metabolic and liver oxidative stress sexual dimorphism. In the liver transcriptomic analysis, we observed diet and age effects in a sex-dependent manner regarding mitochondrial pathways. In our model, we reported the phenotypic characterization of NAFLD in the offspring of obese mothers [10]. The changes observed in MO offspring compared to C offspring were programmed by the mother's consumption of a high-fat diet; since offspring were weaned onto a C diet and did not consume a high-fat diet, the observed changes in the NAFLD phenotype in gene expression and protein concentration were programmed from fetal and neonatal exposure to excess fetal nutrients. Importantly, changes in mitochondrial function have been demonstrated from fetal and neonatal ages, prior to the establishment of NAFLD [31].

The liver is an organ that plays a central role in the body's main metabolic processes, including energy production, and is therefore essential for regulating energy balance [61]. In this regard, oxidative phosphorylation is by far the principal pathway for cellular energy production and is the primary source of ROS production [62]. Aging induces morphological, structural, and functional changes in the liver, as well as increased levels of ROS, oxidative damage, decreased mitochondrial energy production capacity, and dysfunction of the respiratory chain [62–64]. Among the molecular mechanisms of NAFLD programmed by MO, major pathways and genes related to mitochondrial function, such as lysosome, ribosome, peroxisome, TCA cycle, mitophagy, ETC, oxidative stress, and oxidative phosphorylation, are involved in premature aging in males. Therefore, mitochondria and peroxisomes are significant ROS sources [64].

We studied genes involved in oxidative phosphorylation as possible contributors to increased ROS concentrations. During both normal aging and accelerated aging in the offspring of obese mothers, a number of sex-related gene-expression changes were detected. Age-related declines in mitochondrial function and antioxidant enzymes result in a rise in mitochondrial ROS production. Different studies comparing old and young animals have evaluated mitochondrial function and found that the number of mitochondria and the mitochondrial protein concentrations decrease with age in the liver cells of mice, rats, and humans [24]. In addition, the respiratory chain capacity of liver mitochondria in aged rats (720 days) is reduced by 40% compared to young rats (90–120 days) [25]. Mitochondrial dysfunction is one of the hallmarks of aging [22–27,65,66] and is related to the progression of NAFLD.

In males, maternal obesity and aging led to the down-regulation of representative genes for Complexes I, II, IV, and V. These findings are consistent with the decreased immunolocalization of Complexes I and IV, mainly in the MO groups, as well as the decreased immunolocalization of Complexes II and V observed in the MO and aged groups. In fact, the activity of Complexes I and IV decreased with age in the livers of mice and rats; whereas, the activity of Complexes II, III, and IV remained relatively unchanged [25]. In a mouse model of maternal obesity, it has been reported that 105-day-old female offspring reduced the hepatic mitochondrial ETC activity of Complexes I, II/III, and IV [32]. This observation suggests the presence of post-translational mechanisms in ETC-associated gene expression. Maternal obesity also programs increased adiposity in males and females [7], which worsens with age [10]. In this regard, it is known that obesity alone accelerates aging and adipose tissue dysfunction can be observed earlier than in normal aging [67]. In addition, the continued delivery of FFAs to liver mitochondria induces a hypermetabolic state, as occurs with insulin resistance, which further impairs mitochondrial bioenergetics in the adipocytes of diabetic (*db/db*) individuals. This situation may resemble our model in which the offspring of obese mothers accumulated much dysfunctional adipose tissue with signs of insulin resistance in which the suppressed expression of mitochondrial proteins caused mitochondrial loss, decreased fatty acid oxidation, and lowered ATP production [68]. Thus, the loss of mitochondrial function plays an important role in the progression of NAFLD [29].

MO led to the down-regulation of representative genes for Complexes I, II, IV, and V, only in females at 650PND. Nevertheless, the increased immunolocalization of Complexes I and II was mainly observed in aged offspring MO females. These findings suggest an adaptation mechanism for offspring MO females as they age. Compared to males, females have greater respiratory function and mitochondrial biogenesis in several tissues [69]. In addition, females exhibit a tighter regulation of mitochondrial processes than males, which affords them increased protection in the presence of metabolic challenges [70]. In this regard, the ETC can be regulated through the expression of Complexes I and II by tuning the availability of NADH and succinate [71]. In addition, the observed increased immunostaining for Complex II, which catalyzes the oxidation of succinate to fumarate, suggests a mechanism for protecting the integrity of the TCA cycle and oxidative phosphorylation [72]. Regardless of age, the decreased immunolocalization of Complex V was observed mainly in the MO groups for both sexes. The primary function of mitochondria is to generate ATP via oxidative phosphorylation, which is carried out by the four respiratory chain complexes (I–IV) and the ATP synthase (Complex V), which are localized within the mitochondrial inner membrane.

Through the ATP synthase system, the ETC is tightly coupled with the oxidative phosphorylation pathway to enable the production of metabolically useful energy in the form of ATP. The lack of consistency observed between the transcription and expression of mitochondrial complexes in each sex indicates that mitochondrial biogenesis is sex-dependent. The increased expression of *sirt-2* (from the cytoplasm) and *sirt-3* (from the mitochondria) that we observed in females in the offspring of the MO 650PND group may be related to a potential increase in mitochondrial biogenesis as SIRTs are known to indirectly regulate the expression of mitochondrial biogenesis through PGC-1 activation.

NAFLD is graded as simple steatosis, nonalcoholic steatohepatitis (NASH), liver cirrhosis, or hepatocellular cancer [73]. The progression from simple steatosis to NASH involves the generation of reactive oxygen species, lipotoxicity, and inflammatory cytokines [74]. The sirtuins family are highly conserved NAD^+-dependent histone deacetylases that have been related to antioxidant and oxidative stress-related processes and functions like longevity, mitochondrial function, DNA-damage repair, and metabolism [75]. In mammals, seven members (*sirt1-7*) have been identified, with *sirt-2* being the least recognized but highly expressed in metabolically active tissues, including the liver, heart, brain, and adipose tissue [76]. In obese mice, it has been shown that *sirt-2* hepatic overexpression ameliorates insulin sensitivity, oxidative stress, and mitochondrial dysfunction [77]. However, a link between *sirt-2* and NAFLD has not yet been established. In obese *ob/ob* mice and HFD-fed mice, it has been reported that liver Sirt-2 protein levels gradually decreased with age. This reduction was also confirmed in HepG2 cells treated with palmitate in a time- and dose-dependent manner, indicating that hepatic *sirt-2* expression significantly decreased in the context of NAFLD [78]. Our findings showed that maternal obesity decreased liver *sirt-2* expression in offspring in a sex-dependent manner, with the reduction starting at PND110 in MO males and PND650 in females. The *sirt-3* is also highly expressed in the liver and other metabolic tissues with high oxidative capacity. Sirt-3 plays an important role in mitochondrial metabolism through the reversible acetylation of mitochondrial proteins [79]. Low Sirt-3 activity, mitochondrial dysfunction, and protein hyperacetylation were observed in the liver of mice fed a chronic HFD [80]. In a separate study, *sirt-3*-deficient mice fed a chronic HFD developed obesity, insulin resistance, and steatohepatitis more rapidly than wild-type mice [81]. Our findings showed that maternal obesity decreased liver *sirt-3* expression in a sex-dependent manner, with the reduction starting at 110PND in MO males and 650PND in MO females. Therefore, the reduction in *sirt-2* and *sirt-3* expression might be related to the decline in the expression of antioxidant enzyme genes and the increased reactive oxygen species, oxidative stress, and fatty liver accumulation [10]. It is well known that oxidative stress contributes to aging. During the aging process, cells defend themselves against oxidative damage by expressing a variety of non-enzymatic and enzymatic antioxidant defenses that convert ROS into less dangerous byproducts. Sod converts the anion superoxide to hydrogen peroxide and it mitigates the ROS produced by the mitochondria; but, as NAFLD progresses, Sod decreases. In the present study, age and diet reduced *sod* gene expression in both males and females. However, the amount of protein was higher in MO-650PND compared to MO-110PND and the C group. This observation merits further study. It may be due to post-translational changes in protein production. In mice, the deletion of liver *sod-1* accelerates aging, shortens the life span, and results in the development of hepatocellular carcinoma [82].

The observed changes in gene and protein expression associated with the mitochondrial function pathways (Figure 9), together with those previously observed in our experimental model, such as insulin resistance, increased liver fat accumulation, visceral fat and oxidative stress, decreased antioxidant enzymes, and liver morphological alterations in MO offspring, contribute to the programming of the MO offspring fatty liver phenotype. Likewise, the differences in the changes in gene expression observed between the diet, age, and sex comparisons could be associated with the severity of the fatty liver over the life span as the changes observed at 110PND remain at age 650PND. This study links mitochondrial function to signaling pathways that regulate the life span and the aging process; it demonstrates the role and importance of the mitochondria in the predisposition to developing NAFLD.

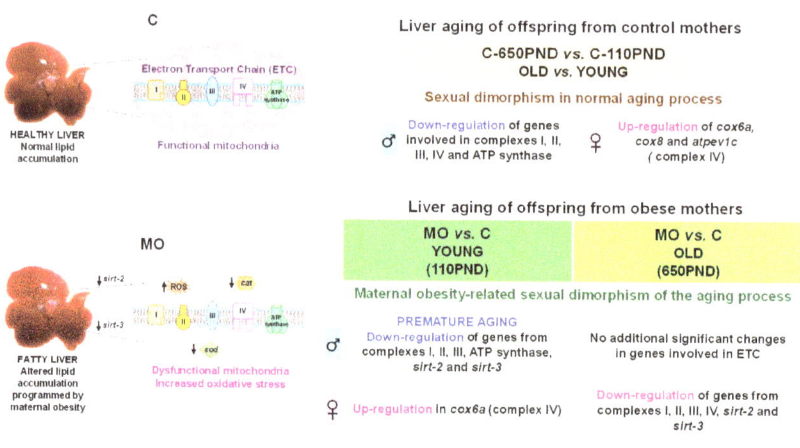

Figure 9. Summary of findings.

5. Conclusions

Maternal obesity programs sex-specific changes associated with the natural aging process leading to liver dysfunction in offspring. In males at 110PND, maternal obesity accelerates the age-associated down-regulation of genes and pathways related to mitochondrial function. In females, these programming effects occur at 650PND. Moreover, maternal obesity programs decreased offspring liver ETC gene expression, especially Complex 1, the major site of ROS production. These changes can lead to metabolic dysfunction and offspring obesity and are potential mechanisms for programming offspring from maternal obesity life-course metabolic dysfunction.

Supplementary Materials: The following supporting information can be downloaded at: https://www.mdpi.com/article/10.3390/biology12091166/s1, Figure S1: Representative IHC micrograph of negative controls (40x), Table S1: Male DEG in common from the comparisons MO-110PND vs C-110PND and C-650PND vs C-110PND in males. Log2Fold change regulation and their statistical significance are shown by *p*-value, Table S2: Male DEG in common from the comparisons MO-110PND vs C-110PND and C-650PND vs C-110PND in males. Log2Fold change regulation and their statistical significance are shown by *p*-value.

Author Contributions: C.L.-S., G.L.R.-G., L.A.R.-C. and C.A.I., researched data, C.L.-S. data analysis. P.W.N. and E.Z. funding acquisition. P.W.N. and E.Z. study design, C.L.-S., G.L.R.-G., P.W.N. and E.Z. preparation and review of the manuscript. E.Z. final approval of the manuscript. All persons designated as authors qualify for authorship and all those who qualify for authorship are listed. All authors have read and agreed to the published version of the manuscript.

Funding: This work was supported by the Newton Fund RCUK-CONACyT (Research Councils UK–Consejo Nacional de Ciencia y Tecnología) I000/726/2016 FONCICYT/49/2016 and the National Institutes of Health U19AG057758.

Institutional Review Board Statement: This study was conducted in accordance with the Declaration of Helsinki and approved by the Animal Experimentation Ethics Committee of the Instituto Nacional de Ciencias Médicas y Nutrición Salvador Zubirán (INCMNSZ), Mexico City, Mexico (CINVA 271 and 1868).

Informed Consent Statement: Not applicable.

Data Availability Statement: The data that support the findings of this study are openly available in NCBI's Gene Expression Omnibus and are accessible through GEO Series accession numbers GSE115535 and GSE160153.

Acknowledgments: Laura A. Cox for the acquisition and analysis of RNA-seq data.

Conflicts of Interest: The authors declare no conflict of interest.

References

1. Tiwari, A.; Balasundaram, P. *Public Health Considerations Regarding Obesity*; StatPearls Publishing: Treasure Island, FL, USA, 2023.
2. Reichetzeder, C. Overweight and obesity in pregnancy: Their impact on epigenetics. *Eur. J. Clin. Nutr.* **2021**, *75*, 1710–1722. [CrossRef] [PubMed]
3. Snelgrove-Clarke, E.; Macdonald, D.; Helwig, M.; Alsius, A. Women's experiences of living with obesity during pregnancy, birthing, and postpartum: A qualitative systematic review protocol. *JBI Evid. Synth.* **2021**, *19*, 3183–3189. [CrossRef]
4. Lomas-Soria, C.; Reyes-Castro, L.A.; Rodriguez-Gonzalez, G.L.; Ibanez, C.A.; Bautista, C.J.; Cox, L.A.; Nathanielsz, P.W.; Zambrano, E. Maternal obesity has sex-dependent effects on insulin, glucose and lipid metabolism and the liver transcriptome in young adult rat offspring. *J. Physiol.* **2018**, *596*, 4611–4628. [CrossRef] [PubMed]
5. Zambrano, E.; Rodriguez-Gonzalez, G.L.; Reyes-Castro, L.A.; Bautista, C.J.; Castro-Rodriguez, D.C.; Juarez-Pilares, G.; Ibanez, C.A.; Hernandez-Rojas, A.; Nathanielsz, P.W.; Montano, S.; et al. DHA Supplementation of Obese Rats throughout Pregnancy and Lactation Modifies Milk Composition and Anxiety Behavior of Offspring. *Nutrients.* **2021**, *13*, 4243. [CrossRef] [PubMed]
6. Rodriguez-Gonzalez, G.L.; De Los Santos, S.; Mendez-Sanchez, D.; Reyes-Castro, L.A.; Ibanez, C.A.; Canto, P.; Zambrano, E. High-fat diet consumption by male rat offspring of obese mothers exacerbates adipose tissue hypertrophy and metabolic alterations in adult life. *Br. J. Nutr.* **2022**, *130*, 783–792. [CrossRef]
7. Ibanez, C.A.; Lira-Leon, G.; Reyes-Castro, L.A.; Rodriguez-Gonzalez, G.L.; Lomas-Soria, C.; Hernandez-Rojas, A.; Bravo-Flores, E.; Solis-Paredes, J.M.; Estrada-Gutierrez, G.; Zambrano, E. Programming Mechanism of Adipose Tissue Expansion in the Rat Offspring of Obese Mothers Occurs in a Sex-Specific Manner. *Nutrients* **2023**, *15*, 2245. [CrossRef]
8. Wankhade, U.D.; Zhong, Y.; Kang, P.; Alfaro, M.; Chintapalli, S.V.; Thakali, K.M.; Shankar, K. Enhanced offspring predisposition to steatohepatitis with maternal high-fat diet is associated with epigenetic and microbiome alterations. *PLoS ONE* **2017**, *12*, e0175675. [CrossRef] [PubMed]

9. Chavira-Suarez, E.; Reyes-Castro, L.A.; Lopez, T., II; Vargas-Hernandez, L.; Rodriguez-Gonzalez, G.L.; Chavira, R.; Zarate-Segura, P.; Dominguez-Lopez, A.; Vadillo-Ortega, F.; Zambrano, E. Sex-differential RXRalpha gene methylation effects on mRNA and protein expression in umbilical cord of the offspring rat exposed to maternal obesity. *Front. Cell Dev. Biol.* **2022**, *10*, 892315. [CrossRef]
10. Rodriguez-Gonzalez, G.L.; Reyes-Castro, L.A.; Bautista, C.J.; Beltran, A.A.; Ibanez, C.A.; Vega, C.C.; Lomas-Soria, C.; Castro-Rodriguez, D.C.; Elias-Lopez, A.L.; Nathanielsz, P.W.; et al. Maternal obesity accelerates rat offspring metabolic ageing in a sex-dependent manner. *J. Physiol.* **2019**, *597*, 5549–5563. [CrossRef]
11. Rodriguez-Gonzalez, G.L.; Vargas-Hernandez, L.; Reyes-Castro, L.A.; Ibanez, C.A.; Bautista, C.J.; Lomas-Soria, C.; Itani, N.; Estrada-Gutierrez, G.; Espejel-Nunez, A.; Flores-Pliego, A.; et al. Resveratrol Supplementation in Obese Pregnant Rats Improves Maternal Metabolism and Prevents Increased Placental Oxidative Stress. *Antioxidants.* **2022**, *11*, 1871. [CrossRef]
12. Anderson, E.L.; Howe, L.D.; Jones, H.E.; Higgins, J.P.; Lawlor, D.A.; Fraser, A. The Prevalence of Non-Alcoholic Fatty Liver Disease in Children and Adolescents: A Systematic Review and Meta-Analysis. *PLoS ONE* **2015**, *10*, e0140908. [CrossRef]
13. Vos, M.B.; Abrams, S.H.; Barlow, S.E.; Caprio, S.; Daniels, S.R.; Kohli, R.; Mouzaki, M.; Sathya, P.; Schwimmer, J.B.; Sundaram, S.S.; et al. NASPGHAN Clinical Practice Guideline for the Diagnosis and Treatment of Nonalcoholic Fatty Liver Disease in Children: Recommendations from the Expert Committee on NAFLD (ECON) and the North American Society of Pediatric Gastroenterology, Hepatology and Nutrition (NASPGHAN). *J. Pediatr. Gastroenterol. Nutr.* **2017**, *64*, 319–334. [CrossRef] [PubMed]
14. Newton, K.P.; Feldman, H.S.; Chambers, C.D.; Wilson, L.; Behling, C.; Clark, J.M.; Molleston, J.P.; Chalasani, N.; Sanyal, A.J.; Fishbein, M.H.; et al. Low and High Birth Weights Are Risk Factors for Nonalcoholic Fatty Liver Disease in Children. *J. Pediatr.* **2017**, *187*, 141–146.e141. [CrossRef]
15. Serafim, T.L.; Cunha-Oliveira, T.; Deus, C.M.; Sardao, V.A.; Cardoso, I.M.; Yang, S.; Odhiambo, J.F.; Ghnenis, A.B.; Smith, A.M.; Li, J.; et al. Maternal obesity in sheep impairs foetal hepatic mitochondrial respiratory chain capacity. *Eur. J. Clin. Investig.* **2021**, *51*, e13375. [CrossRef]
16. Reynolds, R.M.; Allan, K.M.; Raja, E.A.; Bhattacharya, S.; McNeill, G.; Hannaford, P.C.; Sarwar, N.; Lee, A.J.; Bhattacharya, S.; Norman, J.E. Maternal obesity during pregnancy and premature mortality from cardiovascular event in adult offspring: Follow-up of 1 323 275 person years. *BMJ* **2013**, *347*, f4539. [CrossRef] [PubMed]
17. Mennitti, L.V.; Carpenter, A.A.M.; Loche, E.; Pantaleao, L.C.; Fernandez-Twinn, D.S.; Schoonejans, J.M.; Blackmore, H.L.; Ashmore, T.J.; Pisani, L.P.; Tadross, J.A.; et al. Effects of maternal diet-induced obesity on metabolic disorders and age-associated miRNA expression in the liver of male mouse offspring. *Int. J. Obes.* **2022**, *46*, 269–278. [CrossRef]
18. Odhiambo, J.F.; Pankey, C.L.; Ghnenis, A.B.; Ford, S.P. A Review of Maternal Nutritionduring Pregnancy and Impact on the Off-spring through Development: Evidencefrom Animal Models of Over-and Undernutrition. *Int. J. Environ. Res. Public Health* **2020**, *17*, 6926. [CrossRef] [PubMed]
19. Lin, Y.; Feng, X.; Cao, X.; Miao, R.; Sun, Y.; Li, R.; Ye, J.; Zhong, B. Age patterns of nonalcoholic fatty liver disease incidence: Heterogeneous associations with metabolic changes. *Diabetol. Metab. Syndr.* **2022**, *14*, 181. [CrossRef]
20. Guo, J.; Huang, X.; Dou, L.; Yan, M.; Shen, T.; Tang, W.; Li, J. Aging and aging-related diseases: From molecular mechanisms to interventions and treatments. *Signal Transduct. Target. Ther.* **2022**, *7*, 391. [CrossRef]
21. He, F.; Huang, Y.; Song, Z.; Zhou, H.J.; Zhang, H.; Perry, R.J.; Shulman, G.I.; Min, W. Mitophagy-mediated adipose inflammation contributes to type 2 diabetes with hepatic insulin resistance. *J. Exp. Med.* **2021**, *218*, e20201416. [CrossRef]
22. Lopez-Otin, C.; Blasco, M.A.; Partridge, L.; Serrano, M.; Kroemer, G. The hallmarks of aging. *Cell* **2013**, *153*, 1194–1217. [CrossRef] [PubMed]
23. Schmauck-Medina, T.; Moliere, A.; Lautrup, S.; Zhang, J.; Chlopicki, S.; Madsen, H.B.; Cao, S.; Soendenbroe, C.; Mansell, E.; Vestergaard, M.B.; et al. New hallmarks of ageing: A 2022 Copenhagen ageing meeting summary. *Aging* **2022**, *14*, 6829–6839. [CrossRef] [PubMed]
24. Baker, D.J.; Peleg, S. Biphasic Modeling of Mitochondrial Metabolism Dysregulation during Aging. *Trends Biochem. Sci.* **2017**, *42*, 702–711. [CrossRef]
25. Bratic, A.; Larsson, N.G. The role of mitochondria in aging. *J. Clin. Investig.* **2013**, *123*, 951–957. [CrossRef] [PubMed]
26. Chistiakov, D.A.; Sobenin, I.A.; Revin, V.V.; Orekhov, A.N.; Bobryshev, Y.V. Mitochondrial aging and age-related dysfunction of mitochondria. *BioMed Res. Int.* **2014**, *2014*, 238463. [CrossRef]
27. Wang, Y.; Hekimi, S. Mitochondrial dysfunction and longevity in animals: Untangling the knot. *Science* **2015**, *350*, 1204–1207. [CrossRef]
28. Dabravolski, S.A.; Bezsonov, E.E.; Orekhov, A.N. The role of mitochondria dysfunction and hepatic senescence in NAFLD development and progression. *Biomed. Pharmacother.* **2021**, *142*, 112041. [CrossRef]
29. Dornas, W.; Schuppan, D. Mitochondrial oxidative injury: A key player in nonalcoholic fatty liver disease. *Am. J. Physiol. Gastrointest. Liver Physiol.* **2020**, *319*, G400–G411. [CrossRef]
30. Fromenty, B.; Roden, M. Mitochondrial alterations in fatty liver diseases. *J. Hepatol.* **2023**, *78*, 415–429. [CrossRef]
31. Baker, P.R., 2nd; Friedman, J.E. Mitochondrial role in the neonatal predisposition to developing nonalcoholic fatty liver disease. *J. Clin. Investig.* **2018**, *128*, 3692–3703. [CrossRef]
32. Bruce, K.D.; Cagampang, F.R.; Argenton, M.; Zhang, J.; Ethirajan, P.L.; Burdge, G.C.; Bateman, A.C.; Clough, G.F.; Poston, L.; Hanson, M.A.; et al. Maternal high-fat feeding primes steatohepatitis in adult mice offspring, involving mitochondrial dysfunction and altered lipogenesis gene expression. *Hepatology* **2009**, *50*, 1796–1808. [CrossRef] [PubMed]

33. Bayol, S.A.; Simbi, B.H.; Fowkes, R.C.; Stickland, N.C. A maternal "junk food" diet in pregnancy and lactation promotes nonalcoholic Fatty liver disease in rat offspring. *Endocrinology* **2010**, *151*, 1451–1461. [CrossRef] [PubMed]
34. Alfaradhi, M.Z.; Fernandez-Twinn, D.S.; Martin-Gronert, M.S.; Musial, B.; Fowden, A.; Ozanne, S.E. Oxidative stress and altered lipid homeostasis in the programming of offspring fatty liver by maternal obesity. *Am. J. Physiol. Regul. Integr. Comp. Physiol.* **2014**, *307*, R26–R34. [CrossRef] [PubMed]
35. Puppala, S.; Li, C.; Glenn, J.P.; Saxena, R.; Gawrieh, S.; Quinn, A.; Palarczyk, J.; Dick, E.J., Jr.; Nathanielsz, P.W.; Cox, L.A. Primate fetal hepatic responses to maternal obesity: Epigenetic signalling pathways and lipid accumulation. *J. Physiol.* **2018**, *596*, 5823–5837. [CrossRef]
36. Wesolowski, S.R.; Kasmi, K.C.; Jonscher, K.R.; Friedman, J.E. Developmental origins of NAFLD: A womb with a clue. *Nat. Rev. Gastroenterol. Hepatol.* **2017**, *14*, 81–96. [CrossRef]
37. Thompson, M.D. Developmental Programming of NAFLD by Parental Obesity. *Hepatol. Commun.* **2020**, *4*, 1392–1403. [CrossRef]
38. Valentini, F.; Rocchi, G.; Vespasiani-Gentilucci, U.; Guarino, M.P.L.; Altomare, A.; Carotti, S. The Origins of NAFLD: The Potential Implication of Intrauterine Life and Early Postnatal Period. *Cells* **2022**, *11*, 562. [CrossRef]
39. Grundy, D. Principles and standards for reporting animal experiments in The Journal of Physiology and Experimental Physiology. *J. Physiol.* **2015**, *593*, 2547–2549. [CrossRef]
40. Kilkenny, C.; Browne, W.J.; Cuthi, I.; Emerson, M.; Altman, D.G. Improving bioscience research reporting: The ARRIVE guidelines for reporting animal research. *Vet. Clin. Pathol.* **2012**, *41*, 27–31. [CrossRef]
41. Vega, C.C.; Reyes-Castro, L.A.; Bautista, C.J.; Larrea, F.; Nathanielsz, P.W.; Zambrano, E. Exercise in obese female rats has beneficial effects on maternal and male and female offspring metabolism. *Int. J. Obes.* **2015**, *39*, 712–719. [CrossRef]
42. Zhang, B.; Kirov, S.; Snoddy, J. WebGestalt: An integrated system for exploring gene sets in various biological contexts. *Nucleic. Acids. Res.* **2005**, *33*, W741–W748. [CrossRef] [PubMed]
43. Kanehisa, M.; Goto, S. KEGG: Kyoto encyclopedia of genes and genomes. *Nucleic Acids Res.* **2000**, *28*, 27–30. [CrossRef]
44. Brumbaugh, D.E.; Friedman, J.E. Developmental origins of nonalcoholic fatty liver disease. *Pediatr. Res.* **2014**, *75*, 140–147. [CrossRef] [PubMed]
45. Han, S.; Zhu, F.; Huang, X.; Yan, P.; Xu, K.; Shen, F.; Sun, J.; Yang, Z.; Jin, G.; Teng, Y. Maternal obesity accelerated non-alcoholic fatty liver disease in offspring mice by reducing autophagy. *Exp. Ther. Med.* **2021**, *22*, 716. [CrossRef] [PubMed]
46. Thorn, S.R.; Baquero, K.C.; Newsom, S.A.; El Kasmi, K.C.; Bergman, B.C.; Shulman, G.I.; Grove, K.L.; Friedman, J.E. Early life exposure to maternal insulin resistance has persistent effects on hepatic NAFLD in juvenile nonhuman primates. *Diabetes* **2014**, *63*, 2702–2713. [CrossRef] [PubMed]
47. Hagstrom, H.; Simon, T.G.; Roelstraete, B.; Stephansson, O.; Soderling, J.; Ludvigsson, J.F. Maternal obesity increases the risk and severity of NAFLD in offspring. *J. Hepatol.* **2021**, *75*, 1042–1048. [CrossRef]
48. Nathanielsz, P.W.; Huber, H.F.; Li, C.; Clarke, G.D.; Kuo, A.H.; Zambrano, E. The nonhuman primate hypothalamo-pituitary-adrenal axis is an orchestrator of programming-aging interactions: Role of nutrition. *Nutr. Rev.* **2020**, *78*, 48–61. [CrossRef]
49. Zambrano, E.; Reyes-Castro, L.A.; Rodriguez-Gonzalez, G.L.; Chavira, R.; Nathanielsz, P.W. Aging Endocrine and Metabolic Phenotypes Are Programmed by Mother's Age at Conception in a Sex-Dependent Fashion in the Rat. *J. Gerontol. A Biol. Sci. Med. Sci.* **2020**, *75*, 2304–2307. [CrossRef]
50. Aiken, C.E.; Tarry-Adkins, J.L.; Spiroski, A.M.; Nuzzo, A.M.; Ashmore, T.J.; Rolfo, A.; Sutherland, M.J.; Camm, E.J.; Giussani, D.A.; Ozanne, S.E. Chronic gestational hypoxia accelerates ovarian aging and lowers ovarian reserve in next-generation adult rats. *FASEB J.* **2019**, *33*, 7758–7766. [CrossRef]
51. Nathanielsz, P.W. *Life before Birth: The Challenges of Fetal Development*, 1st ed.; Life Course Health Press, LLC.: San Antonio, TX, USA, 2022; p. 351.
52. Lomas-Soria, C.; Cox, L.A.; Nathanielsz, P.W.; Zambrano, E. Sexual dimorphism in liver cell cycle and senescence signalling pathways in young and old rats. *J. Physiol.* **2021**, *599*, 4309–4320. [CrossRef]
53. Cheng, C.J.; Gelfond, J.A.L.; Strong, R.; Nelson, J.F. Genetically heterogeneous mice exhibit a female survival advantage that is age- and site-specific: Results from a large multi-site study. *Aging Cell* **2019**, *18*, e12905. [CrossRef] [PubMed]
54. Bertolotti, M.; Lonardo, A.; Mussi, C.; Baldelli, E.; Pellegrini, E.; Ballestri, S.; Romagnoli, D.; Loria, P. Nonalcoholic fatty liver disease and aging: Epidemiology to management. *World J. Gastroenterol.* **2014**, *20*, 14185–14204. [CrossRef] [PubMed]
55. Capel, F.; Delmotte, M.H.; Brun, M.; Lonchampt, M.; De Fanti, B.; Xuereb, L.; Baschet, L.; Rolland, G.; Galizzi, J.P.; Lockhart, B.; et al. Aging and obesity induce distinct gene expression adaptation in the liver of C57BL/6J mice. *J. Nutrigenet. Nutr.* **2011**, *4*, 154–164. [CrossRef]
56. Chishti, M.A.; Kaya, N.; Binbakheet, A.B.; Al-Mohanna, F.; Goyns, M.H.; Colak, D. Induction of cell proliferation in old rat liver can reset certain gene expression levels characteristic of old liver to those associated with young liver. *Age* **2013**, *35*, 719–732. [CrossRef]
57. White, R.R.; Milholland, B.; MacRae, S.L.; Lin, M.; Zheng, D.; Vijg, J. Comprehensive transcriptional landscape of aging mouse liver. *BMC Genom.* **2015**, *16*, 899. [CrossRef] [PubMed]
58. Bochkis, I.M.; Przybylski, D.; Chen, J.; Regev, A. Changes in nucleosome occupancy associated with metabolic alterations in aged mammalian liver. *Cell Rep.* **2014**, *9*, 996–1006. [CrossRef]

59. Bacalini, M.G.; Franceschi, C.; Gentilini, D.; Ravaioli, F.; Zhou, X.; Remondini, D.; Pirazzini, C.; Giuliani, C.; Marasco, E.; Gensous, N.; et al. Molecular Aging of Human Liver: An Epigenetic/Transcriptomic Signature. *J. Gerontol. A Biol. Sci. Med. Sci.* **2019**, *74*, 1–8. [CrossRef]
60. Riazi, K.; Azhari, H.; Charette, J.H.; Underwood, F.E.; King, J.A.; Afshar, E.E.; Swain, M.G.; Congly, S.E.; Kaplan, G.G.; Shaheen, A.A. The prevalence and incidence of NAFLD worldwide: A systematic review and meta-analysis. *Lancet Gastroenterol. Hepatol.* **2022**, *7*, 851–861. [CrossRef]
61. Rui, L. Energy metabolism in the liver. *Compr. Physiol.* **2014**, *4*, 177–197. [CrossRef]
62. Lozada-Delgado, J.G.; Torres-Ramos, C.A.; Ayala-Peña, S. Aging, oxidative stress, mitochondrial dysfunction, and the liver. In *Aging*; Preedy, V.R., Patel, V.B., Eds.; Academic Press: Cambridge, MA, USA, 2020; pp. 37–46. [CrossRef]
63. Cui, H.; Kong, Y.; Zhang, H. Oxidative stress, mitochondrial dysfunction, and aging. *J. Signal Transduct.* **2012**, *2012*, 646354. [CrossRef]
64. Zhao, Y.; Yang, Y.; Li, Q.; Li, J. Understanding the Unique Microenvironment in the Aging Liver. *Front. Med.* **2022**, *9*, 842024. [CrossRef] [PubMed]
65. Campisi, J.; Kapahi, P.; Lithgow, G.J.; Melov, S.; Newman, J.C.; Verdin, E. From discoveries in ageing research to therapeutics for healthy ageing. *Nature* **2019**, *571*, 183–192. [CrossRef]
66. Goedeke, L.; Murt, K.N.; Di Francesco, A.; Camporez, J.P.; Nasiri, A.R.; Wang, Y.; Zhang, X.M.; Cline, G.W.; de Cabo, R.; Shulman, G.I. Sex- and strain-specific effects of mitochondrial uncoupling on age-related metabolic diseases in high-fat diet-fed mice. *Aging Cell* **2022**, *21*, e13539. [CrossRef] [PubMed]
67. Perez, L.M.; Pareja-Galeano, H.; Sanchis-Gomar, F.; Emanuele, E.; Lucia, A.; Galvez, B.G. 'Adipaging': Ageing and obesity share biological hallmarks related to a dysfunctional adipose tissue. *J. Physiol.* **2016**, *594*, 3187–3207. [CrossRef] [PubMed]
68. Choo, H.J.; Kim, J.H.; Kwon, O.B.; Lee, C.S.; Mun, J.Y.; Han, S.S.; Yoon, Y.S.; Yoon, G.; Choi, K.M.; Ko, Y.G. Mitochondria are impaired in the adipocytes of type 2 diabetic mice. *Diabetologia* **2006**, *49*, 784–791. [CrossRef] [PubMed]
69. Sultanova, R.F.; Schibalski, R.; Yankelevich, I.A.; Stadler, K.; Ilatovskaya, D.V. Sex differences in renal mitochondrial function: A hormone-gous opportunity for research. *Am. J. Physiol. Renal. Physiol.* **2020**, *319*, F1117–F1124. [CrossRef]
70. Von Schulze, A.M.C.; Onyekere, C.; Allen, J.; Geiger, P.; Dorn, G.W., 2nd; Morris, E.M.; Thyfault, J.P. Hepatic mitochondrial adaptations to physical activity: Impact of sexual dimorphism, PGC1α and BNIP3-mediated mitophagy. *J. Physiol.* **2018**, *596*, 6157–6171. [CrossRef]
71. Arnold, P.K.; Finley, L.W.S. Regulation and function of the mammalian tricarboxylic acid cycle. *J. Biol. Chem.* **2023**, *299*, 102838. [CrossRef] [PubMed]
72. Yamada, T.; Murata, D.; Kleiner, D.E.; Anders, R.; Rosenberg, A.Z.; Kaplan, J.; Hamilton, J.P.; Aghajan, M.; Levi, M.; Wang, N.Y.; et al. Prevention and regression of megamitochondria and steatosis by blocking mitochondrial fusion in the liver. *iScience* **2022**, *25*, 103996. [CrossRef]
73. Friedman, S.L.; Neuschwander-Tetri, B.A.; Rinella, M.; Sanyal, A.J. Mechanisms of NAFLD development and therapeutic strategies. *Nat. Med.* **2018**, *24*, 908–922. [CrossRef]
74. Ziolkowska, S.; Binienda, A.; Jablkowski, M.; Szemraj, J.; Czarny, P. The Interplay between Insulin Resistance, Inflammation, Oxidative Stress, Base Excision Repair and Metabolic Syndrome in Nonalcoholic Fatty Liver Disease. *Int. J. Mol. Sci.* **2021**, *22*, 1128. [CrossRef] [PubMed]
75. Nakagawa, T.; Guarente, L. Sirtuins at a glance. *J. Cell Sci.* **2011**, *124*, 833–838. [CrossRef] [PubMed]
76. Gomes, P.; Fleming Outeiro, T.; Cavadas, C. Emerging Role of Sirtuin 2 in the Regulation of Mammalian Metabolism. *Trends. Pharmacol. Sci.* **2015**, *36*, 756–768. [CrossRef] [PubMed]
77. Lemos, V.; de Oliveira, R.M.; Naia, L.; Szego, E.; Ramos, E.; Pinho, S.; Magro, F.; Cavadas, C.; Rego, A.C.; Costa, V.; et al. The NAD+-dependent deacetylase SIRT2 attenuates oxidative stress and mitochondrial dysfunction and improves insulin sensitivity in hepatocytes. *Hum. Mol. Genet.* **2017**, *26*, 4105–4117. [CrossRef]
78. Ren, H.; Hu, F.; Wang, D.; Kang, X.; Feng, X.; Zhang, L.; Zhou, B.; Liu, S.; Yuan, G. Sirtuin 2 Prevents Liver Steatosis and Metabolic Disorders by Deacetylation of Hepatocyte Nuclear Factor 4alpha. *Hepatology.* **2021**, *74*, 723–740. [CrossRef]
79. Nogueiras, R.; Habegger, K.M.; Chaudhary, N.; Finan, B.; Banks, A.S.; Dietrich, M.O.; Horvath, T.L.; Sinclair, D.A.; Pfluger, P.T.; Tschop, M.H. Sirtuin 1 and sirtuin 3: Physiological modulators of metabolism. *Physiol. Rev.* **2012**, *92*, 1479–1514. [CrossRef]
80. Choudhury, M.; Jonscher, K.R.; Friedman, J.E. Reduced mitochondrial function in obesity-associated fatty liver: SIRT3 takes on the fat. *Aging* **2011**, *3*, 175–178. [CrossRef]
81. Hirschey, M.D.; Shimazu, T.; Jing, E.; Grueter, C.A.; Collins, A.M.; Aouizerat, B.; Stancakova, A.; Goetzman, E.; Lam, M.M.; Schwer, B.; et al. SIRT3 deficiency and mitochondrial protein hyperacetylation accelerate the development of the metabolic syndrome. *Mol. Cell* **2011**, *44*, 177–190. [CrossRef]
82. Zhang, Y.; Liu, Y.; Walsh, M.; Bokov, A.; Ikeno, Y.; Jang, Y.C.; Perez, V.I.; Van Remmen, H.; Richardson, A. Liver specific expression of Cu/ZnSOD extends the lifespan of Sod1 null mice. *Mech. Ageing Dev.* **2016**, *154*, 1–8. [CrossRef]

biology

MDPI

Article

Maternal Nutrient Excess Induces Stress Signaling and Decreases Mitochondrial Number in Term Fetal Baboon Skeletal Muscle

Xu Yan [1,2], Carolina Tocantins [3,4,5], Mei-Jun Zhu [1,6], Susana P. Pereira [3,4,7,8,*] and Min Du [1,9,*]

1 Department of Animal Science, University of Wyoming, Laramie, WY 82071, USA; sean.yan@vu.edu.au (X.Y.); meijun.zhu@wsu.edu (M.-J.Z.)
2 Institute for Health and Sport, Victoria University, Melbourne, VIC 8001, Australia
3 CNC-UC, Center for Neuroscience and Cell Biology, University of Coimbra, 3004-531 Coimbra, Portugal; ctsantos@cnc.uc.pt
4 CIBB, Center for Innovative Biomedicine and Biotechnology, University of Coimbra, 3004-531 Coimbra, Portugal
5 PDBEB—Doctoral Programme in Experimental Biology and Biomedicine, Institute for Interdisciplinary Research, University of Coimbra, 3004-517 Coimbra, Portugal
6 School of Food Science, Washington State University, Pullman, WA 99164, USA
7 UCIBIO, Applied Molecular Biosciences Unit, Department of Chemistry, Faculty of Science and Technology, NOVA University Lisbon, 2829-516 Caparica, Portugal
8 Associate Laboratory i4HB-Institute for Health and Bioeconomy, Faculty of Science and Technology, NOVA University Lisbon, 2829-516 Caparica, Portugal
9 Department of Animal Sciences, Washington State University, Pullman, WA 99164, USA
* Correspondence: pereirasusan@gmail.com (S.P.P.); min.du@wsu.edu (M.D.)

Simple Summary: Obesity during pregnancy can impact the development of the fetus and increase the risk of diseases throughout life, beginning from an early stage. We proposed that maternal obesity, caused by excess nutrient intake, affects the offspring's skeletal muscle by causing inflammation and disrupting the normal function of mitochondria, essential structures for producing energy in cells. To investigate this, female baboons were fed either a normal diet or a nutrient-excess diet with increased fat and sugar content before and during pregnancy. Near the end of gestation, muscle samples from baboon fetuses from mothers on the nutrient-excess diet showed increased indicators of inflammation and decreased levels of key players for proper mitochondrial function. These changes suggest that maternal nutrient excess interferes with mitochondrial metabolism, which may raise the risk of metabolic diseases like diabetes early in life.

Abstract: Maternal obesity programs the fetus for increased risk of chronic disease development in early life and adulthood. We hypothesized that maternal nutrient excess leads to fetal inflammation and impairs offspring skeletal muscle mitochondrial biogenesis in non-human primates. At least 12 months before pregnancy, female baboons were fed a normal chow (CTR, 12% energy fat) or a maternal nutrient excess (MNE, 45% energy fat, and ad libitum fructose sodas) diet, with the latter to induce obesity. After 165 days of gestation (0.9 G), offspring baboons were delivered by cesarean section, and the soleus muscle was collected (CTR n = 16, MNE n = 5). At conception, MNE mothers presented increased body fat and weighed more than controls. The soleus muscle of MNE fetuses exhibited increased levels of stress signaling associated with inflammation (TLR4, TNFα, NF-kB p65, and p38), concomitant with reduced expression of key regulators of mitochondrial biogenesis, including PGC1α, both at the protein and transcript levels, as well as downregulation of *PPARGC1B*, *PPARA*, *PPARB*, *CREB1*, *NOS3*, *SIRT1*, *SIRT3*. Decreased transcript levels of *NRF1* were observed alongside diminished mitochondrial DNA copy number, mitochondrial fusion elements (*MFN1*, *MFN2*), cytochrome C protein levels, and cytochrome C oxidase subunits I and II transcripts (*cox1* and *cox2*). MNE coupled to

 https://doi.org/10.3390/biology14070868

MO-induced stress signaling in fetal baboon soleus muscle is associated with impaired mitochondrial biogenesis and lower mitochondrial content, resembling the changes observed in metabolic dysfunctions, such as diabetes. The observed fetal alterations may have important implications for postnatal development and metabolism, potentially increasing the risk of early-onset metabolic disorders and other non-communicable diseases.

Keywords: maternal obesity; fetal programming; skeletal muscle metabolism; cellular bioenergetics; developmental programming; nutrient excess

1. Introduction

Obesity is considered a global epidemic that has alarmingly reached middle- and low-income countries and affects men and women of all ages [1]. The prevalence of obesity in women of childbearing age is increasing [2]. According to the World Health Organization (WHO), 17.9% of women aged 18 and over were obese in 2022, and 44% were overweight [3]. In the United States (US), where obesity has reached staggering proportions, almost 42% of women aged 20 and over are obese, of whom around 40% are women between 20 and 39 years of age [4]. Moreover, the percentage of women in the US with pre-pregnancy obesity increased to 29% in 2019 (26.1% in 2016) [5]. This increasing obesity trend has also been observed among children [6]. The WHO estimated that 35 million children under 5 were overweight in 2024, and more than 390 million children and adolescents (5–19 years of age) were overweight in 2022, of which 160 million were obese [3].

Numerous epidemiological studies have shown that maternal weight and nutrition during pregnancy may have short- and life-long implications for the offspring's health [7–10]. Increased maternal body mass index (BMI), either overweight (BMI $\geq$ 25 kg/m^2) or obesity (BMI $\geq$ 30 kg/m^2) was associated with adverse neonatal outcomes, including large for gestational age, macrosomia, and extreme pre-term birth [7]. Studies also associated maternal obesity (MO) with neonatal hyperinsulinemia [8] and hypoglycemia [8,9], independently of gestational diabetes mellitus. A multi-cohort meta-analysis estimated that up to 41.7% of the children born to mothers with pre-pregnancy overweight or obesity were themselves overweight or obese [8]. Maternal BMI was also strongly associated with early type 2 diabetes (T2D) and cardiovascular disease development in the offspring of the Helsinki Birth Cohort Study [10].

Fetal exposure to an adverse intrauterine environment can induce metabolic programming [11,12]. The skeletal muscle (SM) represents 40–50% of total body mass and has a paramount role in whole body postprandial insulin-stimulated glucose uptake and fatty acid utilization [13]. Given that muscle fibers do not increase in number after birth, poor fetal SM development may result in permanently reduced muscle mass and function, with long-term effects on body energy homeostasis, thus potentially representing an underlying cause for increased T2D predisposition. Lower muscle mass was associated with increased diabetes development [14,15], independent of body fat distribution, in young adults [14]. Considering the volume of epidemiological studies establishing associations regarding maternal nutrition–adverse intrauterine environment– and developmental disease, it has become clear that the molecular pathways underlying offspring disease must be tackled. Non-human primates (NHP) and other precocial species such as sheep [16] are excellent models to achieve the closest translation to human health and disease, given their similarities concerning genetics, physiology, immunology, the reproductive system, and developmental processes [17].

The effects of MO and nutrient-excess diet during pregnancy on fetal SM have started to be explored. Japanese macaques fetuses (130 days of gestation (d)) exposed to MO and western diet consumption during pregnancy (term 173 d) had reduced insulin-stimulated glucose uptake and Akt phosphorylation [18], which we also found in our study in the fetal SM of ewes at 135 d (term 148 d), similarly exposed to a nutrient-excess diet before and during pregnancy [19]. While neither study showed changes in phosphorylated insulin receptor substrate (IRS-1), Omar et al. reported an increased ratio of phosphorylated (inhibited) IRS-1 in the fetal SM of ewes mid-gestation (75 d), along with elevated active c-jun-NH_2 terminal kinase (JNK) levels [20], which we also observed at late ewe gestation [19]. This kinase responds to inflammatory signals and inhibits insulin signaling [21]. Maternal obesity is characterized by a low-grade systemic and placental inflammation state [22]. Indeed, in our ewe model, toll-like receptor (TLR) 4 levels were increased, as well as the levels of phosphorylated TLR ligands activate IkB kinases (IKK) and nuclear factor-kB (NF-kB) p65 in the fetal SM [19], indicating an MO-induced inflammatory environment for this model.

Despite this knowledge, the bridge between fetal SM inflammation and mitochondrial (dys)function is yet to be established. Increasing evidence reports mitochondria, pivotal controllers of oxidative phosphorylation and energy metabolism, as key players in the underlying mechanisms of metabolic syndrome [23], obesity [24], diabetes [25], and other chronic diseases. For example, obese individuals have abnormally shaped and less efficient mitochondria, with compromised bioenergetic capacity and reduced oxidative capacity [24]. Mitochondrial density is reduced, and ATP production is compromised in T2D patients and insulin-resistant individuals [25]. In T2D, skeletal muscle mitochondrial dysfunction is observed through reduced levels of oxidative enzymes, decreased mitochondrial size, and altered mitochondrial morphology, while reduced expression of oxidative metabolism and mitochondrial respiration-related genes are reported as drivers of insulin resistance [26], supporting mitochondrial dysfunction and obesity as risk factors for insulin resistance and T2D development.

We hypothesized that obesity induced by MNE diet, before conception, and continued during pregnancy, alters fetal soleus skeletal muscle development in offspring of a non-human primate model, with consequences for mitochondrial biogenesis.

2. Materials and Methods

2.1. Care and Use of Animals

All animal procedures were approved by the Texas Biomedical Research Institute (TBRI) Institutional Animal Care and Use Committee (protocol number 1675 PC) and conducted in Association for Assessment and Accreditation of Laboratory Animal Care international-approved facilities. The experimental design adhered to the ARRIVE guidelines and incorporated the principles of the 3Rs [27]. Animals were housed in group cages with a floor area of 37 m^2 and 3.5 m in height. Groups of up to 16 non-pregnant, outbred female baboons (*Papio* spp.) were initially housed with a vasectomized male in outdoor gang cages to promote social stability, facilitate natural social behaviors, and ensure unrestricted physical activity. Details of the housing structure and environmental enrichment have been previously published [28]. Maternal morphometric measurements were performed before pregnancy to ensure weight homogeneity and general morphometrics in females randomly assigned to the two groups, as described elsewhere [29]. Nulliparous female baboons of similar age and body weight (10–15 kg) were either assigned to the control (CTR) or maternal nutrient-excess (MNE) group. Females in the CTR group (n = 16) were fed normal chow, the Purina Monkey Diet 5038 (Purina LabDiets, St. Louis, MO, USA), containing stabilized vitamin C and all required vitamins. MNE females (n = 5) had ad libitum access to the same diet as the CTR group and additional ad libitum access to the Purina 5045-6 (Purina LabDiets, St. Louis, MO, USA) high-fat and high-energy diet, as well as free access to fructose sodas [28]. This diet was consumed for at least 12 months before pregnancy to increase body fat (Figure 1). The composition of each diet, along with the basic composition of the biscuit, is presented in Table 1. Of note, the content of protein and essential minerals and vitamins required for the baboon was matched for both CTR and MNE diets. Twelve months after the nutritional intervention, a fertile male was introduced into the group cages. Male baboons used for breeding were maintained on standard chow and were not subjected to any dietary intervention. Female baboons were monitored twice daily for general well-being and three times per week for perineal turgescence and vaginal bleeding to determine the time of conception. Pregnancy was dated initially by the changes in swelling of the sex skin and confirmed at 30 days of gestation by ultrasonography. Only singleton pregnancies were studied.

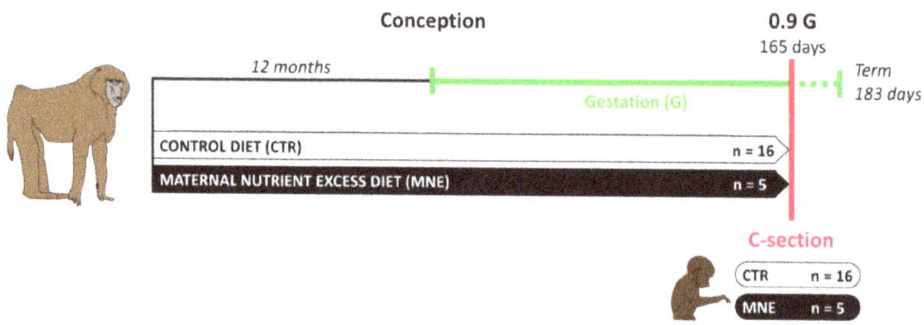

Figure 1. Maternal diet before conception and during pregnancy until cesarean section (C-section) at 90% of the gestation (0.9 G). CTR—control diet; MNE—maternal nutrient-excess diet.

Table 1. Composition of experimental diets and basic biscuit formulation.

Energy Source (%)	Purina Monkey Diet 5038	Purina 5045-6
Fat	12	45
Glucose	0.29	4.62
Fructose	0.32	5.64
Metabolizable Energy Content (kcal/g)	3.07	4.05
Biscuit Basic Composition	Crude protein (≥15%), crude fat (≥5%), crude fiber (≤6%), ash (≤5%), added minerals (≤3%)	

2.2. Cesarean Sections and Tissue Sampling

Surgical procedures and postsurgical care were performed by a fully certified MD or DVM. Cesarean sections were performed at 165 days of gestation (90% of the gestation, 0.9 G, Figure 1) under isoflurane anesthesia (2%, 2 L/min) [28]. Fetuses were euthanized by exsanguination, removed from the uterus, and immediately submitted for morphometric analyses and tissue sampling. Fetal soleus muscle was collected, aliquoted, immediately snap frozen in liquid nitrogen, and stored at −80°. Postoperative maternal analgesia was provided with Buprenorphine hydrochloride 0.015 mg.kg^{-1}.d^{-1} (Reckitt Benckiser Health Care UK Ltd., Hull, UK) during 3 days. After recovering from anesthesia, the baboon mothers were initially housed individually during the post-operative period. Following this, they were group-housed for at least 90 days with a vasectomized male to prevent pregnancy until the surgical site had fully healed [28].

2.3. Dual-Energy X-Ray Absorptiometry (DEXA)

To assess body adiposity before pregnancy, a DEXA scan was conducted in MNE (n = 5) and CTR (n = 7) females after 12 months on the respective diets. For that, a GE Lunar Prodigy 8743 (GE Healthcare, Madison, WI, USA) was used as previously described [30].

2.4. Immunoblotting Analysis

Immunoblotting analyses were conducted according to the procedures previously described [19]. Membranes were visualized using an Odyssey Infrared Imaging System (LI-COR Biosciences, Lincoln, NE, USA). Band density was quantified and normalized to β-tubulin protein levels. Immunoblotting was performed using the antibodies listed in Table S1.

2.5. Analysis of mtDNA Copy Number by Quantitative Real-Time PCR

Total DNA was extracted from the soleus skeletal muscle tissue using the QIAamp DNA mini-kit (#50951304 Qiagen, Düsseldorf, Germany), according to the manufacturer's instructions. The SsoFast Eva Green Supermix (Bio-Rad, Hercules, CA, USA) was used to perform the RT-PCR, with the primers listed in Table S2. DNA amplification was performed with an initial cycle of 2 min at 98 °C, followed by 40 cycles of 5 s at 98 °C plus 5 s at 60 °C. For quality control, melting curves were performed, and no template controls were run.

For absolute quantification and amplification efficiency, standards at known copy numbers were produced by purifying PCR products. After optimizing the annealing temperature, products were amplified for each primer pair using the HotstarTaq Master Mix Kit (#203445 Qiagen). The amplification protocol started with an initial activation step of 15 min at 95 °C, followed by 35 cycles of 1 min at 94 °C plus 1 min at 60 °C, and 1 min at 72 °C, and a final extension step of 10 min at 72 °C. After amplification, the products were purified using the MiniElute PCR purification kit (#280006 Qiagen) following the manufacturer's instructions. All DNA was quantified using a Nanodrop 2000 device (ThermoFisher Scientific, Waltham, MA, USA), and all reactions were performed in a CFX96 real-time PCR system (Bio-Rad). mtDNA copy number was determined by the ratio between the absolute amounts of mitochondrial gene ND1 versus nuclear gene B2M, using the CFX96 Manager software (v. 3.0; Bio-Rad).

2.6. Real-Time Quantitative PCR (RT-PCR)

Total mRNA was extracted from the fetal soleus muscle using TRI reagent (Sigma, St. Louis, MO, USA) and reverse transcribed into cDNA using a kit (Qiagen, Valencia, CA, USA). RT-PCR was performed using the SYBR Green RT-PCR kit from Bio-Rad (Hercules, CA, USA) in a CFX96 real-time PCR system. The reaction was set with the CFX96 Manager software (v. 3.0; Bio-Rad). The list of primers is given in Table S2. Each reaction yielded amplicons between 80–200 bp. PCR conditions were as follows: 10 s at 95 °C, 10 s at 58 °C, and 30 s at 72 °C for 40 cycles. After amplification, a melting curve (0.01 C/s) was used to confirm product purity. The changes in the threshold cycle (CT) values were calculated by the equation CT = CT target − CT input. The fold differences were calculated by the 2−(dCT) method [31]. Results are expressed relative to β-actin.

2.7. Measurement of Citrate Synthase and β-Hydroxyacyl-CoA Dehydrogenase Enzyme Activity

Citrate synthase and β-Hydroxyacyl-CoA dehydrogenase activities were measured by adapting the previously described protocol [32]. The detailed methodology description of each enzymatic activity is provided in the Supplementary Material.

2.8. Statistical Analysis

Each pregnant animal or the respective offspring was considered as an experimental unit. Data were analyzed as a complete randomized design using GLM (General Linear Model of Statistical Analysis System, SAS). For the offspring, the control group was composed of 8 female and 8 male fetuses, and the MNE group of 3 female and 2 male fetuses. The discrepancy of sample size between the two experimental groups resulted from the collection of additional soleus muscle samples from control groups of parallel studies conducted in the same facility, allowing a more robust analysis. Importantly, the variability and main findings remained consistent with results from smaller groups, ensuring reliability. An initial analysis of offspring birth weight and citrate synthase (CS) enzyme activity was performed to assess potential sex differences. CS activity serves as a reliable marker of mitochondrial content and oxidative capacity. Since no differences were observed between female and male fetuses (mean ± SEM: 800.5 ± 34.2 g vs. 859.0 ± 41.7 g in CTR, respectively, and 668.1 ± 64.3 g vs. 686.0 ± 13.0 g in MNE, respectively), data were pooled. Differences in mean values were compared by Tukey's multiple comparison test, which controls for Type I error across pairwise comparisons. Mean ± standard errors of mean (SEM) are reported. Statistical significance was considered as * $p < 0.05$, ** $p < 0.01$ for MNE vs. CTR.

3. Results

In this study, we evaluated the effects of a maternal nutrient-excess diet (MNE) and maternal obesity at conception on fetal soleus muscle at 0.9 G in a baboon model. Maternal obesity was induced through the MNE diet described, starting 12 months before conception and maintained during pregnancy (Figure 1).

3.1. Maternal and Fetal Body Weight

The MNE 12-month diet intervention increased female body weight by 18% at conception compared to females fed a normal chow diet during the same period ($p < 0.05$, Figure 2A). The DEXA scan performed at conception revealed that MNE mothers had a significant increase in overall body adiposity ($p < 0.05$, Figure 3A), especially denoted in the maternal trunk (~30% increase, Figure 3B) but also observed in the legs (~12.5%, Figure 3C) and arms (~10%, Figure 3D). CTR mothers gained on average 1.7 kg (9.4%) during gestation, while MNE mothers lost nearly 0.5 kg (2.5%) ($p < 0.01$, Figure 2C), displaying a similar body weight at cesarean section (Figure 2B). At cesarean section, fetuses of MNE mothers presented a 16% lower body weight compared to CTR fetuses ($p < 0.01$, Figure 2D).

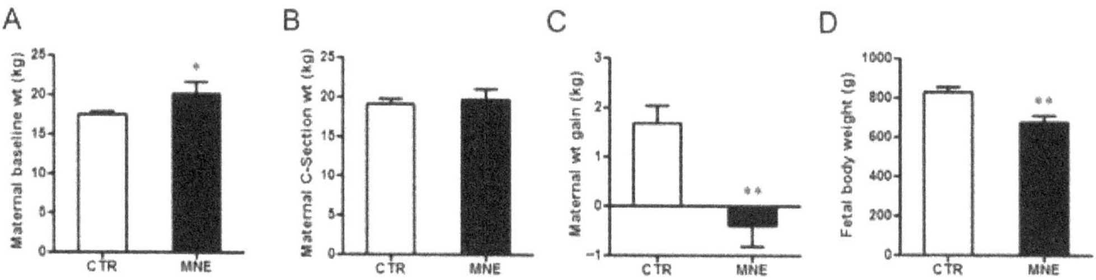

Figure 2. Body weight of mothers subjected to a control (CTR) or maternal nutrient-excess (MNE) diet, and respective fetuses developed in these different maternal conditions. (**A**) Maternal body weight at conception (baseline). (**B**) Maternal body weight at cesarean section (90% of the gestation). (**C**) Maternal weight gain during pregnancy. (**D**) Fetal body weight at cesarean section. CTR: open, n = 16; MNE: closed, n = 5. Data are expressed as mean ± SEM. ** $p < 0.01$, * $p < 0.05$.

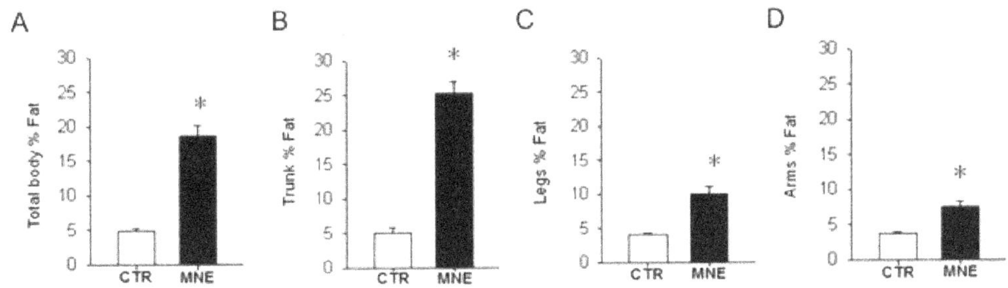

Figure 3. Maternal fat percentage from DEXA scan evaluation after 12 months on the control (CTR) or maternal nutrient-excess (MNE) diet, before conception. (**A**) Total body fat percentage. Fat percentage in the (**B**) trunk, (**C**) legs, and (**D**) arms. CTR: white, n = 7; MNE: black, n = 5. Data are expressed as mean ± SEM; * $p < 0.05$.

3.2. MNE Increased Stress and Pro-Inflammatory Markers in Fetal Soleus Muscle

In light of the characteristic low-grade inflammation associated with obesity, we evaluated the effects of maternal obesity at conception and the MNE diet before and during pregnancy on markers related to inflammation and stress signals within the fetal soleus muscle. The transcript levels of *TNF* and *TLR4* were increased in the soleus muscle of MNE fetuses ($p < 0.05$ and $p < 0.01$, respectively, Figure 4A). A higher WB band density of the proteins encoded by these genes was also observed ($p < 0.05$, Figure 4B). Moreover, the MNE diet contributed to an increased ratio between the phosphorylated form of the NF-kB subunit p65 (Ser536) to total p65 protein content (p-p65/p65, $p < 0.05$, Figure 4C), suggesting the activation of the NF-kB pro-inflammatory pathway in the soleus muscle. A pro-inflammatory environment is further suggested by the observed activation of the p38 MAPK canonical pathway by higher levels of the phosphorylated form of p38 (Thr180/Tyr182) in fetal soleus muscle (p-p38, $p < 0.05$, Figure 4D). Pro-inflammatory signaling is usually associated with altered mitochondria function in several tissues, particularly in the context of chronic diseases, disrupting mitochondrial homeostasis and oxidative capacity [23,24]. Therefore, we next addressed how maternal obesity at conception induced by an MNE diet maintained during pregnancy affected fetal soleus muscle mitochondria quality control.

3.3. Mitochondrial Biogenesis and Mitochondrial Fusion Markers Are Decreased in the Soleus Muscle of MNE Fetuses

The peroxisome proliferator-activated receptors (PPAR) family plays a crucial role in cellular energy homeostasis regulation and metabolic function. In skeletal muscle, PPARs are highly involved in energy utilization and substrate preference but also play a role in inflammation. The relative mRNA levels of *PPARA PPARD* were decreased in the MNE fetal soleus muscle ($p < 0.05$, Figure 5A). Lower levels of the transcriptional co-activators of the PPARγ co-activator family, *PPARGC1A* and *PPARGC1B*, known as the "master regulators" of mitochondrial biogenesis, were also observed ($p < 0.01$ and $p < 0.05$, respectively, Figure 5A). This was accompanied by decreased cAMP responsive element binding protein 1 (*CREB1*) and endothelial nitric oxide synthase (*NOS3* transcript levels ($p < 0.05$, Figure 5C). CREB1 and NO levels, the latter partly regulated by eNOS, are highly involved in cellular signaling, contributing to the transcriptional induction of PGC1α, thus promoting mitochondrial biogenesis [33]. The protein levels of PGC1α were also found to be decreased in the MNE fetal soleus muscle ($p < 0.05$, Figure 5B). Furthermore, the transcript levels of nuclear respiratory factor 1 (*NRF1*), a crucial factor for the transcription of nuclear-encoded mitochondrial genes and whose expression is induced by PGC1α, were also lower in the soleus muscle of MNE fetuses ($p < 0.05$, Figure 5C).

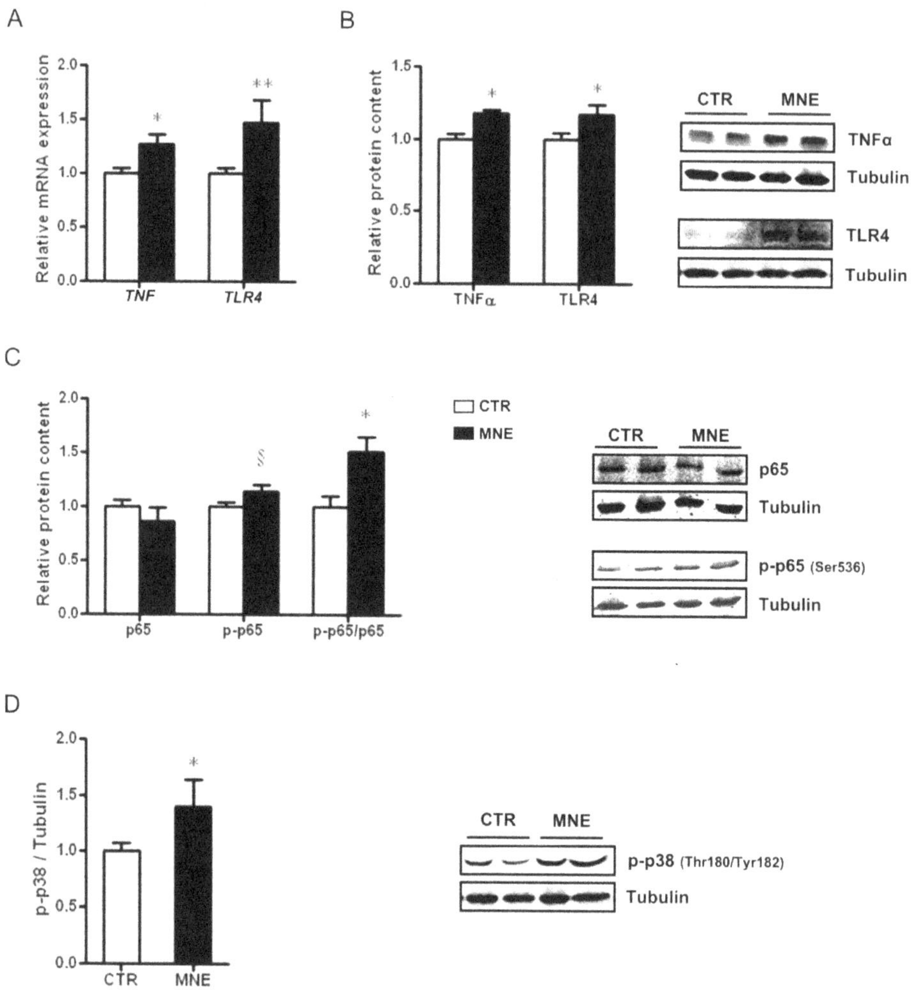

Figure 4. Markers involved in pro-inflammatory pathways and stress responses in fetal baboon soleus muscle at 90% of the gestation were exposed to different maternal conditions, including control (CTR) diet and maternal nutrient-excess (MNE) diet, which included a high-fat, high-sugar diet, and free access to high-fructose sodas. (**A**) Transcript levels of tumor necrosis factor α (*TNF*) and toll-like receptor 4 (*TLR4*). (**B**) Relative protein content of TNFα and TLR4. (**C**) Nuclear factor kappa-light-chain-enhancer of activated B cells (NF-κB) subunit p65, phospho-p65 protein level, and ratio of phosphorylated p65 to total protein. (**D**) Protein levels of phospho-p38 mitogen-activated protein kinase (MAPK). CTR: white, n = 16; MNE: black, n = 5. Data are expressed as mean ± SEM. ** $p < 0.01$, * $p < 0.05$, § $p < 0.10$.

Since mitochondrial quality is also governed by mitochondria's dynamic capacity, i.e., fusion and fission processes, we assessed the levels of two transcripts involved in mitochondrial fusion. The relative mRNA expression of mitofusin 1 and 2 (*MFN1*, *MFN2*) was decreased in the MNE fetal soleus muscle ($p < 0.05$, Figure 5C), suggesting a potential impairment in mitochondrial fusion, which may have implications for mitochondrial quality control and performance.

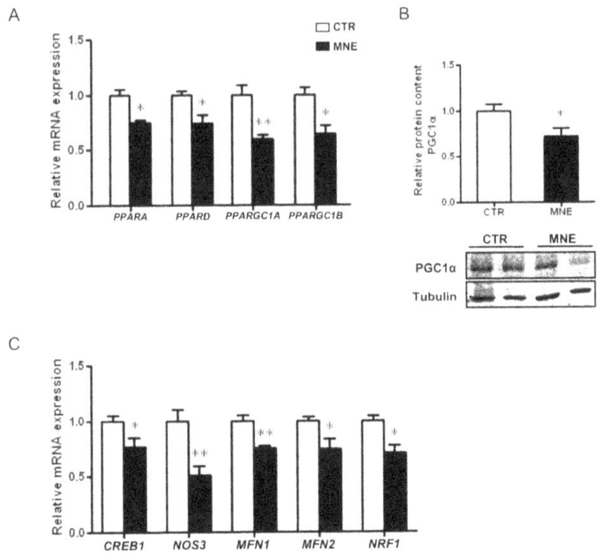

Figure 5. Effects of maternal nutrient excess (MNE) versus control (CTR) conditions on mitochondrial biogenesis and fusion-related markers in the fetal soleus muscle at 90% of the gestation. (**A**) Transcript levels of peroxisome proliferator-activated receptor (PPAR) α (*PPARA*) and *PPARD* and mitochondrial biogenesis-related genes PPARγ coactivator 1 α (*PPARGC1A*) and *PARGC1B*. (**B**) Relative protein levels of PGC1α. (**C**) Transcript levels of cAMP responsive element binding protein 1 (*CREB1*), endothelial nitric oxide synthase (*NOS3*), mitofusin 1 (*MFN1*), *MFN2*, and nuclear respiratory factor 1 (*NRF1*); CTR: white, n = 16; MNE: black, n = 5. Data are expressed as mean ± SEM. ** $p < 0.01$, * $p < 0.05$.

3.4. Fetal Soleus Muscle Expression of SIRT1 and SIRT3

Sirtuins are deacetylases involved in the regulation of various cellular processes, including those related to mitochondrial function, biological responses to stress, metabolism modulation, and development. Sirtuins also play a protective role in several chronic diseases due to their distinct ability to regulate autophagy. While SIRT1 has a diverse subcellular localization pattern, SIRT3 is primarily localized in mitochondria [34,35]. In this study, *SIRT1* and *SIRT3* transcript levels were both lower in the soleus muscle of MNE fetuses ($p < 0.05$, Figure 6A) and while only a decreasing trend was observed for SIRT1 protein levels (Figure 6B), SIRT3 levels were lower in MNE fetal soleus muscle ($p < 0.05$, Figure 6B), with possible implications for mitochondrial oxidative capacity and function regulation.

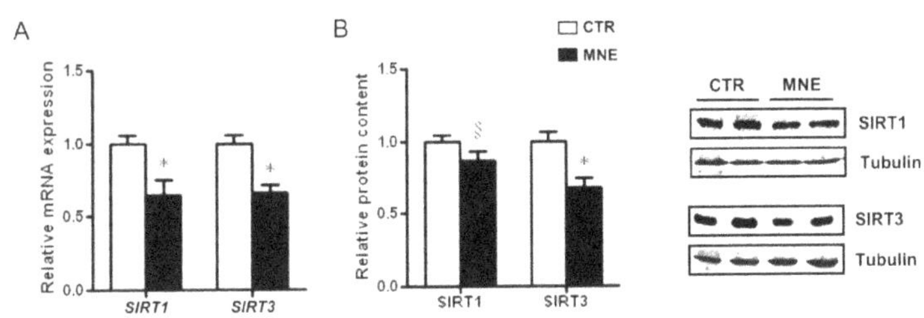

Figure 6. Fetal soleus muscle expression of SIRT1 and SIRT3 at 90% of the gestation as a result of control (CTR) or maternal nutrient-excess (MNE) diets. (**A**) Transcript levels of sirtuin 1 (*SIRT1*) and *SIRT3*. (**B**) Relative protein content of SIRT1 and SIRT3. CTR: white, n = 16; MNE: black, n = 5. Data are expressed as mean ± SEM. * $p < 0.05$, § $p < 0.10$.

3.5. Decreased Fetal Skeletal Muscle Mitochondrial Abundance and Function

Diverse parameters can be used to assess mitochondrial health in frozen tissues. In this work, we determined mitochondrial DNA copy number, often used as a direct indicator of mitochondrial content. In the soleus muscle of MNE fetuses, mtDNA copy number was decreased compared to the levels observed in CTR fetuses ($p < 0.05$, Figure 7A). Alterations in transcripts and protein levels can often manifest as alterations in enzymatic activities. Citrate synthase's (CS) activity, commonly used as a marker to assess mitochondrial content, showed a decreasing trend in the soleus muscle of MNE fetuses (Figure 7B). A similar trend was observed in the activity of a key mitochondrial enzyme involved in the third reaction of β-oxidation, the β-hydroxyacyl-CoA dehydrogenase (BHAD, Figure 7B). Elements of the mitochondrial electron transport chain (ETC) might also be subject to dysregulation due to chronic disease. In the fetuses of MNE mothers, the protein expression of cytochrome C was lower ($p < 0.05$, Figure 7C). Cytochrome C is an ETC essential component that transfers electrons between ubiquinol cytochrome C oxidoreductase (Complex III) and cytochrome C oxidase (Complex IV), the latter being the terminal enzyme of the mitochondrial respiratory chain, as it catalyzes the electron transfer from reduced cytochrome C to molecular oxygen. Three mitochondrial DNA-encoded subunits compose the cytochrome C oxidase catalytic core (COX I, COX II, and COX III). The transcript levels of the I*cox1* and *cox2* subunits were decreased in the soleus skeletal muscle of MNE fetuses ($p < 0.05$, Figure 7D). All in all, these data suggest impaired mitochondrial function in the soleus muscle of fetuses from mothers obese at conception and fed an MNE diet throughout pregnancy.

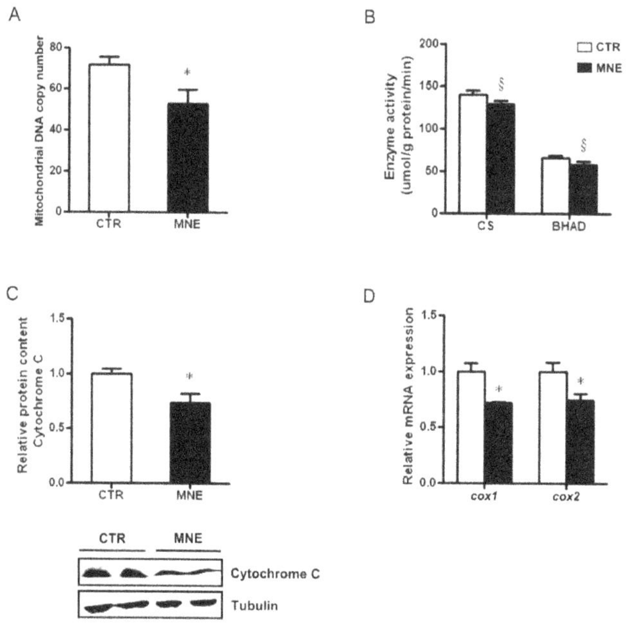

Figure 7. Alterations in fetal soleus muscle mitochondrial content at 90% gestation in mothers on control (CTR) or maternal nutrient-excess (MNE) diets. (**A**) Mitochondrial DNA copy number. (**B**) Enzymatic activities of citrate synthase (CS) and β-hydroxyacyl-CoA dehydrogenase (BHAD). (**C**) Relative protein content of cytochrome C. (**D**) Transcript levels of cytochrome C oxidase subunit 1 (*cox1*) and 2 (*cox2*). Control (CTR): white, n = 16; Maternal nutrient excess (MNE): black, n = 5. Data are expressed as mean ± SEM. * $p < 0.05$, § $p < 0.10$.

4. Discussion

Maternal obesity and nutrient-excess diets are increasingly common and can disrupt fetal metabolism, with lasting effects on offspring health [36]. While adverse intrauterine environments are linked to chronic disease risk, the molecular mechanisms involved remain unclear. Using a non-human primate model (baboon), we show that maternal metabolic stress activates pro-inflammatory and stress factors in the fetal soleus skeletal muscle, affecting mitochondrial content and activity.

Consumption of an MNE diet at least 12 months pre-conception resulted in increased pre-pregnancy body weight in female baboons and increased fat mass, especially in the trunk, denoting a dysfunctional fat distribution. Obesity in humans also portrays an abnormal fat distribution, predominantly in the upper body, with increased visceral fat accumulation [37], which is associated with an increased risk of insulin resistance, dyslipidemia, hypertension, and other irregular metabolic factors observed within the metabolic syndrome cluster [38] and that predispose for T2D and other chronic diseases [39].

In the current study, female baboons on the MNE diet presented reduced gestational weight gain (GWG). Women with pre-pregnancy overweight or obesity have the highest prevalence of excessive GWG [11]. Thus, studies have highly focused on how excessive GWG on obese mothers predisposes them and their offspring to complications (e.g., macrosomia) [40,41]. Some studies suggest that pre-pregnancy weight has a stronger impact on childhood overweight/obesity [8], while emerging evidence links GWG below the guidelines in obese mothers to low birth weight and other offspring complications [42,43], even independently of pre-pregnancy BMI [44]. As previously shown for our model, despite the reduced GWG, MNE mothers show potential metabolic disturbances with increased circulating levels of low-density lipoprotein and triglycerides during pregnancy compared to CTR mothers. The increased triglycerides were still observed at cesarean section and accompanied by increased levels of glucose and insulin [45]. A meta-analysis including only obese women showed that mothers with inadequate GWG had a higher risk of having small for gestational age babies [43]. Indeed, in our study, fetuses of MNE baboons had decreased body weight at term, which could be a consequence of the observed low maternal GWG. A compelling explanation for the observed effects could be the decreased placental efficiency, previously reported in this model [46]. Similar effects were observed in offspring of high-fat fed female mice [47,48]. Our model also previously showed decreased fetal blood levels of amino acids directly involved in one-carbon metabolism, accompanied by a higher Apolipoprotein B to Apolipoprotein A1 ratio, an established marker of atherogenic and cardiovascular risk [46]. Moreover, circulating fetal insulin levels were increased at cesarean section [45]. On another note, a human investigation that included 905 mother-child pairs enrolled in the Hyperglycemia and Adverse Pregnancy Outcome (HAPO) study revealed that independently of pre-pregnancy BMI, both excessive and inadequate GWG were associated with increased offspring hypertension and insulin resistance at 7 years of age [44]. Altered postnatal growth trajectories have already been reported in our model, showing that offspring of obese mothers, with reduced body weight at the fetal stage, had a steeper growth in their first 2 years of life [49].

The maternal obesity-promoted low-grade inflammation generates an intrauterine environment suboptimal for offspring health. One well-known pro-inflammatory cytokine is TNFα, which has been highly associated with obesity and T2D given its implications for insulin signaling and insulin resistance development [50]. Although mostly known as an adipokine, TNFα is also produced in SM [51]. Both transcript and protein TNFα levels were increased in the SM of MNE fetuses, and these were accompanied by increased levels of other proteins involved in inflammatory pathways. We previously showed that TLR4, a key receptor abundantly expressed in the SM and highly involved in immune and inflammatory responses, was upregulated in the sheep fetal SM [19]. Microbial lipopolysaccharides are the main agonists of TLR4, but saturated fatty acids and fibrinogen have been suggested as stimuli for TLR4 dimerization and signaling cascade activation in the context of obesity [21,52]. TLR4 signaling cascade can, through a series of interactions, lead to NF-kB and MAPK activation, ultimately resulting in the transcription of pro-inflammatory factors [52], including TNFα. In this study, both transcript and protein levels of TLR4 were higher in MNE baboon fetal SM, which was accompanied by increased phosphorylation of the NF-kB p65 heterodimer, suggesting activation of the NF-kB pathway, in accordance with our observations in ewes [19]. The increased phosphorylation of p38 MAPK observed further supports this TLR4-induced inflammatory response, given that p38 MAPK can upregulate activator protein 1 (AP1), resulting in pro-inflammatory cytokines transcription.

Nuclear factor-kB activation has been associated with mitochondrial dysfunction in the muscle in response to cellular fuel overload in L6 myotubes, with decreased PGC1α expression, as well as in other genes related to mitochondrial dynamics [53], a similar effect to the one observed in the MNE baboon fetal SM in this study. The group of transcription factors PPAR (PPARα, PPARδ, and PPARγ) has an important role in the SM's metabolic flexibility but also in the regulation of inflammatory responses [54]. Particularly, PPARδ is highly expressed in the SM [55] and has been shown to stimulate PGC1α expression in mice SM, while its ablation induced muscle fiber-type switching, reducing muscle oxidative capacity and consequently predisposing to obesity and diabetes [56]. Indeed, the transcript levels of *PPARB* were lower in the SM of fetal MNE baboon in our study and coupled to the observed reduced transcript levels of *PPARA*, another transcription factor involved in the regulation of lipid metabolism and fatty acid uptake and the second most expressed in the SM [57], these data suggest an impairment in the fetal SM metabolic flexibility, which could have repercussions for MNE offspring future health. Peroxisome proliferator-activated receptors have also been shown to regulate inflammation processes in the SM, and, for instance, PPARα has been shown to inhibit NF-kB transcriptional activity [54].

Several genes involved in mitochondrial dynamics and homeostasis are regulated by PGC1α and PGC1β. Studies have associated mitochondrial alterations in the SM of T2D patients and animal models with altered PGC1α, PGC1β, and Mfn2 levels [58]. In the current study, *PPARGC1A* and *PPARGC1B* transcript levels were reduced, which was previously found in the human SM of not only T2D patients but also of offspring from insulin-resistant individuals [58]. Decreased *PPARGC1B* mRNA levels were also observed in the SM of pig fetuses of high-energy fed mothers [59] and in mice fetal SM of hyperglycemic mothers at late gestation [60]. Moreover, lower levels of the MFN2 and MFN1 transcripts were also observed, suggesting unbalanced mitochondrial dynamics, with impaired fusion events. Multiple studies have reported reduced MFN2 levels in the context of obesity, diabetes, and high-fat diets in the SM, and modulation of its expression can reverse, prevent, or ameliorate SM mitochondrial function [61]. Although these effects do not seem to regularly extend to alterations in MFN1 levels [61], in our study, MFN1 transcript levels were more strongly impacted in the fetal SM of MNE offspring than MFN2 levels, which may represent a specific response of fetal SM programming by maternal obesity at conception and nutrient excess during pregnancy.

The transcription of PGC1α is enhanced by the interaction of multiple factors with the promoter region of its gene. The transcription factor CREB is capable of promoting PGC1α transcription, although mostly studied in response to exercise [62]. Palacios et al. showed that not only exercise, but also nutritional status can influence PGC1α transcription through SIRT3 levels [34]. The study revealed decreased SIRT3 levels due to a high-fat diet and that SIRT3 knockout resulted in decreased CREB phosphorylation and PGC1α transcription [34]. Yan and colleagues reported decreased CREB phosphorylation associated with reduced *Ppargc1α* transcription in the SM of mice fetuses exposed to a hyperglycemic intrauterine environment [60]. In the present study, SIRT3 transcript and protein levels were decreased in the fetal SM of MNE offspring. Although we only measured *CREB1* transcript levels, which were lower in the SM of MNE fetuses, regulation of PGC1α transcription through CREB interaction modulated by diet deserves further attention, especially since it is well described that SIRT3 activity is increased in response to exercise and poor nutrient intake and decreased in diabetic models [35]. Likewise, SIRT1 stimulates PGC1α [63], and exercise training contributes to increased activation of the SIRT1/PGC1α axis with reduced NF-kB signaling in diabetic mice [64], demonstrating a crosstalk between inflammatory mediators and PGC1α. One of the observed effects of PGC1α transcription enhancement by these factors is the upregulation of NRF1 and mitochondrial transcription factor A (TFAM), required for mitochondrial DNA transcription [64]. In this study, the lower *CREB1*, *SIRT1*, and *SIRT3* transcript levels alongside decreased *PPARGC1A* and *NRF1* suggest dysregulation of mitochondrial biogenesis in the SM of fetuses developed in a nutrient-excess environment. Zou et al. reported decreased transcription of *NRF1*, *TFAM*, and *SIRT1* in fetal SM of pigs exposed to maternal high-energy intake, with decreased mRNA levels of DNA polymerase (POLG) and single-strand DNA binding protein 1 (SSBP1), accompanied by lower mtDNA copy number [59]. McCurdy et al. also reported reduced *PGC1α* expression in fetal SM of Japanese macaques exposed to a maternal Western-style diet and obesity. Although *TFAM* and *MFN2* transcript levels were not significantly altered, they observed a reduction in mitochondrial content [65]. In the current study, mtDNA copy number was also found to be decreased in the SM of MNE baboon fetuses. Further supporting the involvement of inflammatory cues in mitochondrial biogenesis dysregulation, a study revealed that lower mRNA expression of *Ppargc1a*, *Nrf1*, and *Tfam*, accompanied by lower expression of eNOS, was ameliorated by TNFα signaling deficiency in the SM of different rodent models of obesity [66]. Accordingly, the transcript levels of *NOS3* in the fetal SM of MNE baboons were substantially lower. On another note, increased NO levels, partly derived from increased eNOS, can lead to increased S-nitrosylation of CREB, stimulating its binding to the PGC1α gene promoter, thus increasing PGC1α transcription [33].

Unsurprisingly, some of the studies mentioned above reported that alterations in mitochondrial-related proteins were important for SM mitochondrial oxidative capacity. For instance, in Liu and Chang's work, cytochrome C oxidase activity was lower in diabetic mice, and exercise stimulation contributed to an increase in mRNA levels of mitochondrial complexes subunits, through the induction of PGC1α, NRF1, and TFAM levels [64]. Moreover, Valerio et al. reported decreased protein levels of COX IV and cytochrome C in obese rodents with decreased eNOS expression [66]. Cytochrome C protein levels were lower in the fetal SM of MNE offspring in our study, and we also found implications for COX IV catalytic core subunits COX I and COX II, with lower mDNA copy number, lower mitochondrial CS and BHAD enzymatic activity. In the previously mentioned study using fetal SM from Japanese macaques, mitochondrial electron transport chain activity was elevated, but coupling efficiency was reduced. This was accompanied by lower CS activity and increased markers of oxidative stress [65]. Levels of mtDNA were also reported to be lower in the different rodent models of obesity [66].

Overall, our data show a strong association between maternal obesity at conception and a nutrient-excess diet during pregnancy-induced chronic inflammation in the fetal soleus skeletal muscle, with implications for mitochondrial content and function. Furthermore, PGC1α seems to represent a major interface between inflammatory signaling pathways and SM mitochondrial alterations that are already present at late gestation in a non-human primate model.

5. Conclusions

The underlying mechanisms of the adverse effects of maternal nutrition and health on fetal soleus skeletal muscle development and metabolism are still poorly understood, especially with regard to mitochondrial consequences. Despite the constant emphasis on chronic inflammation induced by maternal obesity or diabetes, there is a lack of molecular studies during the fetal stage and in animal models with high human translational relevance. In this study, we demonstrate that baboon fetuses exposed to an adverse intrauterine environment resulting from maternal obesity at conception and a nutrient-excessive diet during pregnancy exhibit molecular alterations in the soleus muscle. Specifically, we observed altered activity in soleus muscle mitochondria, posing a potential risk for widespread cellular dysfunction and early disease development. Notably, these effects could potentially program the fetus for insulin resistance, a key factor in the development of T2D, thereby increasing the risk of life-long metabolic complications in the postnatal period.

6. Study Limitations

In this study, we only measured the transcript levels of *CREB1*, *NOS3*, *MFN1*, *MFN2*, *NRF1*, *cox1*, and *cox2*. While we observed differences between the groups, it is crucial to recognize that mRNA levels may not accurately reflect protein content or enzymatic activity. For instance, evaluating the activity of CREB1 and eNOS could have provided a more comprehensive understanding of their contributions to the alterations observed in this study, particularly regarding mitochondrial biogenesis, and might have identified alternative pathways worthy of exploration. One limitation of our NHP model, consistent with observations in other NHP studies, is that despite its robust translational value, the small sample size restricted our capability to assess sexual dimorphism. Nevertheless, when dealing with maternal interventions, acknowledging sex-specific responses is imperative in cohorts with larger sample numbers. This is crucial not only because morphometric parameters differ but also due to variations in molecular alterations observed in different tissues based on fetal sex [67–69]. Furthermore, it is important to note that we exclusively used the first cohort of animals, consisting of only 5 MO offspring, paired in time with the respective controls. This limited sample size, along with the potential for individual variation, further restricted our ability to explore more granular aspects of the data, such as sexual dimorphism or the potential for other molecular alterations not captured in this initial analysis.

Supplementary Materials: The following supporting information can be downloaded at: https://www.mdpi.com/article/10.3390/biology14070868/s1, Table S1. List of primary and secondary antibodies used for immunoblotting; Table S2. List of primers used for transcript amplification; Statement of Honor.

Author Contributions: Conceptualization, X.Y., M.D., S.P.P., C.T. and M.-J.Z.; Methodology, X.Y., M.-J.Z. and S.P.P.; Formal analysis, X.Y. and S.P.P.; Writing—original draft preparation, X.Y. and S.P.P.; Writing—review and editing, X.Y., S.P.P., C.T., M.-J.Z. and M.D.; Visualization, X.Y., C.T. and S.P.P.; Funding acquisition, M.D. All authors have read and agreed to the published version of the manuscript.

Funding: This research was funded by NIH, grant numbers HD067449 and HD060076. S.P.P and C.T were funded by the ERDF funds through the Operational Programme for Competitiveness–COMPETE 2020 and national funds by Foundation for Science and Technology under FCT-Post-doctoral Fellowship (SPP, SFRH/BPD/116061/2016) and the FCT-doctoral Fellowship (CT, SFRH/BD/11924/2022), strategic projects UIDB/04539/2020, UIDP/04539/2020, LA/P/0058/2020, UIDP/04378/2020 and UIDB/04378/2020 of the Research Unit on Applied Molecular Biosciences—UCIBIO, and the project LA/P/0140/2020 of the Associate Laboratory Institute for Health and Bioeconomy—i4HB. Views and opinions expressed are, however, those of the author(s) only and do not necessarily reflect those of the European Union or the Health and Digital Executive Agency. Neither the European Union nor the granting authority can be held responsible for them. The funding agencies had no role in study design, data collection and analysis, decision to publish, or preparation of this document.

Institutional Review Board Statement: All animal procedures were approved by the Texas Biomedical Research Institute (TBRI) Institutional Animal Care and Use Committee (protocol number 1675 PC) and conducted in Association for Assessment and Accreditation of Laboratory Animal Care international-approved facilities. The experimental design adhered to the ARRIVE guidelines and incorporated the principles of the 3Rs.

Informed Consent Statement: Not applicable.

Data Availability Statement: The data presented in this study are available on request from the corresponding author.

Acknowledgments: The authors gratefully acknowledge Peter W. Nathanielsz and his team for providing the animal model, samples, and resources that made this work possible.

Conflicts of Interest: The authors declare no conflicts of interest. The funders had no role in the design of the study; in the collection, analyses, or interpretation of data; in the writing of the manuscript; or in the decision to publish the results.

References

1. Blüher, M. Obesity: Global Epidemiology and Pathogenesis. *Nat. Rev. Endocrinol.* **2019**, *15*, 288–298. [CrossRef] [PubMed]
2. Godfrey, K.M.; Reynolds, R.M.; Prescott, S.L.; Nyirenda, M.; Jaddoe, V.W.V.; Eriksson, J.G.; Broekman, B.F.P. Influence of Maternal Obesity on the Long-Term Health of Offspring. *Lancet Diabetes Endocrinol.* **2017**, *5*, 53–64. [CrossRef] [PubMed]
3. World Health Organization. *World Health Statistics 2024: Monitoring Health for the SDGs, Sustainable Development Goals*; World Health Organization: Geneva, Switzerland, 2024.
4. Stierman, B.; Afful, J.; Carroll, M.D.; Chen, T.-C.; Davy, O.; Fink, S.; Fryar, C.D.; Gu, Q.; Hales, C.M.; Hughes, J.P.; et al. National Health and Nutrition Examination Survey 2017–March 2020 Prepandemic Data Files—Development of Files and Prevalence Estimates for Selected Health Outcomes. *Natl. Health Stat. Rep.* **2021**, *158*, 10-15620. [CrossRef]
5. Driscoll, A.K.; Gregory, E.C.W. *Increases in Prepregnancy Obesity: United States, 2016–2019*; NCHS: Hyattsville, MD, USA, 2020.
6. Bass, R.; Eneli, I. Severe Childhood Obesity: An under-Recognised and Growing Health Problem. *Postgrad. Med. J.* **2015**, *91*, 639–645. [CrossRef] [PubMed]
7. Vats, H.; Saxena, R.; Sachdeva, M.P.; Walia, G.K.; Gupta, V. Impact of Maternal Pre-Pregnancy Body Mass Index on Maternal, Fetal and Neonatal Adverse Outcomes in the Worldwide Populations: A Systematic Review and Meta-Analysis. *Obes. Res. Clin. Pract.* **2021**, *15*, 536–545. [CrossRef] [PubMed]
8. Voerman, E.; Santos, S.; Golab, B.P.; Amiano, P.; Ballester, F.; Barros, H.; Bergström, A.; Charles, M.A.; Chatzi, L.; Chevrier, C.; et al. Maternal Body Mass Index, Gestational Weight Gain, and the Risk of Overweight and Obesity across Childhood: An Individual Participant Data Meta-Analysis. *PLoS Med.* **2019**, *16*, e1002744. [CrossRef] [PubMed]
9. Ijäs, H.; Koivunen, S.; Raudaskoski, T.; Kajantie, E.; Gissler, M.; Vääräsmäki, M. Independent and Concomitant Associations of Gestational Diabetes and Maternal Obesity to Perinatal Outcome: A Register-Based Study. *PLoS ONE* **2019**, *14*, e0221549. [CrossRef] [PubMed]
10. Eriksson, J.G.; Sandboge, S.; Salonen, M.K.; Kajantie, E.; Osmond, C. Long-Term Consequences of Maternal Overweight in Pregnancy on Offspring Later Health: Findings from the Helsinki Birth Cohort Study. *Ann. Med.* **2014**, *46*, 434–438. [CrossRef] [PubMed]
11. Grilo, L.F.; Diniz, M.S.; Tocantins, C.; Areia, A.L.; Pereira, S.P. The Endocrine–Metabolic Axis Regulation in Offspring Exposed to Maternal Obesity—Cause or Consequence in Metabolic Disease Programming? *Obesities* **2022**, *2*, 236–255. [CrossRef]
12. Parrettini, S.; Caroli, A.; Torlone, E. Nutrition and Metabolic Adaptations in Physiological and Complicated Pregnancy: Focus on Obesity and Gestational Diabetes. *Front. Endocrinol.* **2020**, *11*, 611929. [CrossRef] [PubMed]
13. Du, M.; Yan, X.; Tong, J.F.; Zhao, J.; Zhu, M.J. Maternal Obesity, Inflammation, and Fetal Skeletal Muscle Development. *Biol. Reprod.* **2010**, *82*, 4–12. [CrossRef] [PubMed]
14. Haines, M.S.; Leong, A.; Porneala, B.C.; Meigs, J.B.; Miller, K.K. Association between Muscle Mass and Diabetes Prevalence Independent of Body Fat Distribution in Adults under 50 Years Old. *Nutr. Diabetes* **2022**, *12*, 29. [CrossRef] [PubMed]
15. Xu, Y.; Hu, T.; Shen, Y.; Wang, Y.; Bao, Y.; Ma, X. Association of Skeletal Muscle Mass and Its Change with Diabetes Occurrence: A Population-Based Cohort Study. *Diabetol. Metab. Syndr.* **2023**, *15*, 53. [CrossRef] [PubMed]

16. Swanson, A.M.; David, A.L. Animal Models of Fetal Growth Restriction: Considerations for Translational Medicine. *Placenta* **2015**, *36*, 623–630. [CrossRef] [PubMed]
17. Tarantal, A.F.; Noctor, S.C.; Hartigan-O'connor, D.J. Nonhuman Primates in Translational Research. *Annu. Rev. Anim. Biosci.* **2022**, *10*, 441–468. [CrossRef] [PubMed]
18. Campodonico-Burnett, W.; Hetrick, B.; Wesolowski, S.R.; Schenk, S.; Takahashi, D.L.; Dean, T.A.; Sullivan, E.L.; Kievit, P.; Gannon, M.; Aagaard, K.; et al. Maternal Obesity and Western-Style Diet Impair Fetal and Juvenile Offspring Skeletal Muscle Insulin-Stimulated Glucose Transport in Nonhuman Primates. *Diabetes* **2020**, *69*, 1389–1400. [CrossRef] [PubMed]
19. Yan, X.; Zhu, M.J.; Xu, W.; Tong, J.F.; Ford, S.P.; Nathanielsz, P.W.; Du, M. Up-Regulation of Toll-like Receptor 4/Nuclear Factor-KB Signaling Is Associated with Enhanced Adipogenesis and Insulin Resistance in Fetal Skeletal Muscle of Obese Sheep at Late Gestation. *Endocrinology* **2010**, *151*, 380–387. [CrossRef] [PubMed]
20. Omar, A.K.; Li Puma, L.C.; Whitcomb, L.A.; Risk, B.D.; Witt, A.C.; Bruemmer, J.E.; Winger, Q.A.; Bouma, G.J.; Chicco, A.J. High-Fat Diet during Pregnancy Promotes Fetal Skeletal Muscle Fatty Acid Oxidation and Insulin Resistance in an Ovine Model. *Am. J. Physiol. Integr. Comp. Physiol.* **2023**, *325*, R523–R533. [CrossRef] [PubMed]
21. Rogero, M.M.; Calder, P.C. Obesity, Inflammation, Toll-like Receptor 4 and Fatty Acids. *Nutrients* **2018**, *10*, 432. [CrossRef] [PubMed]
22. Parisi, F.; Milazzo, R.; Savasi, V.M.; Cetin, I. Maternal Low-Grade Chronic Inflammation and Intrauterine Programming of Health and Disease. *Int. J. Mol. Sci.* **2021**, *22*, 1732. [CrossRef] [PubMed]
23. Prasun, P. Mitochondrial Dysfunction in Metabolic Syndrome. *Biochim. Biophys. Acta-Mol. Basis Dis.* **2020**, *1866*, 165838. [CrossRef] [PubMed]
24. de Mello, A.H.; Costa, A.B.; Engel, J.D.G.; Rezin, G.T. Mitochondrial Dysfunction in Obesity. *Life Sci.* **2018**, *192*, 26–32. [CrossRef] [PubMed]
25. Blake, R.; Trounce, I.A. Mitochondrial Dysfunction and Complications Associated with Diabetes. *Biochim. Biophys. Acta-Gen. Subj.* **2014**, *1840*, 1404–1412. [CrossRef] [PubMed]
26. Pazderska, A.; Wanic, K.; Nolan, J.J. Skeletal Muscle Mitochondrial Dysfunction in Type2 Diabetes. *Expert Rev. Endocrinol. Metab.* **2010**, *5*, 475–477. [CrossRef] [PubMed]
27. du Sert, N.; Hurst, V.; Ahluwalia, A.; Alam, S.; Avey, M.T.; Baker, M.; Browne, W.J.; Clark, A.; Cuthill, I.C.; Dirnagl, U.; et al. The ARRIVE Guidelines 2.0: Updated Guidelines for Reporting Animal Research. *PLoS Biol.* **2020**, *18*, e3000410. [CrossRef]
28. Schlabritz-Loutsevitch, N.E.; Howell, K.; Rice, K.; Glover, E.J.; Nevill, C.H.; Jenkins, S.L.; Cummins, L.B.; Frost, P.A.; McDonald, T.J.; Nathanielsz, P.W. Development of a System for Individual Feeding of Baboons Maintained in an Outdoor Group Social Environment. *J. Med. Primatol.* **2004**, *33*, 117–126. [CrossRef] [PubMed]
29. Maloyan, A.; Muralimanoharan, S.; Huffman, S.; Cox, L.A.; Nathanielsz, P.W.; Myatt, L.; Nijland, M.J. Identification and Comparative Analyses of Myocardial MiRNAs Involved in the Fetal Response to Maternal Obesity. *Physiol. Genom.* **2013**, *45*, 889–900. [CrossRef] [PubMed]
30. Ford, S.P.; Zhang, L.; Zhu, M.; Miller, M.M.; Smith, D.T.; Hess, B.W.; Moss, G.E.; Nathanielsz, P.W.; Nijland, M.J. Maternal Obesity Accelerates Fetal Pancreatic β-Cell but Not α-Cell Development in Sheep: Prenatal Consequences. *Am. J. Physiol.-Regul. Integr. Comp. Physiol.* **2009**, *297*, 835–843. [CrossRef] [PubMed]
31. Livak, K.J.; Schmittgen, T.D. Analysis of Relative Gene Expression Data Using Real-Time Quantitative PCR and the $2-\Delta\Delta CT$ Method. *Methods* **2001**, *25*, 402–408. [CrossRef] [PubMed]
32. Call, J.A.; Voelker, K.A.; Wolff, A.V.; McMillan, R.P.; Evans, N.P.; Hulver, M.W.; Talmadge, R.J.; Grange, R.W. Endurance Capacity in Maturing Mdx Mice Is Markedly Enhanced by Combined Voluntary Wheel Running and Green Tea Extract. *J. Appl. Physiol.* **2008**, *105*, 923–932. [CrossRef] [PubMed]
33. Baldelli, S.; Barbato, D.L.; Tatulli, G.; Aquilano, K.; Ciriolo, M.R. The Role of NNOS and PGC-1α in Skeletal Muscle Cells. *J. Cell Sci.* **2014**, *127*, 4813–4820. [CrossRef] [PubMed]
34. Palacios, O.M.; Carmona, J.J.; Michan, S.; Chen, K.Y.; Manabe, Y.; Ward, J.L.; Goodyear, L.J.; Tong, Q. Diet and Exercise Signals Regulate SIRT3 and Activate AMPK and PGC-1alpha in Skeletal Muscle. *Aging* **2009**, *1*, 771–783. [CrossRef] [PubMed]
35. Lantier, L.; Williams, A.S.; Williams, I.M.; Yang, K.K.; Bracy, D.P.; Goelzer, M.; James, F.D.; Gius, D.; Wasserman, D.H. SIRT3 Is Crucial for Maintaining Skeletal Muscle Insulin Action and Protects against Severe Insulin Resistance in High-Fat-Fed Mice. *Diabetes* **2015**, *64*, 3081–3092. [CrossRef] [PubMed]
36. Tocantins, C.; Diniz, M.S.; Grilo, L.F.; Pereira, S.P. The Birth of Cardiac Disease: Mechanisms Linking Gestational Diabetes Mellitus and Early Onset of Cardiovascular Disease in Offspring. *WIREs Mech. Dis.* **2022**, *14*, e1555. [CrossRef] [PubMed]
37. Hill, J.H.; Solt, C.; Foster, M.T. Obesity Associated Disease Risk: The Role of Inherent Differences and Location of Adipose Depots. *Horm. Mol. Biol. Clin. Investig.* **2018**, *33*, 20180012. [CrossRef] [PubMed]
38. Kwon, H.; Kim, D.; Kim, J.S. Body Fat Distribution and the Risk of Incident Metabolic Syndrome: A Longitudinal Cohort Study. *Sci. Rep.* **2017**, *7*, 10955. [CrossRef] [PubMed]

39. Kang, P.S.; Neeland, I.J. Body Fat Distribution, Diabetes Mellitus, and Cardiovascular Disease: An Update. *Curr. Cardiol. Rep.* **2023**, *25*, 1555–1564. [CrossRef] [PubMed]
40. Gaudet, L.; Ferraro, Z.M.; Wen, S.W.; Walker, M. Maternal Obesity and Occurrence of Fetal Macrosomia: A Systematic Review and Meta-Analysis. *Biomed Res. Int.* **2014**, *2014*, 640291. [CrossRef] [PubMed]
41. Santos, S.; Voerman, E.; Amiano, P.; Barros, H.; Beilin, L.J.; Bergström, A.; Charles, M.A.; Chatzi, L.; Chevrier, C.; Chrousos, G.P.; et al. Impact of Maternal Body Mass Index and Gestational Weight Gain on Pregnancy Complications: An Individual Participant Data Meta-Analysis of European, North American and Australian Cohorts. *BJOG An Int. J. Obstet. Gynaecol.* **2019**, *126*, 984–995. [CrossRef] [PubMed]
42. Champion, M.L.; Harper, L.M. Gestational Weight Gain: Update on Outcomes and Interventions. *Curr. Diab. Rep.* **2020**, *20*, 11. [CrossRef] [PubMed]
43. Xu, Z.; Wen, Z.; Zhou, Y.; Li, D.; Luo, Z. Inadequate Weight Gain in Obese Women and the Risk of Small for Gestational Age (SGA): A Systematic Review and Meta-Analysis. *J. Matern. Neonatal Med.* **2017**, *30*, 357–367. [CrossRef] [PubMed]
44. Tam, C.H.T.; Ma, R.C.W.; Yuen, L.Y.; Ozaki, R.; Li, A.M.; Hou, Y.; Chan, M.H.M.; Ho, C.S.; Yang, X.; Chan, J.C.N.; et al. The Impact of Maternal Gestational Weight Gain on Cardiometabolic Risk Factors in Children. *Diabetologia* **2018**, *61*, 2539–2548. [CrossRef] [PubMed]
45. Puppala, S.; Li, C.; Glenn, J.P.; Saxena, R.; Gawrieh, S.; Quinn, A.; Palarczyk, J.; Dick, E.J.; Nathanielsz, P.W.; Cox, L.A. Primate Fetal Hepatic Responses to Maternal Obesity: Epigenetic Signalling Pathways and Lipid Accumulation. *J. Physiol.* **2018**, *596*, 5823–5837. [CrossRef] [PubMed]
46. Nathanielsz, P.W.; Yan, J.; Green, R.; Nijland, M.; Miller, J.W.; Wu, G.; McDonald, T.J.; Caudill, M.A. Maternal Obesity Disrupts the Methionine Cycle in Baboon Pregnancy. *Physiol. Rep.* **2015**, *3*, e12564. [CrossRef] [PubMed]
47. Sanches, A.P.V.; de Oliveira, J.L.; Ferreira, M.S.; Lima, B.d.S.; Miyamoto, J.É.; Simino, L.A.d.P.; Torsoni, M.A.; Torsoni, A.S.; Milanski, M.; Ignácio-Souza, L. Obesity Phenotype Induced by High-Fat Diet Leads to Maternal-Fetal Constraint, Placental Inefficiency, and Fetal Growth Restriction in Mice. *J. Nutr. Biochem.* **2022**, *104*, 108977. [CrossRef] [PubMed]
48. Mayor, R.S.; Finch, K.E.; Zehr, J.; Morselli, E.; Neinast, M.D.; Frank, A.P.; Hahner, L.D.; Wang, J.; Rakheja, D.; Palmer, B.F.; et al. Maternal High-Fat Diet Is Associated with Impaired Fetal Lung Development. *Am. J. Physiol. Lung Cell. Mol. Physiol.* **2015**, *309*, L360-8. [CrossRef] [PubMed]
49. Li, C.; Jenkins, S.; Considine, M.M.; Cox, L.A.; Gerow, K.G.; Huber, H.F.; Nathanielsz, P.W. Effect of Maternal Obesity on Fetal and Postnatal Baboon (Papio Species) Early Life Phenotype. *J. Med. Primatol.* **2019**, *48*, 90–98. [CrossRef] [PubMed]
50. Jaganathan, R.; Ravindran, R.; Dhanasekaran, S. Emerging Role of Adipocytokines in Type 2 Diabetes as Mediators of Insulin Resistance and Cardiovascular Disease. *Can. J. Diabetes* **2018**, *42*, 446–456.e1. [CrossRef] [PubMed]
51. Li, F.; Li, Y.; Duan, Y.; Hu, C.A.A.; Tang, Y.; Yin, Y. Myokines and Adipokines: Involvement in the Crosstalk between Skeletal Muscle and Adipose Tissue. *Cytokine Growth Factor Rev.* **2017**, *33*, 73–82. [CrossRef] [PubMed]
52. Li, B.; Leung, J.C.K.; Chan, L.Y.Y.; Yiu, W.H.; Tang, S.C.W. A Global Perspective on the Crosstalk between Saturated Fatty Acids and Toll-like Receptor 4 in the Etiology of Inflammation and Insulin Resistance. *Prog. Lipid Res.* **2020**, *77*, 101020. [CrossRef] [PubMed]
53. Nisr, R.B.; Shah, D.S.; Ganley, I.G.; Hundal, H.S. Proinflammatory NFkB Signalling Promotes Mitochondrial Dysfunction in Skeletal Muscle in Response to Cellular Fuel Overloading. *Cell. Mol. Life Sci.* **2019**, *76*, 4887–4904. [CrossRef] [PubMed]
54. Crossland, H.; Constantin-Teodosiu, D.; Greenhaff, P.L. The Regulatory Roles of Ppars in Skeletal Muscle Fuel Metabolism and Inflammation: Impact of Ppar Agonism on Muscle in Chronic Disease, Contraction and Sepsis. *Int. J. Mol. Sci.* **2021**, *22*, 9775. [CrossRef] [PubMed]
55. Manickam, R.; Wahli, W. Roles of Peroxisome Proliferator-Activated Receptor β/δ in Skeletal Muscle Physiology. *Biochimie* **2017**, *136*, 42–48. [CrossRef] [PubMed]
56. Schuler, M.; Ali, F.; Chambon, C.; Duteil, D.; Bornert, J.M.; Tardivel, A.; Desvergne, B.; Wahli, W.; Chambon, P.; Metzger, D. PGC1α Expression Is Controlled in Skeletal Muscles by PPARβ, Whose Ablation Results in Fiber-Type Switching, Obesity, and Type 2 Diabetes. *Cell Metab.* **2006**, *4*, 407–414. [CrossRef] [PubMed]
57. Phua, W.W.T.; Wong, M.X.Y.; Liao, Z.; Tan, N.S. An Apparent Functional Consequence in Skeletal Muscle Physiology via Peroxisome Proliferator-Activated Receptors. *Int. J. Mol. Sci.* **2018**, *19*, 1425. [CrossRef] [PubMed]
58. Zorzano, A.; Hernández-Alvarez, M.I.; Palacín, M.; Mingrone, G. Alterations in the Mitochondrial Regulatory Pathways Constituted by the Nuclear Co-Factors PGC-1α or PGC-1β and Mitofusin 2 in Skeletal Muscle in Type 2 Diabetes. *Biochim. Biophys. Acta-Bioenerg.* **2010**, *1797*, 1028–1033. [CrossRef] [PubMed]
59. Zou, T.D.; Yu, B.; Yu, J.; Mao, X.B.; Zheng, P.; He, J.; Huang, Z.Q.; He, D.T.; Chen, D.W. Mitochondrial Biogenesis Is Decreased in Skeletal Muscle of Pig Fetuses Exposed to Maternal High-Energy Diets. *Animal* **2017**, *11*, 54–60. [CrossRef] [PubMed]
60. Yan, Y.S.; Mo, J.Y.; Huang, Y.T.; Zhu, H.; Wu, H.Y.; Lin, Z.L.; Liu, R.; Liu, X.Q.; Lv, P.P.; Feng, C.; et al. Intrauterine Hyperglycaemia during Late Gestation Caused Mitochondrial Dysfunction in Skeletal Muscle of Male Offspring through CREB/PGC1A Signaling. *Nutr. Diabetes* **2024**, *14*, 56. [CrossRef] [PubMed]

61. Fealy, C.E.; Mulya, A.; Axelrod, C.L.; Kirwan, J.P. Mitochondrial Dynamics in Skeletal Muscle Insulin Resistance and Type 2 Diabetes. *Transl. Res.* **2018**, *202*, 69–82. [CrossRef] [PubMed]
62. Taylor, D.F.; Bishop, D.J. Transcription Factor Movement and Exercise-Induced Mitochondrial Biogenesis in Human Skeletal Muscle: Current Knowledge and Future Perspectives. *Int. J. Mol. Sci.* **2022**, *23*, 1517. [CrossRef] [PubMed]
63. Cantó, C.; Gerhart-Hines, Z.; Feige, J.N.; Lagouge, M.; Noriega, L.; Milne, J.C.; Elliott, P.J.; Puigserver, P.; Auwerx, J. AMPK Regulates Energy Expenditure by Modulating NAD + Metabolism and SIRT1 Activity. *Nature* **2009**, *458*, 1056–1060. [CrossRef] [PubMed]
64. Liu, H.W.; Chang, S.J. Moderate Exercise Suppresses NF-KB Signaling and Activates the SIRT1-AMPK-PGC1α Axis to Attenuate Muscle Loss in Diabetic Db/Db Mice. *Front. Physiol.* **2018**, *9*, 636. [CrossRef] [PubMed]
65. McCurdy, C.E.; Schenk, S.; Hetrick, B.; Houck, J.; Drew, B.G.; Kaye, S.; Lashbrook, M.; Bergman, B.C.; Takahashi, D.L.; Dean, T.A.; et al. Maternal Obesity Reduces Oxidative Capacity in Fetal Skeletal Muscle of Japanese Macaques. *JCI Insight* **2016**, *1*, e86612. [CrossRef] [PubMed]
66. Valerio, A.; Cardile, A.; Cozzi, V.; Bracale, R.; Tedesco, L.; Pisconti, A.; Palomba, L.; Cantoni, O.; Clementi, E.; Moncada, S.; et al. TNF-α Downregulates ENOS Expression and Mitochondrial Biogenesis in Fat and Muscle of Obese Rodents. *J. Clin. Investig.* **2006**, *116*, 2791–2798. [CrossRef] [PubMed]
67. Ampong, I.; Zimmerman, K.D.; Perumalla, D.S.; Wallis, K.E.; Li, G.; Huber, H.F.; Li, C.; Nathanielsz, P.W.; Cox, L.A.; Olivier, M. Maternal Obesity Alters Offspring Liver and Skeletal Muscle Metabolism in Early Post-Puberty despite Maintaining a Normal Post-Weaning Dietary Lifestyle. *FASEB J.* **2022**, *36*, e22644. [CrossRef] [PubMed]
68. Pereira, S.P.; Diniz, M.S.; Tavares, L.C.; Cunha-Oliveira, T.; Li, C.; Cox, L.A.; Nijland, M.J.; Nathanielsz, P.W.; Oliveira, P.J. Characterizing Early Cardiac Metabolic Programming via 30% Maternal Nutrient Reduction during Fetal Development in a Non-Human Primate Model. *Int. J. Mol. Sci.* **2023**, *24*, 15192. [CrossRef] [PubMed]
69. Ceasrine, A.M.; Devlin, B.A.; Bolton, J.L.; Green, L.A.; Jo, Y.C.; Huynh, C.; Patrick, B.; Washington, K.; Sanchez, C.L.; Joo, F.; et al. Maternal Diet Disrupts the Placenta–Brain Axis in a Sex-Specific Manner. *Nat. Metab.* **2022**, *4*, 1732–1745. [CrossRef] [PubMed]

biology

MDPI

Review

Mitochondrial Dysfunction in Endothelial Progenitor Cells: Unraveling Insights from Vascular Endothelial Cells

Azra Kulovic-Sissawo [1,2], Carolina Tocantins [1,2,3,4,5], Mariana S. Diniz [1,2,3,4,5], Elisa Weiss [1,2,*], Andreas Steiner [1,2], Silvija Tokic [6], Corina T. Madreiter-Sokolowski [7], Susana P. Pereira [3,4,8] and Ursula Hiden [1,2,*]

1 Perinatal Research Laboratory, Department of Obstetrics and Gynaecology, Medical University of Graz, Auenbruggerplatz 14, 8036 Graz, Austria; azra.kulovic@medunigraz.at (A.K.-S.); ctsantos@cnc.uc.pt (C.T.); andreas.steiner@stud.medunigraz.at (A.S.)

2 Research Unit Early Life Determinants (ELiD), Medical University of Graz, Auenbruggerplatz 14, 8036 Graz, Austria

3 CNC-UC—Center for Neuroscience and Cell Biology, University of Coimbra, Rua Larga, 3004-504 Coimbra, Portugal

4 Center for Innovative Biomedicine and Biotechnology (CIBB), University of Coimbra, 3000-504 Coimbra, Portugal

5 Doctoral Programme in Experimental Biology and Biomedicine (PDBEB), Institute for Interdisciplinary Research (IIIUC), University of Coimbra, 3004-531 Coimbra, Portugal

6 Research Unit of Analytical Mass Spectrometry, Cell Biology and Biochemistry of Inborn Errors of Metabolism, Department of Paediatrics and Adolescent Medicine, Medical University of Graz, Auenbruggerplatz 34, 8036 Graz, Austria

7 Division of Molecular Biology and Biochemistry, Medical University of Graz, Neue Stiftingtalstraße 6, 8010 Graz, Austria

8 Laboratory of Metabolism and Exercise (LaMetEx), Research Centre in Physical Activity, Health and Leisure (CIAFEL), Laboratory for Integrative and Translational Research in Population Health (ITR), Faculty of Sports, University of Porto, 4200-450 Porto, Portugal

* Correspondence: elisa.weiss@medunigraz.at (E.W.); ursula.hiden@medunigraz.at (U.H.)

Simple Summary: Endothelial cells (ECs) form the inner lining of all blood vessels. This endothelium has vital functions for the body, and endothelial dysfunction is associated with several lifestyle-related diseases, including cardiovascular and neurodegenerative diseases. Therefore, endothelial dysfunction contributes significantly to the global health burden. Mitochondria are the powerhouses of cells and regulate metabolism and cell behavior. The function of ECs is highly dependent on mitochondria. Cardiovascular risk factors (CVRFs), such as obesity, diabetes mellitus (DM), or chronic inflammation, can impair mitochondria and thus ECfunction. Endothelial progenitor cells (EPCs) are a backup for ECscirculating in the bloodstream. They can be recruited from the blood for endothelial repair. After attachment to the vessel wall, EPCs differentiate into ECs. Recent research has shown that, like ECs, EPCs are also sensitive to CVRFs., but the mechanisms of damage, and whether mitochondria play a role, are not yet known. In this review, we describe the role of mitochondria in endothelial dysfunction. Based on recent studies investigating EPCs in diseases and under the influence of CVRFs, we discuss the role of mitochondria in EPC deterioration. Moreover, we address potential therapeutic interventions targeting mitochondrial health to promote endothelial function.

Abstract: Endothelial dysfunction is associated with several lifestyle-related diseases, including cardiovascular and neurodegenerative diseases, and it contributes significantly to the global health burden. Recent research indicates a link between cardiovascular risk factors (CVRFs), excessive production of reactive oxygen species (ROS), mitochondrial impairment, and endothelial dysfunction. Circulating endothelial progenitor cells (EPCs) are recruited into the vessel wall to maintain appropriate endothelial function, repair, and angiogenesis. After attachment, EPCs differentiate into mature endothelial cells (ECs). Like ECs, EPCs are also susceptible to CVRFs, including metabolic dysfunction and chronic inflammation. Therefore, mitochondrial dysfunction of EPCs may have long-term effects on the function of the mature ECs into which EPCs differentiate, particularly in the presence of endothelial damage. However, a link between CVRFs and impaired mitochondrial function in EPCs has hardly been investigated. In this review, we aim to consolidate existing knowledge on the development of mitochondrial and endothelial dysfunction in the vascular endothelium, place it in the context of recent studies investigating the consequences of CVRFs on EPCs, and discuss the role of mitochondrial dysfunction. Thus, we aim to gain a comprehensive understanding of mechanisms involved in EPC deterioration in relation to CVRFs and address potential therapeutic interventions targeting mitochondrial health to promote endothelial function.

Keywords: mitochondrial dysfunction; reactive oxygen species; cardiovascular risk factors; endothelial dysfunction; endothelial progenitor cells; cardiovascular disease; neurodegenerative disorders

1. Introduction

Endothelial cells (ECs) cover the lumen of all blood vessels and fulfill various functions that are essential for the body's homeostasis. For instance, ECs participate in vascular tone regulation, blood clotting, and immune functions. Endothelial dysfunction arises, in particular, under the influence of cardiovascular risk factors (CVRFs), including obesity, physical inactivity, low-grade inflammation, aging, and smoking [1–6]. Endothelial dysfunction is a major contributor to a plethora of cardiovascular disorders [7], which are the leading cause of disease burden worldwide [8]. In particular, oxidative stress plays a key role in endothelial dysfunction and cardiovascular disorders [7,9]. Oxidative stress is characterized by an imbalance between the overproduction and accumulation of reactive oxygen species (ROS) and lower antioxidant defense, which can lead to cell damage by altering proteins, lipids, and nucleic acids [10]. ROS can be formed as signaling molecules generated by enzymes of the redox signaling pathway [11], which is induced by a range of stimuli, including pro-inflammatory cytokines and growth factors [12,13]. ROS are predominantly generated as natural by-products in the mitochondrial electron transport chain (ETC) [9]. Oxidative stress, hypoxia, and metabolic derangements lead to excessive ROS production through oxidative phosphorylation due to uncoupled electron transport in the mitochondrial ETC and adenosine triphosphate (ATP) synthesis [9,14]. Hence, mitochondria are a primary hub in ROS production, ROS signaling, and oxidative stress. Any failure of normal mitochondrial function is referred to as mitochondrial dysfunction and is characterized by a loss of efficiency in energy production paralleled by increased ROS generation [15]. Mitochondrial dysfunction is a characteristic of aging [16] and various chronic diseases [17–19] and is closely linked to endothelial dysfunction and cardiovascular disease (CVD) development [20].

Within the cardiovascular system, cardiomyocytes, in particular, have a high density of mitochondria to respond to the energetic demands of the cardiac muscle [21]. In contrast, endothelial mitochondria are not as abundant or relevant for energy production, as in EC, 75% of energy is obtained through glycolysis [22]. Thus, the potential role of endothelial mitochondrial dysfunction in endothelial pathophysiology and CVD has been unnoticed for a long time. However, endothelial mitochondria can generate ROS and relevant other metabolic intermediates. During inflammation, hypoxia, or stress, ROS may exceed its physiological levels, disturbing endothelial function and thus promoting the progression of CVD. Recent research highlights the mitochondria's central and long-underestimated contribution in endothelial dysfunction [21,22].

In addition to mature ECs, which are part of the vascular endothelium, there is a distinct population of circulating endothelial progenitor cells (EPCs). These cells function as a reserve pool of ECs recruited to repair damaged vascular endothelium or engage in angiogenesis when needed. Upon recruitment into the vascular wall, EPCs differentiate into mature ECs, which is why EPCs are also termed endothelial colony-forming cells (ECFCs) [23]. CVRFs not only adversely affect vascular ECs but also circulating EPCs and trigger reduced EPC numbers and decreased proliferative and angiogenic potential in situations of compromised vascular health [24–26]. While EPCs play a vital role in maintaining the vascular endothelium, their specific involvement in endothelial dysfunction repair remains largely unexplored, and the potential impact of mitochondria on EPC function has received limited attention. Therefore, this review aims to elucidate the significance of mitochondrial (dys)function in vascular ECs. It also discusses the largely unexplored area of mitochondrial dysfunction in EPCs and its potential implications in the context of endothelial dysfunction and associated chronic diseases.

2. Endothelial Function and Dysfunction

ECs play a critical role in the cardiovascular system. ECs form the inner layer of blood vessels, regulate blood flow, function as a semi-permeable barrier between the circulation and surrounding tissues, participate in immune response, regulate blood clotting, and initiate growth and repair of blood vessels, thus ensuring proper vascular function. If dysfunctional, ECs vastly contribute to the development of CVD. The following subsections will introduce the main endothelial functions and alterations leading to a dysfunctional endothelium.

2.1. Endothelial Function Is Versatile

Among their multifaceted features, ECs regulate the vascular tone through the release of vasodilatory and vasoconstrictive molecules, which actively modulate blood vessel diameter. The main vasodilatory molecule released by ECs is nitric oxide (NO), generated by the enzyme endothelial nitric oxide synthase (eNOS). In an immediate response, NO stimulates cyclic guanosine monophosphate (cGMP) production through the enzyme soluble guanylyl cyclase (sGC) in vascular smooth muscle cells (VSMCs), leading to relaxation and vasodilatation [27]. Moreover, NO inhibits the proliferation of VSMCs, prevents platelet and leukocyte adhesion, and inhibits the expression of pro-inflammatory cytokines, thus exhibiting vasodilatory and anti-thrombotic features [3,4]. Other endothelial-derived vasodilating factors are prostacyclin (PGI2) and bradykinin (BK). ECs also secrete balanced levels of vasoconstricting factors, such as endothelin-1 (ET-1), prostaglandin H2 (PGH2), thromboxane A2 (TXA2), or angiotensin II (AngII) [3–5], serving as vascular tone regulators.

Furthermore, the endothelium represents an adjustable, semi-permeable barrier. Therefore, ECs form special structures, so-called junctions, between neighboring cells. Three types of junctions contribute to the controlled transfer of macromolecules and immune cells, intercellular communication, and paracellular permeability [28–30]. Gap junctions (GJs) enable the transport of small molecules between ECs and support intercellular communication, whilst adherence junctions (AJs) and tight junctions (TJs) form structures that determine paracellular permeability. TJs, on the one hand, fulfill a barrier function by controlling permeability for small molecules and ions, whereas AJs, on the other hand, are mainly required for selective transendothelial migration of immune cells [29]. Environmental signals lead to junctional remodeling, thus regulating permeability and the exchange of nutrients and blood cells [28]. In addition to paracellular transport, molecule transport across the endothelium occurs through transcytosis, i.e., the transcellular transport of molecules via vesicles by carrier-mediated active transport through concentration gradient-dependent facilitated transport, or through diffusion [31]. Endothelial barrier function is organ-specific. For instance, in the brain and retina, the endothelial monolayer is tightly connected to maintain a close barrier, even with reduced transcytosis [32]. The essential transport of glucose occurs via facilitated transport through glucose transporters (GLUT), foremost GLUT1 [33]. In contrast, in the liver and kidneys, the endothelium is discontinuous to allow the desired increased exchange of molecules [34].

ECs also actively participate in immune and inflammatory responses as they not only secrete a plethora of cytokines and chemokines but also express specific cell adhesion molecules for immune cells upon activation by inflammatory signals. Thus, ECs mediate the recruitment and transendothelial migration of leukocytes from the circulation to the target tissue [35].

In healthy conditions, ECs act by secreting anti-coagulant factors, such as tissue plasminogen activator (tPA) [4], in an anti-coagulant way to prevent thrombosis and maintain blood fluidity [4,5]. Upon injury, ECs secrete pro-thrombotic factors, including von Willebrand factor (vWF) and plasminogen activator inhibitor-1 (PAI-1), to induce blood clotting [5].

Two other pivotal roles of ECs are vasculogenesis and angiogenesis, which comprise the formation and growth of blood vessels [3,4,36]. The strongest angiogenic trigger is hypoxia, which induces the release of proangiogenic factors, such as vascular endothelial growth factor (VEGF). Upon binding to the VEGF receptor 2 (VEGFR2) on ECs, VEGF activates quiescent ECs and initiates angiogenesis, ensuring the reestablishment of oxygen and nutrients in the tissue [36,37]. However, other bioactive molecules, including growth factors [38], cytokines [39,40], hormones [41], and non-coding RNAs, such as microRNAs (miRNA) and long non-coding RNAs (lncRNA), also regulate angiogenesis [42].

Given the versatility of these multifaceted functions of ECs, the vascular endothelium can emerge as an extensive and dynamic endocrine organ, acting as a vital interface between the circulation and tissues to ensure body homeostasis. By actively participating in immune responses, coagulation processes, and vascular remodeling, ECs maintain vascular health, playing an indispensable role in the cardiovascular system.

2.2. Endothelial Dysfunction: The Central Role of Reactive Oxygen Species

The intricate endothelial functions are crucial for ensuring adequate blood flow and the overall well-being of the heart and vessels, as well as the organs supplied. However, when the endothelium loses balance, a cascade of health issues can unfold, particularly in CVD. This endothelial dysfunction is not an isolated event but rather a consequence of a complex interplay involving various CVRFs. These factors, dependent on lifestyle and health conditions, conspire to activate and inflame ECs, setting the stage for health issues. Obesity, poor dietary habits, physical inactivity, type II diabetes mellitus (T2DM), aging, smoking, chronic inflammation, and even microbial infections are some of the underlying causes, as they create a hostile environment characterized by inflammation and oxidative stress [1–6].

Oxidative stress, driven by ROS, is a key player in endothelial (dys)function. Several ROS sources in ECs contribute to oxidative stress generation, which can eventually lead to mitochondrial dysfunction, inflammation, and endothelial dysfunction, as illustrated in Figure 1.

The majority (~90%) of cellular ROS is generated in mitochondria [43,44]. Key contributors are ETC constituents: complex I at the flavin mononucleotide (FMN) site [45], and complex III at the quinol cycle (Q-cycle) [46,47]. Additional ROS-producing enzymes associated with nutrient metabolism and oxidative phosphorylation are succinate dehydrogenase (complex II), glycerol-3-phosphate dehydrogenase (GPD), 2-oxoglutarate dehydrogenase (OGDH), pyruvate dehydrogenase (PDH) complex, proline dehydrogenase (PRODH), dihydroorotate dehydrogenase (DHODH), branched chain keto acid dehydrogenase (BCKDH) complex, acyl-CoA dehydrogenases (very long-chain acyl-CoA dehydrogenase ACDVL; long-chain acyl-CoA dehydrogenase ACADL) [48], electron transfer flavoprotein dehydrogenase (ETFDH), and sulfide quinone reductase (SQR) [49,50], which constitute significant sources of mitochondrial ROS (mtROS). Mitochondrial dysfunction, due to possible damages in the respiratory chain, loss of cytochrome c (CytC), and imbalanced energy demand, is associated with excessive ROS production [51].

In addition to mtROS generated by ETC, redox signaling also contributes to ROS generation. Redox signaling regulates cell growth, differentiation, senescence, apoptosis, and autophagy and is induced by [52,53] pro-inflammatory cytokines and growth factors [12,13,54,55]. By binding to their receptors, reduced nicotinamide adenine dinucleotide phosphate (NADPH) oxidases 1, 2, 4, and 5 (NOX1,2,4,5) become activated and produce ROS as signaling molecules [55–57]. NOX enzymes are localized in the plasma membrane and thus contribute to cytosolic ROS [58]. However, NOX4 is also localized in other intracellular compartments, including mitochondria, and it also adds to mtROS [59].

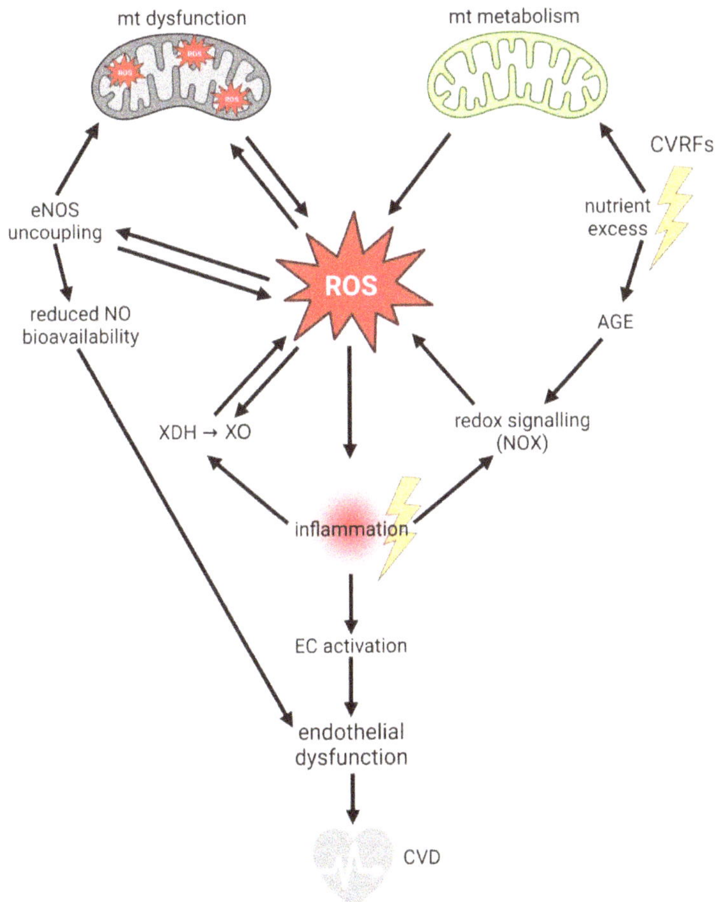

Figure 1. The interplay between metabolism, inflammation, reactive oxygen species, and mitochondrial dysfunction in the development of endothelial dysfunction and cardiovascular disease. Arrows indicate the directionality and stimulation of the respective processes. Influences that represent cardiovascular risk factors (CVRFs), i.e., nutrient excess and inflammation, are marked with yellow flashes. AGE: advanced glycation end products; CVD: cardiovascular disease; EC: endothelial cell; eNOS: endothelial nitric oxide synthase; mt: mitochondrial; NO: nitric oxide; NOX: NADPH oxidases; ROS: reactive oxygen species; XDH: xanthine dehydrogenase; XO: xanthine oxidase. The figure was created using BioRender.com, accessed on 22 January 2024.

The interaction between glucose molecules and essential cellular components leads to the formation of advanced glycation end products (AGE). These AGE-infused structures become agents of chaos, promoting the release of cytokines, enhancing cell adhesion, and even triggering blood coagulation. The downstream effects are several, influencing everything from angiogenesis to overall endothelial function [60–62]. In addition to cytokines and growth factors, the interaction of AGE with their receptor (RAGE) also induces redox signaling by NOX [63].

Another enzyme capable of producing ROS is the purine catabolizing enzyme xanthine dehydrogenase (XDH). Oxidative stress [64,65] or inflammation [66,67] induce post-translational modifications that modify the enzymatic action of XDH to xanthine oxidase (XO) activity, generating superoxide anion ($O_2{\cdot}^-$) [68,69].

Oxidative stress can be self-reinforcing through a process referred to as eNOS uncoupling [70]. Uncoupled eNOS increasingly forms superoxide instead of NO. Superoxide reacts with NO, which is still formed by eNOS at lower levels, to generate peroxynitrite anion (ONOO-) [71]. In mitochondria, peroxynitrite can overwhelm mitochondrial scavenging and repair systems for peroxynitrite-dependent oxidative modifications and, thus, impair mitochondrial energy and calcium (Ca^{2+}) homeostasis and membrane permeability. This contributes to mitochondrial dysfunction and augmented ROS production, perpetuating a dysfunction cycle. Uncoupling of eNOS hence promotes and reinforces oxidative stress and mitochondrial dysfunction, but, at the same time, it causes a reduction in NO bioavailability, with severe effects on endothelial function [72,73].

Besides mitochondria, the endoplasmic reticulum (ER) is a source of ROS under certain conditions: ER stress triggers unfolded protein response (UPR), which activates protein kinase RNA (PKR)-like ER kinase (PERK), inositol-requiring protein-1 (IRE1), and activating transcription factor-6 (ATF6). These three UPR signal transduction mechanisms can activate inflammatory signaling via various pathways, including nuclear factor kappa B (NFκB) signaling, which also increases ROS production [74]. Moreover, an ER enzyme involved in disulfide bond formation within protein folding, i.e., ER oxidoreductin (ERO1), generates hydrogen peroxide (H_2O_2) [75].

In the scope of ROS generators, red blood cells (RBCs) are also considerable contributors [76,77]. The release of ROS is, on the one hand, induced by endogenous factors, including, in particular, the autoxidation of oxyhemoglobin (HbO_2) formed by oxygen binding to ferrous heme (FeII) [76,77]. It is thereby oxidized to its ferric form (FeIII), generating methemoglobin (metHb) and superoxide anion [78], which, via several mechanisms, lead to the formation of H_2O_2, hydroxyl radical ($^{\bullet}OH$), and hydroxyl anion (OH^-) [76,79,80]. Notably, superoxide anion -also rapidly reacts with NO, generating the highly reactive peroxynitrite, a potent inducer of endothelial injury [81]. In T2DM, RBC-released ROS induce endothelial dysfunction via arginase I [82], with peroxinitrite operating as an arginase stimulator and mediating the malfunction of ECs [83]. Similar findings were reported in mice models [84].

On the other hand, oxidative stress in RBCs can be triggered by exogenous metabolites like superoxide anion, peroxynitrite anion, and H_2O_2 from adjacent cells, including endothelial and immune cells [76]. Thus, besides their role in oxygen transportation, RBCs are crucial for redox balance [85,86], and RBC autoxidation is a considerable source of ROS-promoting oxidative stress in the vasculature [76,77].

Oxidative stress is not an isolated phenomenon. It is closely linked to inflammation as increased ROS reinforce inflammation by promoting leukocyte extravasation and by stimulating cytokine production [3–5,87,88]. Pro-inflammatory stimuli destabilize the junctions and thus disrupt the endothelial barrier and increase the permeability [89]. Moreover, oxidative stress per se causes a redistribution of junctional molecules and interferes with signaling pathways associated with barrier function regulation [90].

Under physiological conditions, ROS production and maintenance are regulated through an antioxidant system constituting enzymatic and non-enzymatic factors. The most prominent enzymes are superoxide dismutases (SOD1-3), catalase (CAT), glutathi-one peroxidases (GPX1-7), NAD(P)H quinone dehydrogenase 1 (NQO1), heme oxygenases (HOX1-2), thioredoxin (TXN), and sulfiredoxin 1 (SRXN1). The non-enzymatic system includes uric acid, glutathione, vitamins, and plant secondary metabolites (e.g., polyphenols) [91,92]. These enzymes and antioxidants act in concert to balance the equilibrium between ROS production and oxidative stress.

An imbalance in the antioxidant system and ROS production leads to increased oxidative stress, reduced NO bioavailability, and inflammation as the endothelium shifts to an activated, pro-inflammatory, vasoconstrictive, and pro-thrombotic phenotype with increased cytokine and growth factor release, which promote proliferation, migration, and permeability, as well as imbalanced production of vasodilatory vs. vasoconstrictive factors [3–5,93] (Figure 2). The intricate interplay between oxidative stress, a pro-inflammatory milieu, and EC activation and dysfunction contributes to endothelial dysfunction and cardiovascular disorders. Notably, the significance of mitochondrial dysfunction as a primary source of ROS in endothelial dysfunction has started to gain recognition.

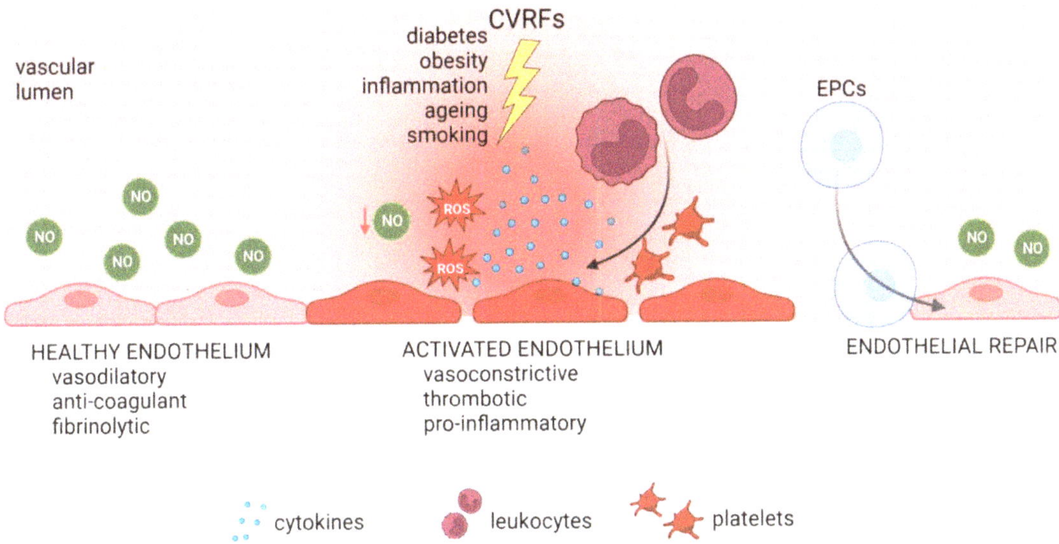

Figure 2. Characteristics of healthy and dysfunctional endothelia and the role of endothelial progenitor cells in repair. Cardiovascular risk factors (CVRFs) disturb normal endothelial function and promote an activated endothelial cell phenotype. A dysfunctional endothelium is accompanied by oxidative stress with increased reactive oxygen species (ROS), inflammation, and reduced nitric oxide (NO) bioavailability. Under healthy conditions, circulating endothelial progenitor cells (EPCs) support, as endothelial colony-forming cells (ECFCs), endothelial repair and recovery. However, it is unclear how CVRFs affect ECFC efficacy and whether the cells remain able to complete repair and restore the endothelium. The figure was created using BioRender.com, accessed on 22 January 2024.

3. Mitochondrial Function in a Healthy Endothelium

Mitochondria are highly dynamic organelles that not only generate energy in form of ATP, but also sense and respond to the surrounding environment. The following subsections will describe the role of mitochondrial dynamics, mitochondrial metabolism, and mtROS in EC function.

3.1. Mitochondrial Structure and Dynamics in Endothelial Cells

Mitochondria, essential powerhouses within cells, possess a distinct structure characterized by outer and inner membranes that enclose the mitochondrial matrix [94]. Mitochondrial function is highly dependent on the ETC system, a compilation of proteins intricately associated with the inner membrane comprising four distinct enzymatic complexes (I–IV) [95]. The electron transport is coupled to proton ejection from the mitochondrial matrix into the intermembrane space in every complex except for complex II [95]. Proton ejection generates an electrochemical gradient, creating a proton-motive force to phosphorylate adenosine diphosphate (ADP) into adenosine triphosphate (ATP) through ATP synthase [96,97]. In the intact endothelium, healthy mitochondria appear to have cylindrical structures with an inner mitochondrial membrane with folded cristae enclosing the mitochondrial matrix [98].

The mitochondrial structure is dynamic and balanced between fission and fusion processes, which determine not only mitochondrial shape but also mitochondrial functions, including performance, ROS production, and quality control [99]. The term 'mitochondrial quality control (MQC) system' has been established for this network, which tightly balances mitochondrial dynamics, i.e., fission and fusion events and mitophagy [100,101]. Mitochondrial fission is mainly regulated by cytoplasmic dynamin-related protein 1 (DRP1) with the assistance of numerous factors, including mitochondrial fission protein 1 (FIS1), mitochondrial fission factor (MFF), and mitochondrial dynamic proteins (MID49 and MID51) located at the outer membrane [102,103]. Mitochondrial fusion is controlled by membrane proteins mitofusin (MFN) 1 and MFN2, together with optic atrophy protein 1 (OPA1) [102,103]. OPA1 furthermore promotes tight folding of cristae, which increases mitochondrial respiratory efficiency and blunts mitochondrial dysfunction [104]. Mitochondrial dynamics, such as migration and proliferation, are essential for EC function [105], highlighting the central role of mitochondrial morphology for endothelial function.

3.2. Mitochondrial Metabolism in Endothelial Cells

The energy metabolism of the vascular endothelium comprises four major metabolic processes: glycolysis, oxidative phosphorylation, fatty acid oxidation (β-oxidation), and glutamine metabolism [106]. Depending on the distinct physiological and pathological stimulations, such as hypoxia and inflammation, cells can adapt their metabolism. This metabolic switch precedes functional changes and disease developments [107,108].

In contrast to neurons and cardiomyocytes, which are highly endowed with mitochondria and perform mitochondrial oxidative phosphorylation and fatty acid oxidation for energy metabolism [109,110], ECs in both macro- and microcirculation depend mainly on glycolysis, which occurs in the cytoplasm [109–115]. On the one hand, using a less energy-efficient metabolic pathway facilitates oxygen diffusion to surrounding cells by consuming minimal oxygen [116]. On the other hand, using glycolysis can reduce ROS generation [116]. In fact, except for ECs from the blood–brain barrier (BBB) [117], ECs have fewer mitochondria and consume lower amounts of oxygen than other cell types, such as neurons and liver and muscle cells [118,119]. Importantly, mitochondria in ECs have functions other than the generation of ATP, such as biomass generation and signaling [120]. Thus, in a healthy state, ECs are quiescent, mainly relying on glycolysis [111], but this steady cellular metabolism changes during cell activation [111]. During vessel growth and sprouting, fatty acids are important for ECs, being metabolized by mitochondrial fatty acid oxidation [112,121] and thereby producing acetyl-coenzyme A (acetyl-CoA), reduced nicotinamide adenine dinucleotide (NADH) and flavin adenine dinucleotide ($FADH_2$) and yielding high amounts of ATP [122]. Also, glutamine metabolism leads into the mitochondrial tricarboxylic acid (TCA) cycle, providing about a third of TCA cycle-derived carbon [123]. However, under normal conditions, ECs do not use fatty acids or glutamine for obtaining energy but mostly for de novo synthesis of nucleotides required for DNA replication and cell proliferation [123,124]. Excess intracellular fatty acids can be stored as cytosolic lipid droplets in ECs [125].

3.3. Mitochondrial ROS Homeostasis in Endothelial Cells

Remarkably, even at physiological levels, mtROS and the proteins orchestrating mitochondrial biogenesis play a central role in the regulation of angiogenesis [126]. ROS activate the promoter of the transcription factor hypoxia-inducible factor-1 α (HIF1α) [126,127], which transactivates genes involved in promoting angiogenesis, including VEGF [128], and reinforces VEGFR2 signaling [129]. In contrast, under hypoxic conditions, HIF plays a critical role in maintaining homeostasis. HIF1α and HIF2α promote the activation of the cytochrome c oxidase 4 isoform 2 (COX4I2) subunit gene transcription, resulting in improved electron transfer within the ETC [130]. HIF1α further contributes to decreased complex I activity through induction of the NADH dehydrogenase (ubiquinone) 1 alpha subcomplex, 4-like 2 (*NDUFA4L2*) gene [131]. As mentioned above, mtROS is mainly formed in ETC complex I and III [45–47,132–134]. Depending on the general cellular conditions, ROS formation can vary between physiological and pathological [132–134]. At complex

I [132], a high NADH/NAD$^+$ ratio results in reduced FMN levels and triggers excessive ROS production. This scenario is induced by damage, ischemia, loss of CytC (apoptosis), and low ATP demand [133,134]. ROS production at complex III mainly happens through auto-oxidation of the Q-cycle intermediate ubisemiquinone [132–134].

Moreover, exposure to H_2O_2 increases mitochondrial Ca^{2+} concentration in ECs and regulates barrier function maintenance and eNOS activity [22,135,136]. Indeed, NO plays a key role in mitochondria and can inhibit mitochondrial respiratory chain complex I (through S-nitrosylation) and complex IV, modulating EC respiration and ATP production [21]. Dysregulation of this mechanism has also been associated with mitochondrial oxidative stress [21]. Consequently, despite their modest presence within EC, mitochondria harbor the latent potential to exceed physiologic ROS formation, with pathologic ROS levels exerting notable disruptions in endothelial function.

4. Unveiling Endothelial Mitochondrial Dysfunction in Pathophysiology

Mitochondrial dysfunction is characterized by a loss of efficiency in the ETC, resulting in reduced synthesis of high-energy molecules, such as ATP [137], increased ROS generation, and oxidative stress [15]. Mitochondrial dysfunction is associated with aging as well as many chronic diseases, including CVD, neurodegenerative disorders (NDDs), metabolic diseases, and chronic infections [16–20,100,138–141]. The following subsections will describe the mechanisms of dysfunction in ECs and the mitochondrial contribution to CVD, NDDs, and DM.

4.1. Mitochondrial Dysfunction in Endothelial Cells

At physiological levels, ROS act as signaling molecules and are beneficial for mitochondria. However, when in excess, ROS are harmful, altering biomolecules and impairing mitochondrial function [142], highlighting the importance of tight mitochondrial regulation of ROS generation. One origin of excess mtROS is damaged mitochondria, which are prone to shifting mitochondrial dynamics to fission, resulting in an overload of mitochondrial fragments. Therefore, a highly efficient mechanism of removing damaged mitochondria exists, i.e., mitophagy, to maintain mitochondrial health, which is of particular value for the cardiovascular system [143,144].

The mitochondrial structure, related to fission and fusion processes, plays a vital role in maintaining the fine-tuning of mitochondrial dynamics and cellular function [145]. In line with this, mitochondrial structural damage has been identified in the context of endothelial dysfunction. For instance, throughout aging, human umbilical vein ECs (HUVECs) present degenerated cristae and swollen regions, along with decreased mitochondrial membrane potential (MMP) and loss of fusion and fission events [146]. Treatment with high glucose and palmitate induces structural changes in rat aortic EC mitochondria, and reduced mitochondrial size is associated with elevated ROS levels and augmented cellular levels of superoxide anion and cytoplasmic H_2O_2. This increased oxidative stress is accompanied by a loss of MMP [147]. Furthermore, ECs reveal pronounced alterations, on the one hand, in mitochondrial dynamics, with increased mitochondrial fission (increased FIS1 and phosphorylated-DRP1/DRP1 ratio) and decreased MFN2. On the other hand, ECs differ in apoptosis, with increased expression of cleaved caspase 3 and caspase 9, CytC release, decreased B-cell lymphoma 2 (BCL2), and increased BCL2-like protein 4 (BAX) levels [147]. These data highlight the link between oxidative stress, altered mitochondrial dynamics, mitochondrial dysfunction, and impaired ECs. Mitochondria from HUVEC subjected to high-glucose treatment show an opening of the mitochondrial permeability transition pore (mPTP) and CytC release. These effects are inhibited by overexpression of uncoupling protein 2 (*UCP2*), a mitochondrial protein able to uncouple the oxidative phosphorylation from ATP synthesis by regulating MMP, modulating ROS generation, and contributing to increased NO levels [148]. UCP2 is often upregulated as an adaptive cellular response to demanding environments, and it has a protective role in high-salt-induced injury in ECs by regulating autophagy. Moreover, *UCP2* overexpression results in a higher number of mitochondria and the upregulation of Parkin (PARK2), a critical protein involved in mitophagy [149].

An inflammatory environment mimicked by stimulation with tumor necrosis factor (TNF)α in primary rat aortic ECs resulted in augmented mitochondrial fission with increased NF-κB activation [150]. This response was found to be mediated by Drp1 [150], and, indeed, pharmacological inhibition of mitochondrial fission with mitochondrial division inhibitor 1 (Mdivi-1) improved endothelial function in these cells [147,150].

But, there is another link between mitochondria and inflammation. Deficiency of isocitrate dehydrogenase $NADP^+$ 2 (IDH2), a TCA cycle enzyme, is associated with increased endothelial inflammation in HUVEC [151] and contributes to enhanced levels of cytokine transcripts, such as TNFα and interleukin (IL) 1β, coincidently with activated p66shc (SHC adaptor protein 1) [151], a protein known to promote oxidative stress in ECs. Furthermore, Idh2 downregulation and increased activation of p66shc in mouse umbilical vein ECs lead to changes in the abundance of ETC complexes, which result in decreased oxygen consumption [151], demonstrating a link between p66shc and mitochondrial endothelial dysfunction. In fact, this damaging role of p66shc is regulated by sirtuin 1 lysine deacetylase (Sirt1) acetylation [152].

Oxidative stress overload also adversely affects mitochondrial DNA (mtDNA) [142]. In general, circular mtDNA is more prone to ROS-induced damage and mutation not only due to the close proximity to one of the ROS sources, i.e., mtROS, but also because of the lack of additional protection from histones compared to genomic DNA [142]. It has been previously described that EC exposed to ROS undergo mtDNA damage [153], which alters mitochondrial gene and protein expression, impairs mitochondrial function, and contributes to vascular disease development [153].

Impaired mitochondria activate innate immune pathways with the release of mtDNA [154] recognized as damage-associated molecular patterns (DAMPs) by pattern recognition receptors (PRR) [155]. Thereby, the nod-like receptor family pyrin domain-containing 3 (NLRP3) inflammasome is triggered. The NLRP3 inflammasome is a protein complex in the cytoplasm that mediates an innate immune response and detects microbial motifs and endogenous danger signals. NLRP3 induction leads to caspase 1 activation and the release of pro-inflammatory molecules, including cytokines IL1β and IL18, and potentially leads to cell death [156–158].

Thus, mitochondrial and endothelial dysfunction are tightly related. Altered and damaging cellular environments, including increased levels of glucose [147,148], palmitate [147], and inflammatory cytokines [150], contribute to endothelial dysfunction, with particular implications for mitochondria-controlled mechanisms. Hyperglycemia, hyperlipidemia, and inflammation represent major CVRFs that ultimately lead to an increased risk for CVD or NDDs (Figure 3). Therefore, tackling the mechanisms involved in mitochondrial dysfunction in ECs can provide critical insights into the development and progression of CVD.

4.2. Endothelial Mitochondrial Dysfunction in Atherosclerosis: A Catalyst for Cardiovascular Diseases

Atherosclerosis is a chronic inflammatory condition and a common precursor of CVD [159]. It is characterized by lipid, mainly cholesterol, and fibrin accumulation in the form of atheroma plaques, accompanied by calcification, endothelial activation, and an inflammatory response within arterial walls [160]. One of the major driving forces of the inflammatory response in ECs is low-density lipoprotein (LDL) in its oxidized form (oxLDL), promoting plaque formation [161–163]. OxLDL binds to the injured vascular endothelium, attracts immune cells, enhances their adhesion, and thereby initiates an immune response [162].

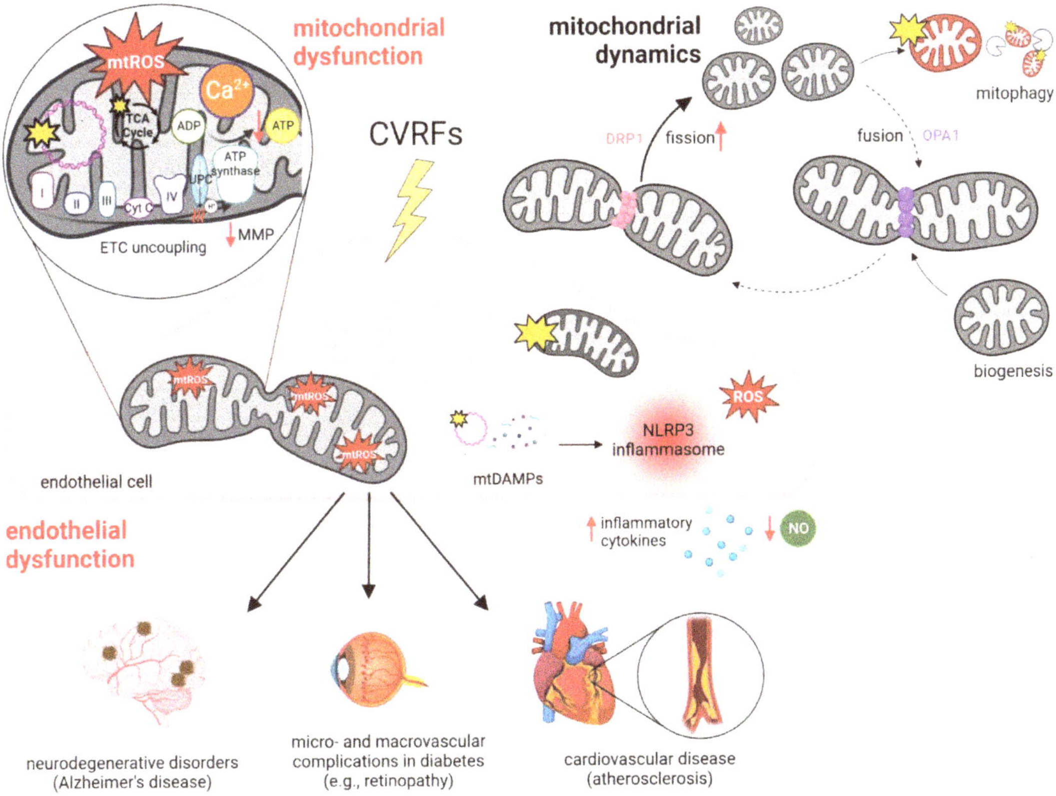

Figure 3. Mitochondria play a decisive role in shaping healthy vs. dysfunctional endothelial phenotypes. Cardiovascular risk factors (CVRFs) trigger detrimental mitochondrial impairment and dysfunction. In this context, impaired or damaged mitochondria discharge reactive oxygen species (mtROS) and mitochondrial-damage-associated molecular patterns (mtDAMPs) into the cytoplasm, which are degraded in the NLRP3 inflammasome. Mitochondrial dynamics shift towards increased fission. Mitophagy, a cellular process that involves the selective removal of damaged or dysfunctional mitochondria, emerges as a guardian of endothelial homeostasis. This process takes on the role of an athero-protective sentinel, as it systematically rids the endothelium of compromised mitochondria, thus safeguarding against the progression of atherosclerosis. Disruption of mitochondrial function and dynamics can pave the way for the onset of endothelial dysfunction and diseases. The figure was created using BioRender.com, accessed on 22 January 2024.

Mitochondrial dysfunction in atherosclerosis was extensively studied in SMCs [164,165] and immune cells, including macrophages [166,167]. Only recently has the significance of mitochondrial damage in ECs been recognized as a pivotal factor contributing to the derangement of the endothelium in atherosclerosis. Consequently, this recognition bears significant new implications for the understanding of CVD development [20,73,168]. The crucial role of properly functioning endothelial mitochondria is highlighted by several publications extensively reviewing its function in the onset and advancement of atherosclerosis [142,145,169–171]. Moreover, the pivotal role of ECs and the result of a damaged endothelium have been widely studied in regard to atherosclerotic progression [172,173].

In fact, endothelial activation [174], accompanied by reduced NO generation [175], initiates atherosclerosis [160], in particular in arterial segments with turbulent flow [174,176] and low wall shear stress [177]. Disturbed flow triggers changes in mitochondrial morphology by stimulating fission, resulting in increased DRP1 levels, excessively fragmented mitochondria, and mtROS release [176]. In vascular pathologies, including atherosclerosis, endothelial mitochondria show functional disturbances and structural changes within the inner arrangement of the mitochondrial membrane and reduced and disorganized cristae [98]. A recent study underlined the importance of mitochondrial dynamics in regard to atherosclerosis progression by investigating the athero-protective role of Opa1 in ECs from LDL receptor (LDLR)-deficient mice [103]. *OPA1* silencing in HUVECs resulted in reduced endothelial migration and increased oxidative stress, highlighting the role of OPA1 in EC response to laminar flow by reducing oxidative stress [103]. When exposed to disturbed flow, *Opa1* expression was reduced in mouse ECs, indicating that endothelial mitochondria indeed tend to fragment under atherosclerotic conditions [103]. An overview of mitochondrial dynamics can be found at the top right in Figure 3.

Endothelial mitochondrial damage can further be induced by *Porphyromonas gingivalis* (*P. gingivalis*), a pathogen found in atherosclerotic plaques, also elevating mtROS [178] and promoting mitochondrial fragmentation in a DRP1-dependent manner [179]. Mitochondrial impairment in *P. gingivalis*-infected ECs is partially regulated by the rat sarcoma (Ras) homolog family member A/Rho associated coiled-coil containing protein kinase 1 (RhoA/ROCK1) pathway activation, resulting in elevated DRP1 phosphorylation levels at Ser616 and promoting DRP1 mitochondrial translocation [180]. Moreover, mitochondria of infected ECs were characterized by a loss of MMP, lower ATP levels [179], and decreased mtDNA copy numbers [180]. These findings emphasize that damaged mitochondria are prone to shifting mitochondrial dynamics to fission.

Besides regulating mitochondrial dynamics [181,182], DRP1 plays an important role in oxLDL-induced endothelial damage, supporting the development of atherosclerosis [183]. The inhibition of this protein by Mdivi-1, studied both in vivo in apolipoprotein E (ApoE)-/- mice [184] and in vitro in HUVECs [185], resulted in athero-protective effects, which suggests its potential as a therapeutic target for multiple CVDs, including atherosclerosis [182,186]. Moreover, oxLDL directly affects the NLRP3 inflammasome in ECs [158,187]. In in vivo studies utilizing endothelial-specific NLRP3 mutant mice, a notable reduction in atherosclerosis severity was observed [187]. The attenuated disease progression was suggested to be due to a lower ROS generation, thus decreasing apoptotic cell death rates [187].

Although the mechanism behind endothelial mechano-transduction remains elusive, recent studies reported oxidative phosphorylation driving mitochondrial ATP generation upon shear stress [188]. Vascular ECs exposed to flow transduce shear stress into mitochondrial ATP synthesis, activating Ca^{2+} influx via purinoceptors, i.e., purinergic receptors [189], with mitochondria regulating Ca^{2+} homeostasis [190]. Elevated intracellular Ca^{2+} levels stimulate NO generation and, therefore, induce flow-dependent vessel relaxation [191]. Thus, changes in shear stress are associated with cardiovascular disorders, i.e., atherosclerosis [192–194]. Ca^{2+} overload initiates the opening of mPTP, causing tissue damage, including ischemia-reperfusion injury [195]. Recently, it was found that the expression of endothelial mitochondrial Ca^{2+} uniporter (MCU) complex in HUVECs is modulated by shear stress both on gene expression and protein levels, with the most prominent change in mitochondrial Ca^{2+} uniporter regulator 1 (MCUR1) expression (downregulation) under atheroprone, i.e., disturbed, flow [196]. It is suggested that MCUR1 levels regulate the sensitivity of mPTP to mitochondrial Ca^{2+} concentration [196].

The effect of shear stress on endothelial mitochondria depends on shear stress properties [197,198]. On the one hand, laminar shear stress promotes an anti-inflammatory phenotype [199,200] and positively influences endothelial mitochondria [201,202], and, on the other hand, oscillatory shear stress shows pro-inflammatory characteristics in ECs [203]. Oscillatory shear stress causes mitochondrial dysfunction, producing excessive ROS and inflammation in vascular ECs, followed by mitochondrial-induced inflammation [197]. It promotes an inflammatory environment [204] and directly influences plaque formation and stability [205]. In line with these findings, oscillatory shear stress enhances fission but does not support mitophagy in mouse aortic ECs [203]. Enlarged and swollen mitochondria with damaged membranes, fewer cristae, and an abnormal internal arrangement were observed in the ECs of human atherosclerotic plaques through transmission electron microscopy [98].

4.3. Endothelial Mitochondrial Dysfunction in Diabetes Mellitus

Hyperglycemia is a main characteristic of DM, and it is considered a major contributor to endothelial dysfunction, a detrimental event in the pathogenesis of DM-associated micro- and macro-vasculopathies [206]. High intracellular glucose increases ROS levels in ECs, ultimately leading to cell and tissue injury [207]. As ECs rely mainly on glycolysis for their energy source, mitochondria are essential for Ca^{2+} homeostasis and ROS generation. Overproduction of ROS by the mitochondrial ETC caused by hyperglycemia affects various aspects of mitochondrial function, as discussed in the Sections 3.3 and 4.1. Hyperglycemia-induced endothelial mitochondrial dysfunction ultimately leads to mitochondria-dependent apoptosis [208].

In fact, mitochondrial fragmentation has been identified in ECs isolated from the arm vein of diabetic patients [209] and in retinal and coronary ECs of diabetic rodents [210,211]. These changes in diabetic patients and mice, which correlated with increased FIS1 and DRP1 levels, respectively [209,211], were also observed in aortic ECs cultured under hyperglycemic conditions [209]. Diabetic retinopathy is also associated with disturbed mitochondrial dynamics in human retinal ECs, where the acetylation of MFN2 protein plays a role [212]. However, hyperglycemia also affects other mitochondrial aspects, such as mtDNA repair mechanisms, which are impaired in hyperglycemia. Moreover, downregulation of the lncRNA *lncCytB* is involved in mitochondrial genomic stability and is reduced in streptozotocin (STZ)-induced diabetic mice and human donors with retinopathy [213].

In addition to these isolated effects of DM on the endothelium, hyperglycemia exacerbates mitochondrial dysfunction in ECs in CVD. Mitochondrial fragmentation occurs in hemorrhagic transformation after middle cerebral artery occlusion, but only under conditions of hyperglycemia, i.e., in STZ-induced diabetic mice [214]. In line with these findings, mtROS production is impaired in saphenous veins of coronary artery disease (CAD) when patients are also diabetic [215]. Thus, the endothelial dysfunction induced by hyperglycemic insults in DM multiplies the patient's cardiovascular risk.

4.4. Endothelial Mitochondrial Dysfunction in Neurodegenerative Disorders

Several NDDs are characterized by endothelial dysfunction [216–219]. Moreover, the risk for dementia is increased by CVRFs, such as obesity, physical inactivity, and smoking [220]. Notably, endothelial mitochondrial dysfunction was associated with the development and progression of several NDDs [19,100,138,218].

The blood brain barrier (BBB) poses a significant challenge in the context of endothelial dysfunction in NDDs, which mediates brain homeostasis [221] and consists of ECs, mural cells, including pericytes and VSMC, and astrocytes [216]. Brain microvascular ECs (BMECs) are directly in contact with circulating factors [221] and, due to their unique features, have a decisive role in maintaining the BBB. Highly developed TJs [222] ensure low BBB permeability and high mitochondria content [138,223,224]. Moreover, BMECs are special regarding their mitochondria. Already in 1977, a distinct difference in endothelial mitochondria abundance, dependent on their properties, was described in rats [224]. The endothelial cytoplasmic volume of the BBB comprises 8–11% of mitochondria, whilst capillary ECs from non-BBB regions have fewer mitochondria, occupying only 2–5% of the cytoplasm [224]. This implicates a higher metabolic activity and capacity and highlights a particular role of mitochondria in the physiology and pathology of ECs from the BBB [224].

In fact, the dominating role of mitochondrial oxidative stress in BMECs and its contribution to BBB damage was recently reviewed by Wang et al. [100]. Mitochondrial ROS [225,226] and oxidized mtDNA [227,228], together with CytC [229], n-formyl peptide [230], and cardiolipins [231] released in the cytoplasm, are recognized as DAMPs and trigger inflammatory responses in BMECs [100,138,232]. The NLRP3 inflammasome is activated by mtROS or mtDNA [227] or through binding to the CD36 membrane receptor, which further activates NF-κB [138]. As an inflammatory response, ECs express cellular adhesion molecules (CAMs), including vascular and intracellular CAMs (VCAM and ICAM), which also stimulate the NLRP3 inflammasome to release pro-inflammatory cytokines, causing BBB injury [138]. The mtDAMP-induced inflammatory response in cerebral ECs (CECs) was also extensively reviewed [138,232]. In addition, lipopolysaccharide (LPS) can efficiently contribute to BBB leakage by triggering an inflammatory response [233] and also by inducing mitochondrial dysfunction [234]. LPS impairs mitochondrial oxidative phosphorylation and reduces mitochondrial function in CECs [234]. Furthermore, by inhibiting oxidative phosphorylation, ECs suffer from TJ disruption [234] and high oxidative stress, promoting mitochondrial fragmentation due to Drp1 activation, which increases BBB permeability [235]. The important role of cerebral endothelial mitochondria for BBB integrity was also shown in vivo through pharmacological mitochondrial inhibition [234]. A disrupted BBB can exacerbate the deposition of disease-specific toxic substances, including amyloid β (Aβ), α-synuclein, fibrin, neurotoxins, and pathogens, with mitochondria being involved in multiple pathological processes leading to unfavorable BBB changes [100].

Alzheimer's disease (AD) is an NDD that progresses with age; it has the strongest causality for dementia. It is characterized by Aβ accumulation, which leads to plaque formation [236]. Mitochondrial dysfunction has also been proposed as the potential primary cause of AD [237].

In fact, among all cellular organelles, mitochondria are most susceptible to Aβ-induced dysfunction [238]. Exposure of mouse brain capillary ECs to Aβ causes increased oxidative phosphorylation, cellular respiration characterized by accelerated oxygen consumption, and mitochondrial superoxide anion generation, potentially generating oxidative damage [239]. All of these changes are accompanied by elevated mitochondrial Ca^{2+} concentration, with the Ca^{2+} influx regulated by multiple pathways stimulating ROS production and, consequently, mitochondrial dysfunction [239]. Complexing Ca^{2+} with EDTA not only abolished mitochondrial activity dysregulation but prevented morphological changes (superoxide anion-induced fragmentation) and apoptotic cell death, indicating the cytotoxic properties of mitochondrial Ca^{2+}-overload [239]. In addition, ECs exposed to Aβ peptides had elevated ROS levels, further contributing to BBB damage [240]. Moreover, Aβ peptides (unmodified, isomerized, and phosphorylated) diversely impact mitochondrial function in vitro, with isomerized Aβ causing the most adverse outcomes: high oxidative stress, cytotoxicity, and increased mitochondrial potential and respiration. This indicates that post-translational Aβ modifications affect endothelial BBB cells [240]. Interestingly, the long-lasting destructive impact of Aβ on mitochondrial respiration capacity is strongest under hypoglycemia in primary human brain ECs, elucidating the underlying mechanism cohering dysglycemia and AD in DM [241]. In Aβ-challenged CECs, H_2O_2 synthesis is upregulated together with mitochondrial membrane depolarization [242]. Aβ uptake in endothelial mitochondria is hindered by Coenzyme Q10 (CoQ10), an antioxidant lipophilic coenzyme showing cytoprotective properties [243]. The detrimental impact of Aβ on mitochondria and BBB was also described in humans [244]. Notably, human cerebral microvasculature is characterized by mitochondrial loss in AD [245]. The first in vivo study with transgenic mice investigating mitochondrial abnormalities occurring close to Aβ plaques was published in 2013 [246], which demonstrated that mitochondria proximal to dense Aβ plaques reveal structural and functional abnormalities, including reduced MMP, swollen and dystrophic morphology, and increased mitochondrial loss and fragmentation [246].

Although AD is probably the most prominent and best-studied example of the relationship between mitochondrial dysfunction in ECs and NDDs, it is not a unique phenomenon. Vascular dementia (VD), for example, is caused by CVRFs and is associated with endothelial dysfunction and cardiovascular problems throughout the body. Also, in VD, an implication of mitochondrial dysfunction in ECs is suggested [218]. These findings emphasize the contribution of endothelial mitochondrial dysfunction to the development and progression of NDDs, and targeting mitochondria in this regard is of relevant therapeutic potential.

5. Endothelial Progenitor Cells in Health and Disease

Due to the limited regenerative potential of mature vascular ECs, circulating EPCs, which mainly derive from hematopoietic stem cells in the bone marrow [247], can be recruited to support endothelial recovery during vascular growth and repair [24]. In vitro, two main types of EPCs are classified. 'Early' EPCs emerge soon after isolation, show a spindle-shaped morphology, proliferate slowly, and have an in vitro life span of only about one month. Early EPCs support the existing endothelium in a paracrine way [23,248]. 'Late' EPCs, i.e., ECFCs, are progenitor-derived cells that grow out in culture after several days and form colonies of mature ECs with a cobblestone morphology. ECFCs can form de novo vessels in vitro and in vivo [23,248]. Regardless of completed differentiation, ECFCs still exhibit progenitor cell features. Despite sharing the same phenotype and morphology with mature ECs, e.g., HUVECs, ECFCs not only proliferate faster but also react more sensitive towards angiogenic factors, highlighting their importance in neovascularization and repair mechanisms [249] (Figure 2). Additionally, ECFCs are characterized by high clonogenic potential (colony-forming ability). Differentiated to mature ECs, ECFCs express endothelial markers including CD31, vWF, vascular endothelial (VE)-Cadherin (CD144), CD146, and VEGFR2, and are negative for the leukocyte and monocyte markers CD45 and CD14. Expression of CD34, a marker for vascular EPCs, diminishes throughout in vitro culture [23,250,251]. ECFCs have the ability to home to ischemic tissue and initiate neovascularization [252]. The angiogenic capacity of ECFCs is facilitated by their ability to form new vessels and to release paracrine factors that promote and support vascular repair [250].

ECFCs can be isolated from peripheral or umbilical cordblood (UCB) by culturing mononuclear cells under endothelial-specific conditions [23,251,252]. The cell number is about 15-fold higher in UCB compared to adult peripheral blood, with neonatal ECFCs also showing faster outgrowth [253]. Due to their minimally invasive isolation method, ECFCs enable personalized patient-related studies on endothelial function and dysfunction [254].

5.1. Endothelial Progenitor Cells and Cardiovascular Risk Factors: Implications for Cardiovascular Disease and Diabetes

Similar to mature vascular ECs, EPCs are susceptible to CVRFs. The number EPC is reduced in peripheral blood in type I and type II DM and exhibit functional abnormalities [255,256], which worsen throughout the course of DM [255]. Moreover, EPCs from diabetic patients differ regarding in vitro cultivation. For instance, isolated ECFCs from T2DM patients show impaired colony outgrowth, less tube formation, decreased proliferation, migration, and impaired in vivo neovascularization (the latter was shown in an animal model) [25,257]. Notably, improved glycemic control also positively impacts EPC numbers and improves the function of differentiated ECFCs [256,258]. Furthermore, the number of EPCs inversely correlates with body mass index (BMI) [259,260] and levels of insulin, leptin, and C-reactive protein (CRP) [260], with ECFCs originating from obese patients showing a slower proliferation rate [260].

These findings indicate that CVRFs have long term effects on circulating EPCs, or even their stem cell precursors (Figure 4). The underlying mechanisms may include epigenetic changes [261,262] as well as covalent modifications of cell components, i.e., oxidative damage of biomolecules, including proteins and lipids, which may lead to potentially irreversible and adverse consequences [263]. Additionally, oxidative DNA damage can induce either permanent genetic or epigenetic changes [264], that might be passed on daughter cells through cell division.

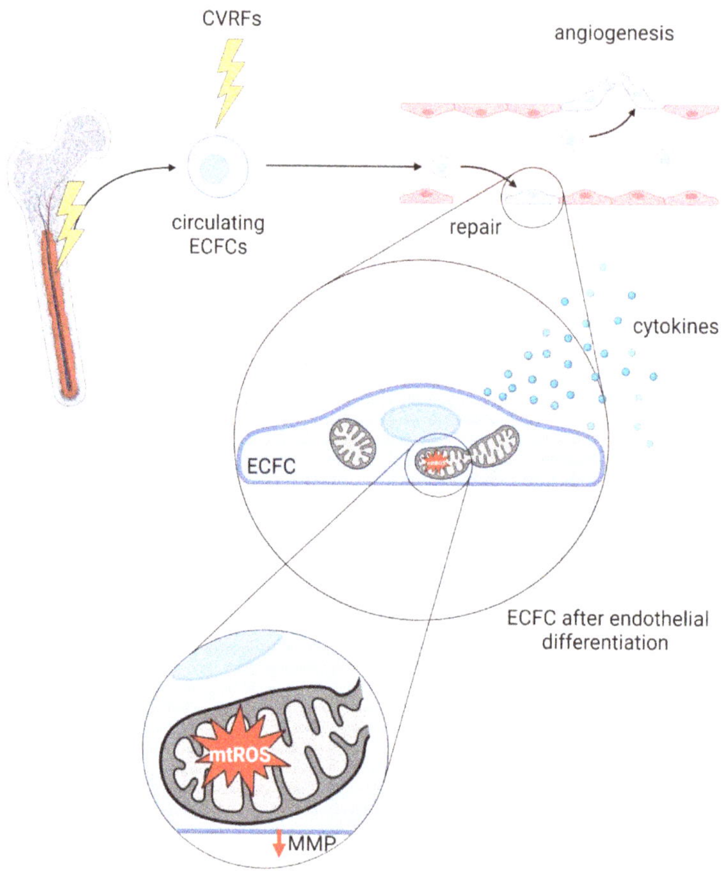

Figure 4. Exposure of endothelial progenitor cells to cardiovascular risk factors disturbs mitochondrial function in the differentiated endothelial cells. Exposure of circulating endothelial progenitor cells (EPCs) and progenitor cells in the bone marrow to cardiovascular risk factors (CVRFs) modulates their mitochondrial function in the long term. Thus, after recruiting the progenitors to the vascular wall, the differentiated endothelial cells remain with dysfunctional mitochondria, elevated reactive oxygen species (ROS) production, reduced mitochondrial membrane potential (MMP), and increased cytokine release. The figure was created using BioRender.com, accessed on 22 January 2024.

5.2. Endothelial Progenitor Cells and Cardiovascular Risk Factors in Pregnancy: Programming of Future Health

In pregnancy, maternal CVRFs may also act on the fetus and affect fetal UCB-derived EPCs. For instance, maternal metabolic state affects EPC function and number. Moreover, maternal pre-pregnancy BMI highjacks the number of fetal UCB-EPCs [265]. Additionally, we have previously demonstrated that during pregnancy, a higher fasting blood glucose within a healthy, non-diabetic range is associated with delayed colony outgrowth of fetal ECFCs [266]. However, there are inconsistencies in the literature regarding the effect of gestational diabetes mellitus (GDM) on fetal EPCs [267]. Several studies reported decreased ECFC colonies with impaired migration and tube formation, accompanied by enhanced cellular senescence and reduced proliferation [26,268]. Others, however, revealed higher proliferation of GDM-derived ECFCs, although with preserved reduced network-formation capacity [269]. In addition, similar outcomes were obtained in fetal EPCs derived from pregnancies complicated by preeclampsia [267]. Findings, such as the developmental programming concept and the Developmental Origins of Health and Disease (DOHaD) paradigm, that describe future susceptibility to disease based on prenatal influences contribute to better understanding of CVD programming in utero.

Thus, circulating EPCs are sensitive to CVRFs, and their acquired impairments may persist even after their recruitment and differentiation to ECs. However, the specific involvement of mitochondria in ECFC dysfunction has remained unexplored.

5.3. *Endothelial Progenitor Cells in Neurodegenerative Disorders*

Early in its disease progression, AD is characterized by the appearance of vascular alterations and BBB disruption [216,244,270,271]. In fact, animal studies in rodents have shown that ECFCs-injections have beneficial effects on plaque deposition and memory [272,273]. Human studies also indicate a role of ECFCs in NDDs, however with variable as well as contradictory results, reporting increased [274], unchanged [275,276], or decreased cell numbers [277,278], possibly due to limited cohort sizes. A new study with over 1500 subjects—currently only published as a preprint—shows a correlation between the number of circulating ECFCs and a reduced risk of AD [279].

ECFC mitochondria in AD have not been investigated so far. As mentioned, CVRFs are affecting ECFCs and therefore, lower cardiovascular risk is associated with slower progression, i.e., cognitive decline, in the general population [280]. Due to the fact that CVRFs cause mitochondrial dysfunction in ECFCs, a link between mitochondrial dysfunction in ECFCs and AD, underlining the importance of future research in this field is suggested.

6. Role of Mitochondria in Endothelial Progenitor Cell Dysfunction

As ECFC number and function are sensitive to CVRFs, CVRFs could—similarly to vascular, mature ECs—disrupt mitochondrial function in ECFCs. In fact, mitochondria of senescent human ECFCs demonstrate an elongated shape associated with increased oxidative stress, reduced ATP levels, and decreased mitochondrial fission, as observed by lower FIS1 levels. The same senescent phenotype was induced by *FIS1* silencing in young (low-passage) ECFCs, which demonstrate reduced proliferation activity, denoting the role of FIS1 in mitochondrial and endothelial dysfunction in an aging model [281].

Besides the role of mitochondria in ECFC aging, studies show mitochondrial alterations in ECFCs in patients or animal models with endothelial dysfunction. ECFCs of patients suffering from recurrent venous thromboembolic disease, a condition characterized by impaired endothelial function, reveal elevated ROS levels, cytokine release, and abnormalities in the organization of mitochondrial cristae, with no changes in network formation [282]. ECFCs of hypertensive patients with capillary rarefaction show swollen mitochondria with a loss of mitochondrial cristae, molecularly accompanied by increased ROS and NADH levels. Additionally, mitochondrial bioenergetics are impaired, with decreased oxygen consumption rates (OCR) and reduced MMP. These alterations are paralleled by impaired migration and adhesion of ECFCs and less CXCR4/JAK2/SIRT5 signaling, a pathway involved in mitochondrial metabolic function [283]. Similar results were found in ECFCs differentiated from bone-marrow-derived EPCs of an atherosclerotic mouse model evidencing mitochondrial dysfunction, as revealed by increased size with distorted cristae and elevated mitochondrial superoxide anion generation [284]. Altered mitochondrial function has also been observed in ECFCs isolated from patients with CAD, as demonstrated by higher superoxide anion production. ECFCs derived from CAD patients also possess increased network formation on Matrigel besides migratory and proliferative capacities compared to ECFCs from individuals without CAD [285], highlighting the relationship between mitochondrial and endothelial function. Mitochondrial morphology was, however, not investigated in that study. ECFCs of type II diabetic patients show increased mitochondrial fragmentation and dysregulation of proteins involved in mitochondrial dynamics [286]. Furthermore, and as mentioned before, diabetic ECFCs are functionally compromised, with reduced proliferation, tube formation, and weakened survival capacities [25,257]. However, upregulated expression of nuclear factor erythroid 2–related factor 2 (*NRF2*), a transcription factor involved in redox balance, seems to counteract these DM-induced effects in ECFCs from diabetic patients. and in ECFCs differentiated from bone-marrow-derived EPCs of diabetic mice by regulating the transcription of *IDH2* [286]. The relationship between the metabolic state and mitochondrial function of ECFCs is further highlighted by a study using db/db diabetic mice, a model of T2DM. The study investigated mitochondrial function, i.e., MMP, of bone marrow-derived ECFCs in the bone marrow as a source, in the circulation, and in the retina, where ECFCs are potentially recruited to repair and counteract retinopathy. The decreased MMP of diabetic mice ECFCs is paralleled by impaired peroxisome proliferator-activated receptor alpha (PPARα) levels [287]. The link between the action of CVRFs, circulating EPCs, and mitochondrial dysfunction in the differentiated ECFCs is illustrated in Figure 4.

Further evidence highlighting the relationship between metabolism, oxidative stress, and ECFC function comes from studies investigating the effect of hyperlipidemia on ECFCs. Increased Nox-derived ROS production is characteristic of hyperlipidemic rats and was associated with reduced ECFC adhesion and migration [288]. This link between NOX activity, ROS, and reduced ECFC function was also found in hyperlipidemic patients, where NOX2 and NOX4 RNA expression and protein levels are increased in ECFCs, which is associated with reduced ECFC adhesion, migration, and tube formation [289].

Apart from the earlier described detrimental effects that pathologies cause in the mitochondrial function of ECFCs, in vitro experiments also highlight the interplay of mitochondrial function and ROS with ECFC function [290] in physiology. For instance, in vitro experiments have demonstrated that the pulsatile pressure within the blood vessels promotes vascular homing of ECFCs, both by stimulating adhesion and endothelial differentiation. Cyclic stretch, when applied to ECFCs, decreases the content of long-chain fatty acids (LCFAs) and induces the expression of long-chain fatty acyl-CoA synthetase 1 (*ACSL1*), which facilitates the catabolism of LCFAs in mitochondria via fatty acid oxidation and oxidative phosphorylation [290]. Transplantation of ECFCs overexpressing *ACSL1* into a rat carotid artery injury model enhances ECFC adhesion and endothelialization. Furthermore, ROS signaling within the physiological range has positive effects on ECFC function: Action of NOX4, the major ROS-producing enzyme in ECFCs, stimulates angiogenesis in these cells by upregulating pro-angiogenic factors linked with eNOS signaling [291], highlighting the importance of fine-tuning mitochondrial metabolism for ECFC function.

The role of mitochondria in the angiogenesis of rat ECFCs has been further emphasized by the fact that pyruvate kinase M2 (Pkm2), a protein responsible for energy metabolism and mitochondrial morphology, promotes ECFC angiogenesis through modulation of glycolysis, mitochondrial fission, and fusion [292]. Further evidence relating mitochondrial function to angiogenesis of ECFCs comes from a study using very low-density lipoprotein receptor knockout mice as a model of ocular neovascularisation induced by Wnt signaling overactivation. The study revealed that circulating EPCs of this mouse model possess higher MMP, with isolated ECFCs showing increased mitochondrial function and biogenesis, as well as a more active state towards endothelial differentiation [293].

As pointed out in this critical review, recent studies clearly show that despite the relatively low number of mitochondria in ECs, mitochondrial dysfunction and ROS are major contributors to endothelial dysfunction. In regard to EPCs and ECFCs, respectively, there are less data available, but these also suggest that mitochondrial function is essential for ECFC physiology and pathology. In summary, the evidence supports the proposition that mitochondrial dysfunction in ECFCs and ECs is intricately linked to endothelial dysfunction and CVD pathogenesis. However, whether this also applies to NDDs, such as AD, remains to be investigated.

7. Mitochondria-Targeted Therapeutic Strategies to Improve Endothelial Function

In recent years, several strategies aiming to restore optimal mitochondrial function have emerged. Notable approaches include using mitochondrial-targeted antioxidants, mitophagy inducers, and mitochondrial biogenesis enhancers. The mitochondrial-targeted antioxidants are compounds specifically targeting mtROS and counteracting oxidative stress. By restoring redox balance, these compounds hold promise for mitigating mitochondrial impairment in ECFCs and ECs, thus ultimately thwarting CVD progression. MtROS overproduction can be hindered, for example, by mitoquinone (MitoQ) [294], a mitochondria-targeting antioxidant accumulating within the organelle and neutralizing oxidative stress [294]. Findings from a randomized controlled trial revealed that acute oral intake of MitoQ restored mitochondrial function and improved endothelial function in patients suffering from peripheral artery disease [295]. Acute and, importantly, chronic intake of MitoQ delivered promising results in elderly adults [296]. In an ex vivo model, exposure of human aortic ECs (HAECs) to plasma from MitoQ-treated adults reduced mtROS, lowered circulating oxLDL levels, and improved endothelial properties [206]. Other promising mitotropic molecules are SkQ1 [297–300], MitoTEMPO [301], SS-31 [302,303], and AntiOxCIN4 [304–306]. As discussed, enhancing mitophagy can prevent the accumulation of dysfunctional mitochondria, preserve cellular health, and improve EPC and EC function. Rapamycin [307,308], urolithin A [309], carbonyl cyanide m-chlorophenyl hydrazone (CCCP) [310], and PTEN-induced kinase 1 (PINK1)/parkin pathway activators [311] were described as potential mitophagy inducers. Another therapeutic strategy is using mitochondrial biogenesis enhancers to facilitate mitochondrial function. That would allow for replenishing the pool of functional mitochondria, bolstering cellular energy production, and combating dysfunction. Resveratrol, PPARγ, Adenosine monophosphate (AMP)-activated protein kinase (AMPK) activators, carnitine, berberine, exercise, and starvation have been described as mitochondrial biogenesis activators [312–318].

Implementing these strategies carries profound implications for comprehending the pathogenesis of CVD and NDDs and formulating therapeutic approaches. Directing attention toward mitigating mitochondrial dysfunction provides an innovative perspective for addressing the fundamental mechanisms fueling endothelial dysfunction. By reinstating optimal mitochondrial function within EPCs and ECs, the progression of endothelial dysfunction, atherosclerosis, other cardiovascular complications, and NDDs may potentially be abated.

8. Conclusions and Future Perspectives

Endothelial dysfunction resulting from the action of CVRFs underlies and contributes to various non-communicable and age-related diseases, including CVD, NDDs, and metabolic diseases. CVD, for instance, has been categorized by the WHO as the disease with the highest mortality worldwide [319]. The relationship between CVRFs, mitochondrial and endothelial dysfunction highlights that a profound understanding of endothelial mitochondrial damage is crucial to improve the prevention and treatment of CVD and NDDs. Until now the role of ECFCs in CVD and NDDs is not yet fully understood. However, the fact that not only ECs but also circulating ECFCs and even their precursors located, for instance, in the bone marrow, are damaged by CVRFs demonstrates the harm that CVRFs exert on the vasculature. Circulating ECFCs would normally be responsible for endothelial repair and recovery. It is, therefore, all the more important to understand the cellular processes of CVD and other non-communicable diseases to develop possible therapies.

Within the framework of the DOHaD concept, an intriguing question surfaces: Can mitochondrial dysfunction be orchestrated by early influential factors in utero? This perspective aligns with the notion that events occurring during critical developmental stages might exert a lasting impact on mitochondrial health, consequently contributing to the trajectory of endothelial, cardiovascular, and neuronal health or susceptibility to disease later in life [320]. This introduces an additional layer of complexity when striving to address CVD. It is imperative to account for the fact that a significant proportion of the proposed strategies to enhance mitochondrial function have not undergone testing during pregnancy, except for exercise [321–326] and MitoQ [327–329], nor has the particular effect on ECs or EPCs been evaluated.

Future research endeavors should delve deeper into the mechanisms that contribute to mitochondrial dysfunction in EPCs and ECs. Additionally, clinical translation of these strategies requires rigorous testing in preclinical models and human trials to validate their efficacy, safety, and long-term benefits. As our understanding of mitochondrial involvement in endothelial dysfunction deepens, successfully translating these approaches could revolutionize cardiovascular therapeutics, potentially leading to more effective strategies for managing and preventing CVD and NDDs.

Author Contributions: Writing—original draft preparation, all authors; writing—review and editing, all authors; visualization, A.K.-S., E.W., U.H. All authors have read and agreed to the published version of the manuscript.

Funding: A.K.-S. and E.W. were funded by the Austrian Science Fund (FWF) by the project KLI 1023 (to UH). C.T., M.S.D. and S.P.P. were funded by the ERDF funds through the Operational Programme for Competitiveness-COMPETE 2020 and national funds from the Foundation for Science and Technology under the FCT—doctoral Fellowship (CT, SFRH/BD/11924/2022), (MSD, SFRH/BD/11934/2022), FCT—Post-doctoral Fellowship (SPP, SFRH/BPD/116061/2016), project grant HORIZON-HLTH-2022-STAYHLTH-101080329; PTDC/DTP-DES/1082/2014 (POCI-01-0145-FEDER-016657), and strategic projects UIDB/04539/2020, UIDP/04539/2020, LA/P/0058/2020, UIDB/00617/2020: doi:10.54499/UIDB/00617/2020, and UIDP/00617/2020: doi: 10.54499/UIDP/00617/2020. C.T.M.-S. was funded by the Austrian Science Fund (FWF) (P 36235, P 36591, FG 24, WKP 235). The views and opinions expressed are, however, those of the author(s) only and do not necessarily reflect those of the European Union or the Health and Digital Executive Agency. Neither the European Union nor the granting authority can be held responsible for them. The funding agencies had no role in the study design, data collection and analysis, decision to publish, or preparation of this document.

Institutional Review Board Statement: Not applicable.

Informed Consent Statement: Not applicable.

Data Availability Statement: Not applicable.

Conflicts of Interest: The authors declare no conflicts of interest.

Abbreviations

OGDH—2-oxoglutarate dehydrogenase; acetyl-CoA—acetyl-coenzyme A; ATF6—activating transcription factor-6; ADP—adenosine diphosphate; AMP—Adenosine monophosphate; ATP—adenosine triphosphate; AJs—adherence junctions; AGE—advanced glycation end products; RAGE—AGE receptor; AD—Alzheimer's disease; AMPK—AMP-activated protein kinase; Aβ—amyloid β; AngII—angiotensin II; BCL2—B-cell lymphoma 2; BAX—BCL2-like protein 4; BBB—blood-brain barrier; BMI—body mass index; BK—bradykinin; BMECs—Brain microvascular ECs; BCKDH—branched chain keto acid dehydrogenase; Ca^{2+}—calcium; CCCP—carbonyl cyanide m-chlorophenyl hydrazone; CVD—cardiovascular disease; CVRFs—cardiovascular risk factors; CAT—catalase; CAMs—cellular adhesion molecules; CECs—cerebral ECs; CoQ10—Coenzyme Q10; CAD—coronary artery disease; CRP—C-reactive protein; cGMP—cyclic guanosine monophosphate; CytC—cytochrome C; COX4I2—cytochrome c oxidase 4 isoform 2; DAMPs—damage-associated molecular patterns; DOHaD—Developmental Origins of Health and Disease; DM—diabetes mellitus; DHODH—dihydroorotate dehydrogenase; DRP1—dynamin-related protein 1; ETFDH—electron transfer flavoprotein dehydrogenase; ETC—electron transport chain; ER—endoplasmic reticulum; ECs—Endothelial cells; ECFCs—endothelial colony-forming cells; eNOS—endothelial nitric oxide synthase; EPCs—Endothelial progenitor cells; ET-1—endothelin-1; ERO1—ER oxidoreductin; FeIII—ferric iron; FeII—ferrous iron; FADH2—flavin adenine dinucleotide; FMN—flavin mononucleotide; GJs—Gap junctions; GDM—gestational diabetes mellitus; GLUT—glucose transporters; GPX1-7—glutathione peroxidases; GPD—glycerol-3-phosphate dehydrogenase; HOX1-2—heme oxygenases; HUVECs—human umbilical vein ECs; H2O2—hydrogen peroxide; OH^-—hydroxyl anion; $^{\bullet}OH$—hydroxyl radical; HIF1a—hypoxia-inducible factor-1 a; IRE1—inositol-requiring protein-1; IL—interleukin; ICAM—intracellular CAM; IDH2—isocitrate dehydrogenase $NADP^+$ 2; LDLR—LDL receptor; LPS—lipopolysaccharide; lncRNA—long non-coding RNAs; ACADL—

long-chain acyl-CoA dehydrogenase; LCFAs—long-chain fatty acids; ACSL1—long-chain fatty acyl-CoA synthetase 1; LDL—low-density lipoprotein; MFN—membrane proteins mitofusin; metHb—methemoglobin; miRNA—microRNAs; MCU—mitochondrial Ca^{2+} uniporter; MCUR1—mitochondrial Ca^{2+} uniporter regulator 1; Mdivi-1—mitochondrial division inhibitor 1; mtDNA—mitochondrial DNA; MID—mitochondrial dynamic proteins; MFF—mitochondrial fission factor; FIS1—mitochondrial fission protein 1; MMP—mitochondrial membrane potential; mPTP—mitochondrial permeability transition pore; MQC—mitochondrial quality control; mtROS—mitochondrial ROS; MitoQ—mitoquinone; NQO1—NADPH quinone dehydrogenase 1; NDUFA4L2—NADH dehydrogenase ubiquinone 1 alpha subcomplex, 4-like 2; NOX—NADPH oxidase; NDDs—neurodegenerative disorders; NADH—nicotinamide adenine dinucleotide; NADPH—nicotinamide adenine dinucleotide phosphate; NO—nitric oxide; NLRP3—nod-like receptor family pyrin domain-containing 3; NRF2—nuclear factor erythroid 2-related factor 2; NFκB—nuclear factor kappa B; OPA1—optic atrophy protein 1; oxLDL—oxidized LDL; OCR—oxygen consumption rates; HbO2—oxyhemoglobin HbO2; PARK2—Parkin; PRR—pattern recognition receptors; PPAR α/γ—Peroxisome Proliferator-Activated Receptor PPAR Alpha/Gamma; $ONOO^-$—peroxynitrite anion; PAI-1—plasminogen activator inhibitor-1; *P. gingivalis*—*Porphyromonas gingivalis*; PRODH—proline dehydrogenase; PGI2—prostacyclin; PGH2—prostaglandin H2; PERK—protein kinase RNA PKR-like ER kinase; PINK1—PTEN-induced kinase 1; PDH—pyruvate dehydrogenase; Pkm2—pyruvate kinase M2; Q-cycle—quinol cycle; RhoA—Ras homolog family member A; Ras—rat sarcoma; ROS—reactive oxygen species; RBCs—red blood cells; ROCK1—Rho associated coiled-coil containing protein kinase 1; Sirt1—sirtuin 1 lysine deacetylase; SMCs—smooth muscle cells; sGC—soluble guanylyl cyclase; STZ—streptozotocin; SRXN1—sulfiredoxin 1; $O_2^{\bullet-}$—superoxide anion; SOD—superoxide dismutase; TXN—thioredoxin; TXA2—thromboxane A2; TJs—tight junctions; tPA—tissue plasminogen activator; TCA—tricarboxylic acid; TNFα—tumor necrosis factor alpha; T2DM—type II DM; UCB—Umbilical cordblood; UCP2—uncoupling protein 2; UPR—unfolded protein response; VCAM—vascular CAM; VD—Vascular dementia; (VE)-Cadherin—vascular endothelial Cadherin; VEGF—vascular endothelial growth factor; VSMCs—vascular SMCs; VEGFR2—VEGF receptor 2; ACDVL—very long-chain acyl-CoA dehydrogenase; vWF—von Willebrand factor; XDH—xanthine dehydrogenase; XO—xanthine oxidase.

References

1. Koenig, W. Low-Grade Inflammation Modifies Cardiovascular Risk Even at Very Low LDL-C Levels: Are We Aiming for a Dual Target Concept? *Circulation* **2018**, *138*, 150–153. [CrossRef]
2. Rodgers, J.L.; Jones, J.; Bolleddu, S.I.; Vanthenapalli, S.; Rodgers, L.E.; Shah, K.; Karia, K.; Panguluri, S.K. Cardiovascular Risks Associated with Gender and Aging. *J. Cardiovasc. Dev. Dis.* **2019**, *6*, 19. [CrossRef] [PubMed]
3. Benincasa, G.; Coscioni, E.; Napoli, C. Cardiovascular risk factors and molecular routes underlying endothelial dysfunction: Novel opportunities for primary prevention. *Biochem. Pharmacol.* **2022**, *202*, 115108. [CrossRef]
4. Incalza, M.A.; D'Oria, R.; Natalicchio, A.; Perrini, S.; Laviola, L.; Giorgino, F. Oxidative stress and reactive oxygen species in endothelial dysfunction associated with cardiovascular and metabolic diseases. *Vascul. Pharmacol.* **2018**, *100*, 1–19. [CrossRef]
5. Rajendran, P.; Rengarajan, T.; Thangavel, J.; Nishigaki, Y.; Sakthisekaran, D.; Sethi, G.; Nishigaki, I. The vascular endothelium and human diseases. *Int. J. Biol. Sci.* **2013**, *9*, 1057–1069. [CrossRef] [PubMed]
6. Dal Canto, E.; Ceriello, A.; Ryden, L.; Ferrini, M.; Hansen, T.B.; Schnell, O.; Standl, E.; Beulens, J.W. Diabetes as a cardiovascular risk factor: An overview of global trends of macro and micro vascular complications. *Eur. J. Prev. Cardiol.* **2019**, *26*, 25–32. [CrossRef]
7. Higashi, Y.; Maruhashi, T.; Noma, K.; Kihara, Y. Oxidative stress and endothelial dysfunction: Clinical evidence and therapeutic implications. *Trends Cardiovasc. Med.* **2014**, *24*, 165–169. [CrossRef]
8. Roth, G.A.; Mensah, G.A.; Johnson, C.O.; Addolorato, G.; Ammirati, E.; Baddour, L.M.; Barengo, N.C.; Beaton, A.Z.; Benjamin, E.J.; Benziger, C.P.; et al. Global Burden of Cardiovascular Diseases and Risk Factors, 1990–2019: Update From the GBD 2019 Study. *J. Am. Coll. Cardiol.* **2020**, *76*, 2982–3021. [CrossRef]
9. Zhang, D.X.; Gutterman, D.D. Mitochondrial reactive oxygen species-mediated signaling in endothelial cells. *Am. J. Physiol. Heart Circ. Physiol.* **2007**, *292*, H2023–H2031. [CrossRef] [PubMed]
10. Juan, C.A.; Perez de la Lastra, J.M.; Plou, F.J.; Perez-Lebena, E. The Chemistry of Reactive Oxygen Species (ROS) Revisited: Outlining Their Role in Biological Macromolecules (DNA, Lipids and Proteins) and Induced Pathologies. *Int. J. Mol. Sci.* **2021**, *22*, 4642. [CrossRef]
11. Schieber, M.; Chandel, N.S. ROS function in redox signaling and oxidative stress. *Curr. Biol.* **2014**, *24*, R453–R462. [CrossRef] [PubMed]

12. Heinrich, J. Cardiotocography practice. Case 16. *Zentralbl. Gynakol.* **1988**, *110*, 1604–1605. [PubMed]
13. Ward, J.P.T. From Physiological Redox Signalling to Oxidant Stress. *Adv. Exp. Med. Biol.* **2017**, *967*, 335–342. [CrossRef]
14. Magnani, N.D.; Marchini, T.; Calabro, V.; Alvarez, S.; Evelson, P. Role of Mitochondria in the Redox Signaling Network and Its Outcomes in High Impact Inflammatory Syndromes. *Front. Endocrinol.* **2020**, *11*, 568305. [CrossRef] [PubMed]
15. Galati, D.; Srinivasan, S.; Raza, H.; Prabu, S.K.; Hardy, M.; Chandran, K.; Lopez, M.; Kalyanaraman, B.; Avadhani, N.G. Role of nuclear-encoded subunit Vb in the assembly and stability of cytochrome c oxidase complex: Implications in mitochondrial dysfunction and ROS production. *Biochem. J.* **2009**, *420*, 439–449. [CrossRef]
16. Miwa, S.; Kashyap, S.; Chini, E.; von Zglinicki, T. Mitochondrial dysfunction in cell senescence and aging. *J. Clin. Investig.* **2022**, *132*, e158447. [CrossRef]
17. Wada, J.; Nakatsuka, A. Mitochondrial Dynamics and Mitochondrial Dysfunction in Diabetes. *Acta Med. Okayama* **2016**, *70*, 151–158. [CrossRef] [PubMed]
18. De Mello, A.H.; Costa, A.B.; Engel, J.D.G.; Rezin, G.T. Mitochondrial dysfunction in obesity. *Life Sci.* **2018**, *192*, 26–32. [CrossRef]
19. Parodi-Rullan, R.; Sone, J.Y.; Fossati, S. Endothelial Mitochondrial Dysfunction in Cerebral Amyloid Angiopathy and Alzheimer's Disease. *J. Alzheimer's Dis.* **2019**, *72*, 1019–1039. [CrossRef]
20. Chistiakov, D.A.; Shkurat, T.P.; Melnichenko, A.A.; Grechko, A.V.; Orekhov, A.N. The role of mitochondrial dysfunction in cardiovascular disease: A brief review. *Ann. Med.* **2018**, *50*, 121–127. [CrossRef]
21. Kluge, M.A.; Fetterman, J.L.; Vita, J.A. Mitochondria and endothelial function. *Circ. Res.* **2013**, *112*, 1171–1188. [CrossRef] [PubMed]
22. Davidson, S.M.; Duchen, M.R. Endothelial mitochondria: Contributing to vascular function and disease. *Circ. Res.* **2007**, *100*, 1128–1141. [CrossRef] [PubMed]
23. Wang, X.; Wang, R.; Jiang, L.; Xu, Q.; Guo, X. Endothelial repair by stem and progenitor cells. *J. Mol. Cell. Cardiol.* **2022**, *163*, 133–146. [CrossRef] [PubMed]
24. Shantsila, E.; Watson, T.; Lip, G.Y. Endothelial progenitor cells in cardiovascular disorders. *J. Am. Coll. Cardiol.* **2007**, *49*, 741–752. [CrossRef] [PubMed]
25. Leicht, S.F.; Schwarz, T.M.; Hermann, P.C.; Seissler, J.; Aicher, A.; Heeschen, C. Adiponectin pretreatment counteracts the detrimental effect of a diabetic environment on endothelial progenitors. *Diabetes* **2011**, *60*, 652–661. [CrossRef]
26. Gui, J.; Rohrbach, A.; Borns, K.; Hillemanns, P.; Feng, L.; Hubel, C.A.; von Versen-Hoynck, F. Vitamin D rescues dysfunction of fetal endothelial colony forming cells from individuals with gestational diabetes. *Placenta* **2015**, *36*, 410–418. [CrossRef] [PubMed]
27. Cooke, J.P.; Dzau, V.J. Nitric oxide synthase: Role in the genesis of vascular disease. *Annu. Rev. Med.* **1997**, *48*, 489–509. [CrossRef]
28. Komarova, Y.A.; Kruse, K.; Mehta, D.; Malik, A.B. Protein Interactions at Endothelial Junctions and Signaling Mechanisms Regulating Endothelial Permeability. *Circ. Res.* **2017**, *120*, 179–206. [CrossRef]
29. Bazzoni, G.; Dejana, E. Endothelial cell-to-cell junctions: Molecular organization and role in vascular homeostasis. *Physiol. Rev.* **2004**, *84*, 869–901. [CrossRef]
30. Sluiter, T.J.; van Buul, J.D.; Huveneers, S.; Quax, P.H.A.; de Vries, M.R. Endothelial Barrier Function and Leukocyte Transmigration in Atherosclerosis. *Biomedicines* **2021**, *9*, 328. [CrossRef]
31. Pulgar, V.M. Transcytosis to Cross the Blood Brain Barrier, New Advancements and Challenges. *Front. Neurosci.* **2018**, *12*, 1019. [CrossRef] [PubMed]
32. Ayloo, S.; Gu, C. Transcytosis at the blood-brain barrier. *Curr. Opin. Neurobiol.* **2019**, *57*, 32–38. [CrossRef]
33. Patching, S.G. Glucose Transporters at the Blood-Brain Barrier: Function, Regulation and Gateways for Drug Delivery. *Mol. Neurobiol.* **2017**, *54*, 1046–1077. [CrossRef] [PubMed]
34. Dejana, E.; Hirschi, K.K.; Simons, M. The molecular basis of endothelial cell plasticity. *Nat. Commun.* **2017**, *8*, 14361. [CrossRef] [PubMed]
35. Vestweber, D. How leukocytes cross the vascular endothelium. *Nat. Rev. Immunol.* **2015**, *15*, 692–704. [CrossRef]
36. Wong, B.W.; Marsch, E.; Treps, L.; Baes, M.; Carmeliet, P. Endothelial cell metabolism in health and disease: Impact of hypoxia. *EMBO J.* **2017**, *36*, 2187–2203. [CrossRef] [PubMed]
37. Eelen, G.; Treps, L.; Li, X.; Carmeliet, P. Basic and Therapeutic Aspects of Angiogenesis Updated. *Circ. Res.* **2020**, *127*, 310–329. [CrossRef] [PubMed]
38. Simo, R.; Carrasco, E.; Garcia-Ramirez, M.; Hernandez, C. Angiogenic and antiangiogenic factors in proliferative diabetic retinopathy. *Curr. Diabetes Rev.* **2006**, *2*, 71–98. [CrossRef]
39. Geindreau, M.; Bruchard, M.; Vegran, F. Role of Cytokines and Chemokines in Angiogenesis in a Tumor Context. *Cancers* **2022**, *14*, 2446. [CrossRef]
40. Boomsma, R.A.; Geenen, D.L. Mesenchymal stem cells secrete multiple cytokines that promote angiogenesis and have contrasting effects on chemotaxis and apoptosis. *PLoS ONE* **2012**, *7*, e35685. [CrossRef]
41. Lee, W.S.; Lu, Y.C.; Kuo, C.T.; Chen, C.T.; Tang, P.H. Effects of female sex hormones on folic acid-induced anti-angiogenesis. *Acta Physiol.* **2018**, *222*, e13001. [CrossRef] [PubMed]
42. Hernandez-Romero, I.A.; Guerra-Calderas, L.; Salgado-Albarran, M.; Maldonado-Huerta, T.; Soto-Reyes, E. The Regulatory Roles of Non-coding RNAs in Angiogenesis and Neovascularization From an Epigenetic Perspective. *Front. Oncol.* **2019**, *9*, 1091. [CrossRef] [PubMed]

43. Zorov, D.B.; Juhaszova, M.; Sollott, S.J. Mitochondrial reactive oxygen species (ROS) and ROS-induced ROS release. *Physiol. Rev.* **2014**, *94*, 909–950. [CrossRef] [PubMed]
44. Balaban, R.S.; Nemoto, S.; Finkel, T. Mitochondria, oxidants, and aging. *Cell* **2005**, *120*, 483–495. [CrossRef] [PubMed]
45. Hirst, J.; King, M.S.; Pryde, K.R. The production of reactive oxygen species by complex I. *Biochem. Soc. Trans.* **2008**, *36*, 976–980. [CrossRef]
46. Tirichen, H.; Yaigoub, H.; Xu, W.; Wu, C.; Li, R.; Li, Y. Mitochondrial Reactive Oxygen Species and Their Contribution in Chronic Kidney Disease Progression through Oxidative Stress. *Front. Physiol.* **2021**, *12*, 627837. [CrossRef]
47. Selivanov, V.A.; Votyakova, T.V.; Pivtoraiko, V.N.; Zeak, J.; Sukhomlin, T.; Trucco, M.; Roca, J.; Cascante, M. Reactive oxygen species production by forward and reverse electron fluxes in the mitochondrial respiratory chain. *PLoS Comput. Biol.* **2011**, *7*, e1001115. [CrossRef]
48. Mailloux, R.J. An Update on Mitochondrial Reactive Oxygen Species Production. *Antioxidants* **2020**, *9*, 472. [CrossRef]
49. Mailloux, R.J.; Craig Ayre, D.; Christian, S.L. Induction of mitochondrial reactive oxygen species production by GSH mediated S-glutathionylation of 2-oxoglutarate dehydrogenase. *Redox Biol.* **2016**, *8*, 285–297. [CrossRef]
50. Mailloux, R.J. Teaching the fundamentals of electron transfer reactions in mitochondria and the production and detection of reactive oxygen species. *Redox Biol.* **2015**, *4*, 381–398. [CrossRef]
51. Murphy, M.P. How mitochondria produce reactive oxygen species. *Biochem. J.* **2009**, *417*, 1–13. [CrossRef] [PubMed]
52. Sena, L.A.; Chandel, N.S. Physiological roles of mitochondrial reactive oxygen species. *Mol. Cell* **2012**, *48*, 158–167. [CrossRef] [PubMed]
53. Breton-Romero, R.; Lamas, S. Hydrogen peroxide signaling in vascular endothelial cells. *Redox Biol.* **2014**, *2*, 529–534. [CrossRef]
54. Roberge, S.; Roussel, J.; Andersson, D.C.; Meli, A.C.; Vidal, B.; Blandel, F.; Lanner, J.T.; Le Guennec, J.Y.; Katz, A.; Westerblad, H.; et al. TNF-α-mediated caspase-8 activation induces ROS production and TRPM2 activation in adult ventricular myocytes. *Cardiovasc. Res.* **2014**, *103*, 90–99. [CrossRef]
55. Frey, R.S.; Ushio-Fukai, M.; Malik, A.B. NADPH oxidase-dependent signaling in endothelial cells: Role in physiology and pathophysiology. *Antioxid. Redox Signal.* **2009**, *11*, 791–810. [CrossRef] [PubMed]
56. Ilatovskaya, D.V.; Pavlov, T.S.; Levchenko, V.; Staruschenko, A. ROS production as a common mechanism of ENaC regulation by EGF, insulin, and IGF-1. *Am. J. Physiol. Cell Physiol.* **2013**, *304*, C102–C111. [CrossRef]
57. Dikalov, S.I.; Nazarewicz, R.R.; Bikineyeva, A.; Hilenski, L.; Lassegue, B.; Griendling, K.K.; Harrison, D.G.; Dikalova, A.E. Nox2-induced production of mitochondrial superoxide in angiotensin II-mediated endothelial oxidative stress and hypertension. *Antioxid. Redox Signal.* **2014**, *20*, 281–294. [CrossRef]
58. Brandes, R.P.; Weissmann, N.; Schroder, K. Nox family NADPH oxidases: Molecular mechanisms of activation. *Free Radic. Biol. Med.* **2014**, *76*, 208–226. [CrossRef]
59. Vendrov, A.E.; Vendrov, K.C.; Smith, A.; Yuan, J.; Sumida, A.; Robidoux, J.; Runge, M.S.; Madamanchi, N.R. NOX4 NADPH Oxidase-Dependent Mitochondrial Oxidative Stress in Aging-Associated Cardiovascular Disease. *Antioxid. Redox Signal.* **2015**, *23*, 1389–1409. [CrossRef]
60. Basta, G.; Lazzerini, G.; Massaro, M.; Simoncini, T.; Tanganelli, P.; Fu, C.; Kislinger, T.; Stern, D.M.; Schmidt, A.M.; De Caterina, R. Advanced glycation end products activate endothelium through signal-transduction receptor RAGE: A mechanism for amplification of inflammatory responses. *Circulation* **2002**, *105*, 816–822. [CrossRef]
61. Rowan, S.; Bejarano, E.; Taylor, A. Mechanistic targeting of advanced glycation end-products in age-related diseases. *Biochim. Biophys. Acta (BBA) Mol. Basis Dis.* **2018**, *1864*, 3631–3643. [CrossRef] [PubMed]
62. Katakami, N. Mechanism of Development of Atherosclerosis and Cardiovascular Disease in Diabetes Mellitus. *J. Atheroscler. Thromb.* **2018**, *25*, 27–39. [CrossRef] [PubMed]
63. Cepas, V.; Collino, M.; Mayo, J.C.; Sainz, R.M. Redox Signaling and Advanced Glycation Endproducts (AGEs) in Diet-Related Diseases. *Antioxidants* **2020**, *9*, 142. [CrossRef] [PubMed]
64. Kelley, E.E.; Hock, T.; Khoo, N.K.; Richardson, G.R.; Johnson, K.K.; Powell, P.C.; Giles, G.I.; Agarwal, A.; Lancaster, J.R., Jr.; Tarpey, M.M. Moderate hypoxia induces xanthine oxidoreductase activity in arterial endothelial cells. *Free Radic. Biol. Med.* **2006**, *40*, 952–959. [CrossRef] [PubMed]
65. Bortolotti, M.; Polito, L.; Battelli, M.G.; Bolognesi, A. Xanthine oxidoreductase: One enzyme for multiple physiological tasks. *Redox Biol.* **2021**, *41*, 101882. [CrossRef]
66. Zhang, C.; Hein, T.W.; Wang, W.; Ren, Y.; Shipley, R.D.; Kuo, L. Activation of JNK and xanthine oxidase by TNF-α impairs nitric oxide-mediated dilation of coronary arterioles. *J. Mol. Cell. Cardiol.* **2006**, *40*, 247–257. [CrossRef] [PubMed]
67. Dupont, G.P.; Huecksteadt, T.P.; Marshall, B.C.; Ryan, U.S.; Michael, J.R.; Hoidal, J.R. Regulation of xanthine dehydrogenase and xanthine oxidase activity and gene expression in cultured rat pulmonary endothelial cells. *J. Clin. Investig.* **1992**, *89*, 197–202. [CrossRef]
68. Kelley, E.E. A new paradigm for XOR-catalyzed reactive species generation in the endothelium. *Pharmacol. Rep.* **2015**, *67*, 669–674. [CrossRef]
69. Ben-Mahdi, M.H.; Dang, P.M.; Gougerot-Pocidalo, M.A.; O'Dowd, Y.; El-Benna, J.; Pasquier, C. Xanthine Oxidase-Derived ROS Display a Biphasic Effect on Endothelial Cells Adhesion and FAK Phosphorylation. *Oxid. Med. Cell. Longev.* **2016**, *2016*, 9346242. [CrossRef]

70. Forstermann, U.; Sessa, W.C. Nitric oxide synthases: Regulation and function. *Eur. Heart J.* **2012**, *33*, 829–837, 837a–837d. [CrossRef]
71. Forstermann, U.; Li, H. Therapeutic effect of enhancing endothelial nitric oxide synthase (eNOS) expression and preventing eNOS uncoupling. *Br. J. Pharmacol.* **2011**, *164*, 213–223. [CrossRef] [PubMed]
72. Janaszak-Jasiecka, A.; Siekierzycka, A.; Ploska, A.; Dobrucki, I.T.; Kalinowski, L. Endothelial Dysfunction Driven by Hypoxia-The Influence of Oxygen Deficiency on NO Bioavailability. *Biomolecules* **2021**, *11*, 982. [CrossRef] [PubMed]
73. Kirkman, D.L.; Robinson, A.T.; Rossman, M.J.; Seals, D.R.; Edwards, D.G. Mitochondrial contributions to vascular endothelial dysfunction, arterial stiffness, and cardiovascular diseases. *Am. J. Physiol. Heart Circ. Physiol.* **2021**, *320*, H2080–H2100. [CrossRef] [PubMed]
74. Chipurupalli, S.; Samavedam, U.; Robinson, N. Crosstalk between ER Stress, Autophagy and Inflammation. *Front. Med.* **2021**, *8*, 758311. [CrossRef] [PubMed]
75. Shergalis, A.G.; Hu, S.; Bankhead, A., 3rd; Neamati, N. Role of the ERO1-PDI interaction in oxidative protein folding and disease. *Pharmacol. Ther.* **2020**, *210*, 107525. [CrossRef] [PubMed]
76. Moller, M.N.; Orrico, F.; Villar, S.F.; Lopez, A.C.; Silva, N.; Donze, M.; Thomson, L.; Denicola, A. Oxidants and Antioxidants in the Redox Biochemistry of Human Red Blood Cells. *ACS Omega* **2023**, *8*, 147–168. [CrossRef] [PubMed]
77. Orrico, F.; Laurance, S.; Lopez, A.C.; Lefevre, S.D.; Thomson, L.; Moller, M.N.; Ostuni, M.A. Oxidative Stress in Healthy and Pathological Red Blood Cells. *Biomolecules* **2023**, *13*, 1262. [CrossRef] [PubMed]
78. Tsuruga, M.; Shikama, K. Biphasic nature in the autoxidation reaction of human oxyhemoglobin. *Biochim. Biophys. Acta (BBA) Protein Struct. Mol. Enzymol.* **1997**, *1337*, 96–104. [CrossRef]
79. Wang, Y.; Branicky, R.; Noe, A.; Hekimi, S. Superoxide dismutases: Dual roles in controlling ROS damage and regulating ROS signaling. *J. Cell Biol.* **2018**, *217*, 1915–1928. [CrossRef]
80. Kehrer, J.P. The Haber-Weiss reaction and mechanisms of toxicity. *Toxicology* **2000**, *149*, 43–50. [CrossRef]
81. Beckman, J.S.; Beckman, T.W.; Chen, J.; Marshall, P.A.; Freeman, B.A. Apparent hydroxyl radical production by peroxynitrite: Implications for endothelial injury from nitric oxide and superoxide. *Proc. Natl. Acad. Sci. USA* **1990**, *87*, 1620–1624. [CrossRef] [PubMed]
82. Zhou, Z.; Mahdi, A.; Tratsiakovich, Y.; Zahoran, S.; Kovamees, O.; Nordin, F.; Uribe Gonzalez, A.E.; Alvarsson, M.; Ostenson, C.G.; Andersson, D.C.; et al. Erythrocytes from Patients with Type 2 Diabetes Induce Endothelial Dysfunction Via Arginase I. *J. Am. Coll. Cardiol.* **2018**, *72*, 769–780. [CrossRef] [PubMed]
83. Mahdi, A.; Tengbom, J.; Alvarsson, M.; Wernly, B.; Zhou, Z.; Pernow, J. Red Blood Cell Peroxynitrite Causes Endothelial Dysfunction in Type 2 Diabetes Mellitus via Arginase. *Cells* **2020**, *9*, 1712. [CrossRef] [PubMed]
84. Zhuge, Z.; McCann Haworth, S.; Nihlen, C.; Carvalho, L.; Heuser, S.K.; Kleschyov, A.L.; Nasiell, J.; Cortese-Krott, M.M.; Weitzberg, E.; Lundberg, J.O.; et al. Red blood cells from endothelial nitric oxide synthase-deficient mice induce vascular dysfunction involving oxidative stress and endothelial arginase I. *Redox Biol.* **2023**, *60*, 102612. [CrossRef] [PubMed]
85. Pernow, J.; Mahdi, A.; Yang, J.; Zhou, Z. Red blood cell dysfunction: A new player in cardiovascular disease. *Cardiovasc. Res.* **2019**, *115*, 1596–1605. [CrossRef] [PubMed]
86. Mahdi, A.; Cortese-Krott, M.M.; Kelm, M.; Li, N.; Pernow, J. Novel perspectives on redox signaling in red blood cells and platelets in cardiovascular disease. *Free Radic. Biol. Med.* **2021**, *168*, 95–109. [CrossRef]
87. Mittal, M.; Siddiqui, M.R.; Tran, K.; Reddy, S.P.; Malik, A.B. Reactive oxygen species in inflammation and tissue injury. *Antioxid. Redox Signal.* **2014**, *20*, 1126–1167. [CrossRef]
88. Naik, E.; Dixit, V.M. Mitochondrial reactive oxygen species drive proinflammatory cytokine production. *J. Exp. Med.* **2011**, *208*, 417–420. [CrossRef]
89. Chistiakov, D.A.; Orekhov, A.N.; Bobryshev, Y.V. Endothelial Barrier and Its Abnormalities in Cardiovascular Disease. *Front. Physiol.* **2015**, *6*, 365. [CrossRef]
90. Boueiz, A.; Hassoun, P.M. Regulation of endothelial barrier function by reactive oxygen and nitrogen species. *Microvasc. Res.* **2009**, *77*, 26–34. [CrossRef]
91. De Almeida, A.; de Oliveira, J.; da Silva Pontes, L.V.; de Souza Junior, J.F.; Goncalves, T.A.F.; Dantas, S.H.; de Almeida Feitosa, M.S.; Silva, A.O.; de Medeiros, I.A. ROS: Basic Concepts, Sources, Cellular Signaling, and its Implications in Aging Pathways. *Oxid. Med. Cell. Longev.* **2022**, *2022*, 1225578. [CrossRef] [PubMed]
92. Gulcin, I. Antioxidants and antioxidant methods: An updated overview. *Arch. Toxicol.* **2020**, *94*, 651–715. [CrossRef] [PubMed]
93. Sun, H.J.; Wu, Z.Y.; Nie, X.W.; Bian, J.S. Role of Endothelial Dysfunction in Cardiovascular Diseases: The Link between Inflammation and Hydrogen Sulfide. *Front. Pharmacol.* **2019**, *10*, 1568. [CrossRef] [PubMed]
94. Nunnari, J.; Suomalainen, A. Mitochondria: In sickness and in health. *Cell* **2012**, *148*, 1145–1159. [CrossRef] [PubMed]
95. Teodoro, J.S.; Palmeira, C.M.; Rolo, A.P. Determination of oxidative phosphorylation complexes activities. *Methods Mol. Biol.* **2015**, *1241*, 71–84. [CrossRef] [PubMed]
96. Murphy, M.P.; Hartley, R.C. Mitochondria as a therapeutic target for common pathologies. *Nat. Rev. Drug Discov.* **2018**, *17*, 865–886. [CrossRef] [PubMed]
97. Moreno, A.J.; Santos, D.L.; Magalhaes-Novais, S.; Oliveira, P.J. Measuring Mitochondrial Membrane Potential with a Tetraphenylphosphonium-Selective Electrode. *Curr. Protoc. Toxicol.* **2015**, *65*, 25.5.1–25.5.16. [CrossRef]

98. Perrotta, I. The microscopic anatomy of endothelial cells in human atherosclerosis: Focus on ER and mitochondria. *J. Anat.* **2020**, *237*, 1015–1025. [CrossRef]
99. Sabouny, R.; Shutt, T.E. Reciprocal Regulation of Mitochondrial Fission and Fusion. *Trends Biochem. Sci.* **2020**, *45*, 564–577. [CrossRef]
100. Wang, Y.; Wu, J.; Wang, J.; He, L.; Lai, H.; Zhang, T.; Wang, X.; Li, W. Mitochondrial oxidative stress in brain microvascular endothelial cells: Triggering blood-brain barrier disruption. *Mitochondrion* **2023**, *69*, 71–82. [CrossRef]
101. Wang, J.; Zhou, H. Mitochondrial quality control mechanisms as molecular targets in cardiac ischemia-reperfusion injury. *Acta Pharm. Sin. B* **2020**, *10*, 1866–1879. [CrossRef] [PubMed]
102. Vasquez-Trincado, C.; Garcia-Carvajal, I.; Pennanen, C.; Parra, V.; Hill, J.A.; Rothermel, B.A.; Lavandero, S. Mitochondrial dynamics, mitophagy and cardiovascular disease. *J. Physiol.* **2016**, *594*, 509–525. [CrossRef] [PubMed]
103. Chehaitly, A.; Guihot, A.L.; Proux, C.; Grimaud, L.; Aurriere, J.; Legouriellec, B.; Rivron, J.; Vessieres, E.; Tetaud, C.; Zorzano, A.; et al. Altered Mitochondrial Opa1-Related Fusion in Mouse Promotes Endothelial Cell Dysfunction and Atherosclerosis. *Antioxidants* **2022**, *11*, 1078. [CrossRef] [PubMed]
104. Varanita, T.; Soriano, M.E.; Romanello, V.; Zaglia, T.; Quintana-Cabrera, R.; Semenzato, M.; Menabo, R.; Costa, V.; Civiletto, G.; Pesce, P.; et al. The OPA1-dependent mitochondrial cristae remodeling pathway controls atrophic, apoptotic, and ischemic tissue damage. *Cell Metab.* **2015**, *21*, 834–844. [CrossRef] [PubMed]
105. Wang, L.T.; He, P.C.; Li, A.Q.; Cao, K.X.; Yan, J.W.; Guo, S.; Jiang, L.; Yao, L.; Dai, X.Y.; Feng, D.; et al. Caffeine promotes angiogenesis through modulating endothelial mitochondrial dynamics. *Acta Pharmacol. Sin.* **2021**, *42*, 2033–2045. [CrossRef] [PubMed]
106. Eelen, G.; de Zeeuw, P.; Treps, L.; Harjes, U.; Wong, B.W.; Carmeliet, P. Endothelial Cell Metabolism. *Physiol. Rev.* **2018**, *98*, 3–58. [CrossRef] [PubMed]
107. Lai, L.; Reineke, E.; Hamilton, D.J.; Cooke, J.P. Glycolytic Switch Is Required for Transdifferentiation to Endothelial Lineage. *Circulation* **2019**, *139*, 119–133. [CrossRef]
108. Rafikova, O.; Meadows, M.L.; Kinchen, J.M.; Mohney, R.P.; Maltepe, E.; Desai, A.A.; Yuan, J.X.; Garcia, J.G.; Fineman, J.R.; Rafikov, R.; et al. Metabolic Changes Precede the Development of Pulmonary Hypertension in the Monocrotaline Exposed Rat Lung. *PLoS ONE* **2016**, *11*, e0150480. [CrossRef]
109. Magistretti, P.J.; Allaman, I. A cellular perspective on brain energy metabolism and functional imaging. *Neuron* **2015**, *86*, 883–901. [CrossRef]
110. Kolwicz, S.C., Jr.; Purohit, S.; Tian, R. Cardiac metabolism and its interactions with contraction, growth, and survival of cardiomyocytes. *Circ. Res.* **2013**, *113*, 603–616. [CrossRef]
111. De Zeeuw, P.; Wong, B.W.; Carmeliet, P. Metabolic adaptations in diabetic endothelial cells. *Circ. J.* **2015**, *79*, 934–941. [CrossRef] [PubMed]
112. De Bock, K.; Georgiadou, M.; Schoors, S.; Kuchnio, A.; Wong, B.W.; Cantelmo, A.R.; Quaegebeur, A.; Ghesquiere, B.; Cauwenberghs, S.; Eelen, G.; et al. Role of PFKFB3-driven glycolysis in vessel sprouting. *Cell* **2013**, *154*, 651–663. [CrossRef] [PubMed]
113. Schoonjans, C.A.; Mathieu, B.; Joudiou, N.; Zampieri, L.X.; Brusa, D.; Sonveaux, P.; Feron, O.; Gallez, B. Targeting Endothelial Cell Metabolism by Inhibition of Pyruvate Dehydrogenase Kinase and Glutaminase-1. *J. Clin. Med.* **2020**, *9*, 3308. [CrossRef] [PubMed]
114. Koneru, S.; Penumathsa, S.V.; Thirunavukkarasu, M.; Samuel, S.M.; Zhan, L.; Han, Z.; Maulik, G.; Das, D.K.; Maulik, N. Redox regulation of ischemic preconditioning is mediated by the differential activation of caveolins and their association with eNOS and GLUT-4. *Am. J. Physiol. Heart Circ. Physiol.* **2007**, *292*, H2060–H2072. [CrossRef] [PubMed]
115. Paik, J.Y.; Lee, K.H.; Ko, B.H.; Choe, Y.S.; Choi, Y.; Kim, B.T. Nitric oxide stimulates 18F-FDG uptake in human endothelial cells through increased hexokinase activity and GLUT1 expression. *J. Nucl. Med.* **2005**, *46*, 365–370.
116. Rohlenova, K.; Veys, K.; Miranda-Santos, I.; De Bock, K.; Carmeliet, P. Endothelial Cell Metabolism in Health and Disease. *Trends Cell Biol.* **2018**, *28*, 224–236. [CrossRef]
117. Cruys, B.; Wong, B.W.; Kuchnio, A.; Verdegem, D.; Cantelmo, A.R.; Conradi, L.C.; Vandekeere, S.; Bouche, A.; Cornelissen, I.; Vinckier, S.; et al. Glycolytic regulation of cell rearrangement in angiogenesis. *Nat. Commun.* **2016**, *7*, 12240. [CrossRef]
118. Davidson, S.M. Endothelial mitochondria and heart disease. *Cardiovasc. Res.* **2010**, *88*, 58–66. [CrossRef]
119. Groschner, L.N.; Waldeck-Weiermair, M.; Malli, R.; Graier, W.F. Endothelial mitochondria—Less respiration, more integration. *Pflugers Arch.* **2012**, *464*, 63–76. [CrossRef]
120. Potente, M.; Carmeliet, P. The Link between Angiogenesis and Endothelial Metabolism. *Annu. Rev. Physiol.* **2017**, *79*, 43–66. [CrossRef]
121. Patella, F.; Schug, Z.T.; Persi, E.; Neilson, L.J.; Erami, Z.; Avanzato, D.; Maione, F.; Hernandez-Fernaud, J.R.; Mackay, G.; Zheng, L.; et al. Proteomics-based metabolic modeling reveals that fatty acid oxidation (FAO) controls endothelial cell (EC) permeability. *Mol. Cell. Proteom.* **2015**, *14*, 621–634. [CrossRef] [PubMed]
122. Adeva-Andany, M.M.; Carneiro-Freire, N.; Seco-Filgueira, M.; Fernandez-Fernandez, C.; Mourino-Bayolo, D. Mitochondrial beta-oxidation of saturated fatty acids in humans. *Mitochondrion* **2019**, *46*, 73–90. [CrossRef] [PubMed]
123. Schoors, S.; Bruning, U.; Missiaen, R.; Queiroz, K.C.; Borgers, G.; Elia, I.; Zecchin, A.; Cantelmo, A.R.; Christen, S.; Goveia, J.; et al. Fatty acid carbon is essential for dNTP synthesis in endothelial cells. *Nature* **2015**, *520*, 192–197. [CrossRef] [PubMed]

124. Cory, J.G.; Cory, A.H. Critical roles of glutamine as nitrogen donors in purine and pyrimidine nucleotide synthesis: Asparaginase treatment in childhood acute lymphoblastic leukemia. *In Vivo* **2006**, *20*, 587–589. [PubMed]
125. Kuo, A.; Lee, M.Y.; Sessa, W.C. Lipid Droplet Biogenesis and Function in the Endothelium. *Circ. Res.* **2017**, *120*, 1289–1297. [CrossRef]
126. Fukai, T.; Ushio-Fukai, M. Cross-Talk between NADPH Oxidase and Mitochondria: Role in ROS Signaling and Angiogenesis. *Cells* **2020**, *9*, 1849. [CrossRef]
127. Bonello, S.; Zahringer, C.; BelAiba, R.S.; Djordjevic, T.; Hess, J.; Michiels, C.; Kietzmann, T.; Gorlach, A. Reactive oxygen species activate the HIF-1α promoter via a functional NFκB site. *Arterioscler. Thromb. Vasc. Biol.* **2007**, *27*, 755–761. [CrossRef]
128. Mazure, N.M.; Chen, E.Y.; Laderoute, K.R.; Giaccia, A.J. Induction of vascular endothelial growth factor by hypoxia is modulated by a phosphatidylinositol 3-kinase/Akt signaling pathway in Ha-ras-transformed cells through a hypoxia inducible factor-1 transcriptional element. *Blood* **1997**, *90*, 3322–3331. [CrossRef]
129. Kim, Y.M.; Kim, S.J.; Tatsunami, R.; Yamamura, H.; Fukai, T.; Ushio-Fukai, M. ROS-induced ROS release orchestrated by Nox4, Nox2, and mitochondria in VEGF signaling and angiogenesis. *Am. J. Physiol. Cell Physiol.* **2017**, *312*, C749–C764. [CrossRef]
130. Fukuda, R.; Zhang, H.; Kim, J.W.; Shimoda, L.; Dang, C.V.; Semenza, G.L. HIF-1 regulates cytochrome oxidase subunits to optimize efficiency of respiration in hypoxic cells. *Cell* **2007**, *129*, 111–122. [CrossRef]
131. Tello, D.; Balsa, E.; Acosta-Iborra, B.; Fuertes-Yebra, E.; Elorza, A.; Ordonez, A.; Corral-Escariz, M.; Soro, I.; Lopez-Bernardo, E.; Perales-Clemente, E.; et al. Induction of the mitochondrial NDUFA4L2 protein by HIF-1α decreases oxygen consumption by inhibiting Complex I activity. *Cell Metab.* **2011**, *14*, 768–779. [CrossRef] [PubMed]
132. Tahara, E.B.; Navarete, F.D.; Kowaltowski, A.J. Tissue-, substrate-, and site-specific characteristics of mitochondrial reactive oxygen species generation. *Free Radic. Biol. Med.* **2009**, *46*, 1283–1297. [CrossRef] [PubMed]
133. Kussmaul, L.; Hirst, J. The mechanism of superoxide production by NADH:ubiquinone oxidoreductase (complex I) from bovine heart mitochondria. *Proc. Natl. Acad. Sci. USA* **2006**, *103*, 7607–7612. [CrossRef] [PubMed]
134. Kushnareva, Y.; Murphy, A.N.; Andreyev, A. Complex I-mediated reactive oxygen species generation: Modulation by cytochrome c and NAD(P)+ oxidation-reduction state. *Biochem. J.* **2002**, *368*, 545–553. [CrossRef] [PubMed]
135. Dalal, P.J.; Muller, W.A.; Sullivan, D.P. Endothelial Cell Calcium Signaling during Barrier Function and Inflammation. *Am. J. Pathol.* **2020**, *190*, 535–542. [CrossRef] [PubMed]
136. Jornot, L.; Maechler, P.; Wollheim, C.B.; Junod, A.F. Reactive oxygen metabolites increase mitochondrial calcium in endothelial cells: Implication of the Ca^{2+}/Na^{+} exchanger. *J. Cell Sci.* **1999**, *112 Pt 7*, 1013–1022. [CrossRef]
137. Atamna, H.; Mackey, J.; Dhahbi, J.M. Mitochondrial pharmacology: Electron transport chain bypass as strategies to treat mitochondrial dysfunction. *Biofactors* **2012**, *38*, 158–166. [CrossRef]
138. Parodi-Rullan, R.M.; Javadov, S.; Fossati, S. Dissecting the Crosstalk between Endothelial Mitochondrial Damage, Vascular Inflammation, and Neurodegeneration in Cerebral Amyloid Angiopathy and Alzheimer's Disease. *Cells* **2021**, *10*, 2903. [CrossRef]
139. Malpartida, A.B.; Williamson, M.; Narendra, D.P.; Wade-Martins, R.; Ryan, B.J. Mitochondrial Dysfunction and Mitophagy in Parkinson's Disease: From Mechanism to Therapy. *Trends Biochem. Sci.* **2021**, *46*, 329–343. [CrossRef]
140. Moon, H.E.; Paek, S.H. Mitochondrial Dysfunction in Parkinson's Disease. *Exp. Neurobiol.* **2015**, *24*, 103–116. [CrossRef]
141. Nicolson, G.L. Mitochondrial Dysfunction and Chronic Disease: Treatment with Natural Supplements. *Integr. Med.* **2014**, *13*, 35–43.
142. Salnikova, D.; Orekhova, V.; Grechko, A.; Starodubova, A.; Bezsonov, E.; Popkova, T.; Orekhov, A. Mitochondrial Dysfunction in Vascular Wall Cells and Its Role in Atherosclerosis. *Int. J. Mol. Sci.* **2021**, *22*, 8990. [CrossRef] [PubMed]
143. Bravo-San Pedro, J.M.; Kroemer, G.; Galluzzi, L. Autophagy and Mitophagy in Cardiovascular Disease. *Circ. Res.* **2017**, *120*, 1812–1824. [CrossRef] [PubMed]
144. Zhang, Y.; Weng, J.; Huan, L.; Sheng, S.; Xu, F. Mitophagy in atherosclerosis: From mechanism to therapy. *Front. Immunol.* **2023**, *14*, 1165507. [CrossRef] [PubMed]
145. Qu, K.; Yan, F.; Qin, X.; Zhang, K.; He, W.; Dong, M.; Wu, G. Mitochondrial dysfunction in vascular endothelial cells and its role in atherosclerosis. *Front. Physiol.* **2022**, *13*, 1084604. [CrossRef] [PubMed]
146. Jendrach, M.; Pohl, S.; Voth, M.; Kowald, A.; Hammerstein, P.; Bereiter-Hahn, J. Morpho-dynamic changes of mitochondria during ageing of human endothelial cells. *Mech. Ageing Dev.* **2005**, *126*, 813–821. [CrossRef]
147. Liu, N.; Wu, J.; Zhang, L.; Gao, Z.; Sun, Y.; Yu, M.; Zhao, Y.; Dong, S.; Lu, F.; Zhang, W. Hydrogen Sulphide modulating mitochondrial morphology to promote mitophagy in endothelial cells under high-glucose and high-palmitate. *J. Cell. Mol. Med.* **2017**, *21*, 3190–3203. [CrossRef]
148. He, Y.; Luan, Z.; Fu, X.; Xu, X. Overexpression of uncoupling protein 2 inhibits the high glucose-induced apoptosis of human umbilical vein endothelial cells. *Int. J. Mol. Med.* **2016**, *37*, 631–638. [CrossRef]
149. Forte, M.; Bianchi, F.; Cotugno, M.; Marchitti, S.; Stanzione, R.; Maglione, V.; Sciarretta, S.; Valenti, V.; Carnevale, R.; Versaci, F.; et al. An interplay between UCP2 and ROS protects cells from high-salt-induced injury through autophagy stimulation. *Cell Death Dis.* **2021**, *12*, 919. [CrossRef]
150. Forrester, S.J.; Preston, K.J.; Cooper, H.A.; Boyer, M.J.; Escoto, K.M.; Poltronetti, A.J.; Elliott, K.J.; Kuroda, R.; Miyao, M.; Sesaki, H.; et al. Mitochondrial Fission Mediates Endothelial Inflammation. *Hypertension* **2020**, *76*, 267–276. [CrossRef]

151. Choi, S.J.; Piao, S.; Nagar, H.; Jung, S.B.; Kim, S.; Lee, I.; Kim, S.M.; Song, H.J.; Shin, N.; Kim, D.W.; et al. Isocitrate dehydrogenase 2 deficiency induces endothelial inflammation via p66sh-mediated mitochondrial oxidative stress. *Biochem. Biophys. Res. Commun.* **2018**, *503*, 1805–1811. [CrossRef] [PubMed]
152. Kumar, S.; Kim, Y.R.; Vikram, A.; Naqvi, A.; Li, Q.; Kassan, M.; Kumar, V.; Bachschmid, M.M.; Jacobs, J.S.; Kumar, A.; et al. Sirtuin1-regulated lysine acetylation of p66Shc governs diabetes-induced vascular oxidative stress and endothelial dysfunction. *Proc. Natl. Acad. Sci. USA* **2017**, *114*, 1714–1719. [CrossRef] [PubMed]
153. Ballinger, S.W.; Patterson, C.; Yan, C.N.; Doan, R.; Burow, D.L.; Young, C.G.; Yakes, F.M.; Van Houten, B.; Ballinger, C.A.; Freeman, B.A.; et al. Hydrogen peroxide- and peroxynitrite-induced mitochondrial DNA damage and dysfunction in vascular endothelial and smooth muscle cells. *Circ. Res.* **2000**, *86*, 960–966. [CrossRef] [PubMed]
154. Yu, C.H.; Davidson, S.; Harapas, C.R.; Hilton, J.B.; Mlodzianoski, M.J.; Laohamonthonkul, P.; Louis, C.; Low, R.R.J.; Moecking, J.; De Nardo, D.; et al. TDP-43 Triggers Mitochondrial DNA Release via mPTP to Activate cGAS/STING in ALS. *Cell* **2020**, *183*, 636–649 e618. [CrossRef]
155. Zhang, Q.; Raoof, M.; Chen, Y.; Sumi, Y.; Sursal, T.; Junger, W.; Brohi, K.; Itagaki, K.; Hauser, C.J. Circulating mitochondrial DAMPs cause inflammatory responses to injury. *Nature* **2010**, *464*, 104–107. [CrossRef]
156. Liu, Q.; Zhang, D.; Hu, D.; Zhou, X.; Zhou, Y. The role of mitochondria in NLRP3 inflammasome activation. *Mol. Immunol.* **2018**, *103*, 115–124. [CrossRef] [PubMed]
157. He, Y.; Hara, H.; Nunez, G. Mechanism and Regulation of NLRP3 Inflammasome Activation. *Trends Biochem. Sci.* **2016**, *41*, 1012–1021. [CrossRef]
158. Jin, H.; Zhu, Y.; Wang, X.D.; Luo, E.F.; Li, Y.P.; Wang, B.L.; Chen, Y.F. BDNF corrects NLRP3 inflammasome-induced pyroptosis and glucose metabolism reprogramming through KLF2/HK1 pathway in vascular endothelial cells. *Cell Signal.* **2021**, *78*, 109843. [CrossRef]
159. Bjorkegren, J.L.M.; Lusis, A.J. Atherosclerosis: Recent developments. *Cell* **2022**, *185*, 1630–1645. [CrossRef]
160. Jebari-Benslaiman, S.; Galicia-Garcia, U.; Larrea-Sebal, A.; Olaetxea, J.R.; Alloza, I.; Vandenbroeck, K.; Benito-Vicente, A.; Martin, C. Pathophysiology of Atherosclerosis. *Int. J. Mol. Sci.* **2022**, *23*, 3346. [CrossRef]
161. Dwivedi, A.; Anggard, E.E.; Carrier, M.J. Oxidized LDL-mediated monocyte adhesion to endothelial cells does not involve NFκB. *Biochem. Biophys. Res. Commun.* **2001**, *284*, 239–244. [CrossRef] [PubMed]
162. Mundi, S.; Massaro, M.; Scoditti, E.; Carluccio, M.A.; van Hinsbergh, V.W.M.; Iruela-Arispe, M.L.; De Caterina, R. Endothelial permeability, LDL deposition, and cardiovascular risk factors—A review. *Cardiovasc. Res.* **2018**, *114*, 35–52. [CrossRef] [PubMed]
163. Rhoads, J.P.; Major, A.S. How Oxidized Low-Density Lipoprotein Activates Inflammatory Responses. *Crit. Rev. Immunol.* **2018**, *38*, 333–342. [CrossRef] [PubMed]
164. He, L.; Zhou, Q.; Huang, Z.; Xu, J.; Zhou, H.; Lv, D.; Lu, L.; Huang, S.; Tang, M.; Zhong, J.; et al. PINK1/Parkin-mediated mitophagy promotes apelin-13-induced vascular smooth muscle cell proliferation by AMPKα and exacerbates atherosclerotic lesions. *J. Cell. Physiol.* **2019**, *234*, 8668–8682. [CrossRef] [PubMed]
165. Huynh, D.T.N.; Heo, K.S. Role of mitochondrial dynamics and mitophagy of vascular smooth muscle cell proliferation and migration in progression of atherosclerosis. *Arch. Pharm. Res.* **2021**, *44*, 1051–1061. [CrossRef]
166. Duan, M.; Chen, H.; Yin, L.; Zhu, X.; Novak, P.; Lv, Y.; Zhao, G.; Yin, K. Mitochondrial apolipoprotein A-I binding protein alleviates atherosclerosis by regulating mitophagy and macrophage polarization. *Cell Commun. Signal.* **2022**, *20*, 60. [CrossRef]
167. Dumont, A.; Lee, M.; Barouillet, T.; Murphy, A.; Yvan-Charvet, L. Mitochondria orchestrate macrophage effector functions in atherosclerosis. *Mol. Asp. Med.* **2021**, *77*, 100922. [CrossRef]
168. Stamerra, C.A.; Di Giosia, P.; Giorgini, P.; Ferri, C.; Sukhorukov, V.N.; Sahebkar, A. Mitochondrial Dysfunction and Cardiovascular Disease: Pathophysiology and Emerging Therapies. *Oxid. Med. Cell. Longev.* **2022**, *2022*, 9530007. [CrossRef]
169. Peng, W.; Cai, G.; Xia, Y.; Chen, J.; Wu, P.; Wang, Z.; Li, G.; Wei, D. Mitochondrial Dysfunction in Atherosclerosis. *DNA Cell Biol.* **2019**, *38*, 597–606. [CrossRef]
170. Suarez-Rivero, J.M.; Pastor-Maldonado, C.J.; Povea-Cabello, S.; Alvarez-Cordoba, M.; Villalon-Garcia, I.; Talaveron-Rey, M.; Suarez-Carrillo, A.; Munuera-Cabeza, M.; Sanchez-Alcazar, J.A. From Mitochondria to Atherosclerosis: The Inflammation Path. *Biomedicines* **2021**, *9*, 258. [CrossRef]
171. Shemiakova, T.; Ivanova, E.; Grechko, A.V.; Gerasimova, E.V.; Sobenin, I.A.; Orekhov, A.N. Mitochondrial Dysfunction and DNA Damage in the Context of Pathogenesis of Atherosclerosis. *Biomedicines* **2020**, *8*, 166. [CrossRef] [PubMed]
172. Gimbrone, M.A., Jr.; Garcia-Cardena, G. Endothelial Cell Dysfunction and the Pathobiology of Atherosclerosis. *Circ. Res.* **2016**, *118*, 620–636. [CrossRef] [PubMed]
173. Sitia, S.; Tomasoni, L.; Atzeni, F.; Ambrosio, G.; Cordiano, C.; Catapano, A.; Tramontana, S.; Perticone, F.; Naccarato, P.; Camici, P.; et al. From endothelial dysfunction to atherosclerosis. *Autoimmun. Rev.* **2010**, *9*, 830–834. [CrossRef] [PubMed]
174. Liao, J.K. Linking endothelial dysfunction with endothelial cell activation. *J. Clin. Investig.* **2013**, *123*, 540–541. [CrossRef]
175. Oemar, B.S.; Tschudi, M.R.; Godoy, N.; Brovkovich, V.; Malinski, T.; Luscher, T.F. Reduced endothelial nitric oxide synthase expression and production in human atherosclerosis. *Circulation* **1998**, *97*, 2494–2498. [CrossRef]
176. Hong, S.G.; Shin, J.; Choi, S.Y.; Powers, J.C.; Meister, B.M.; Sayoc, J.; Son, J.S.; Tierney, R.; Recchia, F.A.; Brown, M.D.; et al. Flow pattern-dependent mitochondrial dynamics regulates the metabolic profile and inflammatory state of endothelial cells. *JCI Insight* **2022**, *7*, e159286. [CrossRef]

177. Zhang, B.; Gu, J.; Qian, M.; Niu, L.; Zhou, H.; Ghista, D. Correlation between quantitative analysis of wall shear stress and intima-media thickness in atherosclerosis development in carotid arteries. *Biomed. Eng. Online* **2017**, *16*, 137. [CrossRef]
178. Xie, M.; Tang, Q.; Nie, J.; Zhang, C.; Zhou, X.; Yu, S.; Sun, J.; Cheng, X.; Dong, N.; Hu, Y.; et al. BMAL1-Downregulation Aggravates *Porphyromonas Gingivalis*-Induced Atherosclerosis by Encouraging Oxidative Stress. *Circ. Res.* **2020**, *126*, e15–e29. [CrossRef]
179. Xu, T.; Dong, Q.; Luo, Y.; Liu, Y.; Gao, L.; Pan, Y.; Zhang, D. *Porphyromonas gingivalis* infection promotes mitochondrial dysfunction through Drp1-dependent mitochondrial fission in endothelial cells. *Int. J. Oral Sci.* **2021**, *13*, 28. [CrossRef]
180. Dong, Q.; Luo, Y.; Yin, Y.; Ma, Y.; Yu, Y.; Wang, L.; Yang, H.; Pan, Y.; Zhang, D. RhoA/ROCK1 regulates the mitochondrial dysfunction through Drp1 induced by *Porphyromonas gingivalis* in endothelial cells. *J. Cell. Mol. Med.* **2023**, *27*, 2123–2135. [CrossRef]
181. Crola Da Silva, C.; Baetz, D.; Vedere, M.; Lo-Grasso, M.; Wehbi, M.; Chouabe, C.; Bidaux, G.; Ferrera, R. Isolated Mitochondria State after Myocardial Ischemia-Reperfusion Injury and Cardioprotection: Analysis by Flow Cytometry. *Life* **2023**, *13*, 707. [CrossRef] [PubMed]
182. Jin, J.Y.; Wei, X.X.; Zhi, X.L.; Wang, X.H.; Meng, D. Drp1-dependent mitochondrial fission in cardiovascular disease. *Acta Pharmacol. Sin.* **2021**, *42*, 655–664. [CrossRef]
183. Liu, S.; Zhao, Y.; Yao, H.; Zhang, L.; Chen, C.; Zheng, Z.; Jin, S. DRP1 knockdown and atorvastatin alleviate ox-LDL-induced vascular endothelial cells injury: DRP1 is a potential target for preventing atherosclerosis. *Exp. Cell Res.* **2023**, *429*, 113688. [CrossRef] [PubMed]
184. Su, Z.D.; Li, C.Q.; Wang, H.W.; Zheng, M.M.; Chen, Q.W. Inhibition of DRP1-dependent mitochondrial fission by Mdivi-1 alleviates atherosclerosis through the modulation of M1 polarization. *J. Transl. Med.* **2023**, *21*, 427. [CrossRef] [PubMed]
185. Zeng, Z.; Zheng, Q.; Chen, J.; Tan, X.; Li, Q.; Ding, L.; Zhang, R.; Lin, X. FGF21 mitigates atherosclerosis via inhibition of NLRP3 inflammasome-mediated vascular endothelial cells pyroptosis. *Exp. Cell Res.* **2020**, *393*, 112108. [CrossRef] [PubMed]
186. Zerihun, M.; Sukumaran, S.; Qvit, N. The Drp1-Mediated Mitochondrial Fission Protein Interactome as an Emerging Core Player in Mitochondrial Dynamics and Cardiovascular Disease Therapy. *Int. J. Mol. Sci.* **2023**, *24*, 5785. [CrossRef] [PubMed]
187. Huang, D.; Gao, W.; Zhong, X.; Ge, J. NLRP3 activation in endothelia promotes development of diabetes-associated atherosclerosis. *Aging (Albany NY)* **2020**, *12*, 18181–18191. [CrossRef]
188. Yamamoto, K.; Nogimori, Y.; Imamura, H.; Ando, J. Shear stress activates mitochondrial oxidative phosphorylation by reducing plasma membrane cholesterol in vascular endothelial cells. *Proc. Natl. Acad. Sci. USA* **2020**, *117*, 33660–33667. [CrossRef]
189. Yamamoto, K.; Imamura, H.; Ando, J. Shear stress augments mitochondrial ATP generation that triggers ATP release and Ca^{2+} signaling in vascular endothelial cells. *Am. J. Physiol. Heart Circ. Physiol.* **2018**, *315*, H1477–H1485. [CrossRef]
190. O-Uchi, J.; Pan, S.; Sheu, S.S. Perspectives on: SGP symposium on mitochondrial physiology and medicine: Molecular identities of mitochondrial Ca^{2+} influx mechanism: Updated passwords for accessing mitochondrial Ca^{2+}-linked health and disease. *J. Gen. Physiol.* **2012**, *139*, 435–443. [CrossRef]
191. Yamamoto, K.; Sokabe, T.; Matsumoto, T.; Yoshimura, K.; Shibata, M.; Ohura, N.; Fukuda, T.; Sato, T.; Sekine, K.; Kato, S.; et al. Impaired flow-dependent control of vascular tone and remodeling in P2X4-deficient mice. *Nat. Med.* **2006**, *12*, 133–137. [CrossRef] [PubMed]
192. Koskinas, K.C.; Feldman, C.L.; Chatzizisis, Y.S.; Coskun, A.U.; Jonas, M.; Maynard, C.; Baker, A.B.; Papafaklis, M.I.; Edelman, E.R.; Stone, P.H. Natural history of experimental coronary atherosclerosis and vascular remodeling in relation to endothelial shear stress: A serial, in vivo intravascular ultrasound study. *Circulation* **2010**, *121*, 2092–2101. [CrossRef]
193. Scharf, S.J.; Bowcock, A.M.; McClure, G.; Klitz, W.; Yandell, D.W.; Erlich, H.A. Amplification and characterization of the retinoblastoma gene VNTR by PCR. *Am. J. Hum. Genet.* **1992**, *50*, 371–381. [PubMed]
194. Cecchi, E.; Giglioli, C.; Valente, S.; Lazzeri, C.; Gensini, G.F.; Abbate, R.; Mannini, L. Role of hemodynamic shear stress in cardiovascular disease. *Atherosclerosis* **2011**, *214*, 249–256. [CrossRef]
195. Seidlmayer, L.K.; Juettner, V.V.; Kettlewell, S.; Pavlov, E.V.; Blatter, L.A.; Dedkova, E.N. Distinct mPTP activation mechanisms in ischaemia-reperfusion: Contributions of Ca^{2+}, ROS, pH, and inorganic polyphosphate. *Cardiovasc. Res.* **2015**, *106*, 237–248. [CrossRef] [PubMed]
196. Patel, A.; Pietromicca, J.G.; Venkatesan, M.; Maity, S.; Bard, J.E.; Madesh, M.; Alevriadou, B.R. Modulation of the mitochondrial Ca^{2+} uniporter complex subunit expression by different shear stress patterns in vascular endothelial cells. *Physiol. Rep.* **2023**, *11*, e15588. [CrossRef]
197. Cheng, H.; Zhong, W.; Wang, L.; Zhang, Q.; Ma, X.; Wang, Y.; Wang, S.; He, C.; Wei, Q.; Fu, C. Effects of shear stress on vascular endothelial functions in atherosclerosis and potential therapeutic approaches. *Biomed. Pharmacother.* **2023**, *158*, 114198. [CrossRef]
198. Souilhol, C.; Serbanovic-Canic, J.; Fragiadaki, M.; Chico, T.J.; Ridger, V.; Roddie, H.; Evans, P.C. Endothelial responses to shear stress in atherosclerosis: A novel role for developmental genes. *Nat. Rev. Cardiol.* **2020**, *17*, 52–63. [CrossRef]
199. Traub, O.; Berk, B.C. Laminar shear stress: Mechanisms by which endothelial cells transduce an atheroprotective force. *Arterioscler. Thromb. Vasc. Biol.* **1998**, *18*, 677–685. [CrossRef]
200. Parmar, K.M.; Larman, H.B.; Dai, G.; Zhang, Y.; Wang, E.T.; Moorthy, S.N.; Kratz, J.R.; Lin, Z.; Jain, M.K.; Gimbrone, M.A., Jr.; et al. Integration of flow-dependent endothelial phenotypes by Kruppel-like factor 2. *J. Clin. Investig.* **2006**, *116*, 49–58. [CrossRef]
201. Wu, L.H.; Chang, H.C.; Ting, P.C.; Wang, D.L. Laminar shear stress promotes mitochondrial homeostasis in endothelial cells. *J. Cell. Physiol.* **2018**, *233*, 5058–5069. [CrossRef] [PubMed]

202. Li, R.; Beebe, T.; Cui, J.; Rouhanizadeh, M.; Ai, L.; Wang, P.; Gundersen, M.; Takabe, W.; Hsiai, T.K. Pulsatile shear stress increased mitochondrial membrane potential: Implication of Mn-SOD. *Biochem. Biophys. Res. Commun.* **2009**, *388*, 406–412. [CrossRef] [PubMed]
203. Coon, B.G.; Timalsina, S.; Astone, M.; Zhuang, Z.W.; Fang, J.; Han, J.; Themen, J.; Chung, M.; Yang-Klingler, Y.J.; Jain, M.; et al. A mitochondrial contribution to anti-inflammatory shear stress signaling in vascular endothelial cells. *J. Cell Biol.* **2022**, *221*, e202109144. [CrossRef]
204. Huang, H.; Ren, P.; Zhao, Y.; Weng, H.; Jia, C.; Yu, F.; Nie, Y. Low shear stress induces inflammatory response via CX3CR1/NF-κB signal pathway in human umbilical vein endothelial cells. *Tissue Cell.* **2023**, *82*, 102043. [CrossRef] [PubMed]
205. Pfenniger, A.; Meens, M.J.; Pedrigi, R.M.; Foglia, B.; Sutter, E.; Pelli, G.; Rochemont, V.; Petrova, T.V.; Krams, R.; Kwak, B.R. Shear stress-induced atherosclerotic plaque composition in ApoE$^{-/-}$ mice is modulated by connexin37. *Atherosclerosis* **2015**, *243*, 1–10. [CrossRef] [PubMed]
206. Murray, K.O.; Ludwig, K.R.; Darvish, S.; Coppock, M.E.; Seals, D.R.; Rossman, M.J. Chronic mitochondria antioxidant treatment in older adults alters the circulating milieu to improve endothelial cell function and mitochondrial oxidative stress. *Am. J. Physiol. Heart Circ. Physiol.* **2023**, *325*, H187–H194. [CrossRef] [PubMed]
207. Zhang, J.; Guo, Y.; Ge, W.; Zhou, X.; Pan, M. High glucose induces apoptosis of HUVECs in a mitochondria-dependent manner by suppressing hexokinase 2 expression. *Exp. Ther. Med.* **2019**, *18*, 621–629. [CrossRef]
208. Tang, X.; Luo, Y.X.; Chen, H.Z.; Liu, D.P. Mitochondria, endothelial cell function, and vascular diseases. *Front. Physiol.* **2014**, *5*, 175. [CrossRef]
209. Shenouda, S.M.; Widlansky, M.E.; Chen, K.; Xu, G.; Holbrook, M.; Tabit, C.E.; Hamburg, N.M.; Frame, A.A.; Caiano, T.L.; Kluge, M.A.; et al. Altered mitochondrial dynamics contributes to endothelial dysfunction in diabetes mellitus. *Circulation* **2011**, *124*, 444–453. [CrossRef]
210. Kim, D.; Roy, S. Effects of Diabetes on Mitochondrial Morphology and Its Implications in Diabetic Retinopathy. *Investig. Ophthalmol. Vis. Sci.* **2020**, *61*, 10. [CrossRef]
211. Makino, A.; Scott, B.T.; Dillmann, W.H. Mitochondrial fragmentation and superoxide anion production in coronary endothelial cells from a mouse model of type 1 diabetes. *Diabetologia* **2010**, *53*, 1783–1794. [CrossRef] [PubMed]
212. Alka, K.; Kumar, J.; Kowluru, R.A. Impaired mitochondrial dynamics and removal of the damaged mitochondria in diabetic retinopathy. *Front. Endocrinol.* **2023**, *14*, 1160155. [CrossRef]
213. Kumar, J.; Mohammad, G.; Alka, K.; Kowluru, R.A. Mitochondrial Genome-Encoded Long Noncoding RNA and Mitochondrial Stability in Diabetic Retinopathy. *Diabetes* **2023**, *72*, 520–531. [CrossRef] [PubMed]
214. Mishiro, K.; Imai, T.; Sugitani, S.; Kitashoji, A.; Suzuki, Y.; Takagi, T.; Chen, H.; Oumi, Y.; Tsuruma, K.; Shimazawa, M.; et al. Diabetes mellitus aggravates hemorrhagic transformation after ischemic stroke via mitochondrial defects leading to endothelial apoptosis. *PLoS ONE* **2014**, *9*, e103818. [CrossRef]
215. Mackenzie, R.M.; Salt, I.P.; Miller, W.H.; Logan, A.; Ibrahim, H.A.; Degasperi, A.; Dymott, J.A.; Hamilton, C.A.; Murphy, M.P.; Delles, C.; et al. Mitochondrial reactive oxygen species enhance AMP-activated protein kinase activation in the endothelium of patients with coronary artery disease and diabetes. *Clin. Sci.* **2013**, *124*, 403–411. [CrossRef] [PubMed]
216. Sweeney, M.D.; Sagare, A.P.; Zlokovic, B.V. Blood-brain barrier breakdown in Alzheimer disease and other neurodegenerative disorders. *Nat. Rev. Neurol.* **2018**, *14*, 133–150. [CrossRef] [PubMed]
217. Tajes, M.; Ramos-Fernandez, E.; Weng-Jiang, X.; Bosch-Morato, M.; Guivernau, B.; Eraso-Pichot, A.; Salvador, B.; Fernandez-Busquets, X.; Roquer, J.; Munoz, F.J. The blood-brain barrier: Structure, function and therapeutic approaches to cross it. *Mol. Membr. Biol.* **2014**, *31*, 152–167. [CrossRef]
218. Wu, S.; Huang, R.; Zhang, R.; Xiao, C.; Wang, L.; Luo, M.; Song, N.; Zhang, J.; Yang, F.; Liu, X.; et al. Gastrodin and Gastrodigenin Improve Energy Metabolism Disorders and Mitochondrial Dysfunction to Antagonize Vascular Dementia. *Molecules* **2023**, *28*, 2598. [CrossRef]
219. Gray, M.T.; Woulfe, J.M. Striatal blood-brain barrier permeability in Parkinson's disease. *J. Cereb. Blood Flow Metab.* **2015**, *35*, 747–750. [CrossRef]
220. Fillit, H.; Nash, D.T.; Rundek, T.; Zuckerman, A. Cardiovascular risk factors and dementia. *Am. J. Geriatr. Pharmacother.* **2008**, *6*, 100–118. [CrossRef]
221. Tyagi, A.; Mirita, C.; Shah, I.; Reddy, P.H.; Pugazhenthi, S. Effects of Lipotoxicity in Brain Microvascular Endothelial Cells During Sirt3 Deficiency-Potential Role in Comorbid Alzheimer's Disease. *Front. Aging Neurosci.* **2021**, *13*, 716616. [CrossRef] [PubMed]
222. Hawkins, B.T.; Davis, T.P. The blood-brain barrier/neurovascular unit in health and disease. *Pharmacol. Rev.* **2005**, *57*, 173–185. [CrossRef] [PubMed]
223. Zlokovic, B.V. Neurovascular pathways to neurodegeneration in Alzheimer's disease and other disorders. *Nat. Rev. Neurosci.* **2011**, *12*, 723–738. [CrossRef] [PubMed]
224. Oldendorf, W.H.; Cornford, M.E.; Brown, W.J. The large apparent work capability of the blood-brain barrier: A study of the mitochondrial content of capillary endothelial cells in brain and other tissues of the rat. *Ann. Neurol.* **1977**, *1*, 409–417. [CrossRef]
225. Patergnani, S.; Bouhamida, E.; Leo, S.; Pinton, P.; Rimessi, A. Mitochondrial Oxidative Stress and "Mito-Inflammation": Actors in the Diseases. *Biomedicines* **2021**, *9*, 216. [CrossRef] [PubMed]

226. Long, Y.; Liu, X.; Tan, X.Z.; Jiang, C.X.; Chen, S.W.; Liang, G.N.; He, X.M.; Wu, J.; Chen, T.; Xu, Y. ROS-induced NLRP3 inflammasome priming and activation mediate PCB 118- induced pyroptosis in endothelial cells. *Ecotoxicol. Environ. Saf.* **2020**, *189*, 109937. [CrossRef]
227. Zhong, Z.; Liang, S.; Sanchez-Lopez, E.; He, F.; Shalapour, S.; Lin, X.J.; Wong, J.; Ding, S.; Seki, E.; Schnabl, B.; et al. New mitochondrial DNA synthesis enables NLRP3 inflammasome activation. *Nature* **2018**, *560*, 198–203. [CrossRef]
228. Shimada, K.; Crother, T.R.; Karlin, J.; Dagvadorj, J.; Chiba, N.; Chen, S.; Ramanujan, V.K.; Wolf, A.J.; Vergnes, L.; Ojcius, D.M.; et al. Oxidized mitochondrial DNA activates the NLRP3 inflammasome during apoptosis. *Immunity* **2012**, *36*, 401–414. [CrossRef]
229. Eleftheriadis, T.; Pissas, G.; Liakopoulos, V.; Stefanidis, I. Cytochrome c as a Potentially Clinical Useful Marker of Mitochondrial and Cellular Damage. *Front. Immunol.* **2016**, *7*, 279. [CrossRef]
230. Raoof, M.; Zhang, Q.; Itagaki, K.; Hauser, C.J. Mitochondrial peptides are potent immune activators that activate human neutrophils via FPR-1. *J. Trauma* **2010**, *68*, 1328–1332, discussion 1332–1324. [CrossRef]
231. Iyer, S.S.; He, Q.; Janczy, J.R.; Elliott, E.I.; Zhong, Z.; Olivier, A.K.; Sadler, J.J.; Knepper-Adrian, V.; Han, R.; Qiao, L.; et al. Mitochondrial cardiolipin is required for Nlrp3 inflammasome activation. *Immunity* **2013**, *39*, 311–323. [CrossRef]
232. Yoo, S.M.; Park, J.; Kim, S.H.; Jung, Y.K. Emerging perspectives on mitochondrial dysfunction and inflammation in Alzheimer's disease. *BMB Rep.* **2020**, *53*, 35–46. [CrossRef] [PubMed]
233. Banks, W.A.; Erickson, M.A. The blood-brain barrier and immune function and dysfunction. *Neurobiol. Dis.* **2010**, *37*, 26–32. [CrossRef] [PubMed]
234. Doll, D.N.; Hu, H.; Sun, J.; Lewis, S.E.; Simpkins, J.W.; Ren, X. Mitochondrial crisis in cerebrovascular endothelial cells opens the blood-brain barrier. *Stroke* **2015**, *46*, 1681–1689. [CrossRef] [PubMed]
235. Haileselassie, B.; Joshi, A.U.; Minhas, P.S.; Mukherjee, R.; Andreasson, K.I.; Mochly-Rosen, D. Mitochondrial dysfunction mediated through dynamin-related protein 1 (Drp1) propagates impairment in blood brain barrier in septic encephalopathy. *J. Neuroinflamm.* **2020**, *17*, 36. [CrossRef]
236. 2021 Alzheimer's disease facts and figures. *Alzheimer's Dement.* **2021**, *17*, 327–406. [CrossRef]
237. Ashleigh, T.; Swerdlow, R.H.; Beal, M.F. The role of mitochondrial dysfunction in Alzheimer's disease pathogenesis. *Alzheimer's Dement.* **2023**, *19*, 333–342. [CrossRef]
238. Salmina, A.B.; Kharitonova, E.V.; Gorina, Y.V.; Teplyashina, E.A.; Malinovskaya, N.A.; Khilazheva, E.D.; Mosyagina, A.I.; Morgun, A.V.; Shuvaev, A.N.; Salmin, V.V.; et al. Blood-Brain Barrier and Neurovascular Unit In Vitro Models for Studying Mitochondria-Driven Molecular Mechanisms of Neurodegeneration. *Int. J. Mol. Sci.* **2021**, *22*, 4661. [CrossRef]
239. Quintana, D.D.; Garcia, J.A.; Anantula, Y.; Rellick, S.L.; Engler-Chiurazzi, E.B.; Sarkar, S.N.; Brown, C.M.; Simpkins, J.W. Amyloid-beta Causes Mitochondrial Dysfunction via a Ca^{2+}-Driven Upregulation of Oxidative Phosphorylation and Superoxide Production in Cerebrovascular Endothelial Cells. *J. Alzheimer's Dis.* **2020**, *75*, 119–138. [CrossRef]
240. Petrovskaya, A.V.; Tverskoi, A.M.; Barykin, E.P.; Varshavskaya, K.B.; Dalina, A.A.; Mitkevich, V.A.; Makarov, A.A.; Petrushanko, I.Y. Distinct Effects of Beta-Amyloid, Its Isomerized and Phosphorylated Forms on the Redox Status and Mitochondrial Functioning of the Blood-Brain Barrier Endothelium. *Int. J. Mol. Sci.* **2022**, *24*, 183. [CrossRef]
241. Sakamuri, S.; Sure, V.N.; Wang, X.; Bix, G.; Fonseca, V.A.; Mostany, R.; Katakam, P.V.G. Amyloid β (1–42) peptide impairs mitochondrial respiration in primary human brain microvascular endothelial cells: Impact of dysglycemia and pre-senescence. *GeroScience* **2022**, *44*, 2721–2739. [CrossRef] [PubMed]
242. Solesio, M.E.; Peixoto, P.M.; Debure, L.; Madamba, S.M.; de Leon, M.J.; Wisniewski, T.; Pavlov, E.V.; Fossati, S. Carbonic anhydrase inhibition selectively prevents amyloid beta neurovascular mitochondrial toxicity. *Aging Cell* **2018**, *17*, e12787. [CrossRef]
243. Frontinan-Rubio, J.; Rabanal-Ruiz, Y.; Duran-Prado, M.; Alcain, F.J. The Protective Effect of Ubiquinone against the Amyloid Peptide in Endothelial Cells Is Isoprenoid Chain Length-Dependent. *Antioxidants* **2021**, *10*, 1806. [CrossRef] [PubMed]
244. Kurz, C.; Walker, L.; Rauchmann, B.S.; Perneczky, R. Dysfunction of the blood-brain barrier in Alzheimer's disease: Evidence from human studies. *Neuropathol. Appl. Neurobiol.* **2022**, *48*, e12782. [CrossRef] [PubMed]
245. Claudio, L. Ultrastructural features of the blood-brain barrier in biopsy tissue from Alzheimer's disease patients. *Acta Neuropathol.* **1996**, *91*, 6–14. [CrossRef] [PubMed]
246. Xie, H.; Guan, J.; Borrelli, L.A.; Xu, J.; Serrano-Pozo, A.; Bacskai, B.J. Mitochondrial alterations near amyloid plaques in an Alzheimer's disease mouse model. *J. Neurosci.* **2013**, *33*, 17042–17051. [CrossRef] [PubMed]
247. Urbich, C.; Dimmeler, S. Endothelial progenitor cells: Characterization and role in vascular biology. *Circ. Res.* **2004**, *95*, 343–353. [CrossRef] [PubMed]
248. Keighron, C.; Lyons, C.J.; Creane, M.; O'Brien, T.; Liew, A. Recent Advances in Endothelial Progenitor Cells Toward Their Use in Clinical Translation. *Front. Med.* **2018**, *5*, 354. [CrossRef]
249. Bompais, H.; Chagraoui, J.; Canron, X.; Crisan, M.; Liu, X.H.; Anjo, A.; Tolla-Le Port, C.; Leboeuf, M.; Charbord, P.; Bikfalvi, A.; et al. Human endothelial cells derived from circulating progenitors display specific functional properties compared with mature vessel wall endothelial cells. *Blood* **2004**, *103*, 2577–2584. [CrossRef]
250. Dight, J.; Zhao, J.; Styke, C.; Khosrotehrani, K.; Patel, J. Resident vascular endothelial progenitor definition and function: The age of reckoning. *Angiogenesis* **2022**, *25*, 15–33. [CrossRef]
251. O'Neill, C.L.; McLoughlin, K.J.; Chambers, S.E.J.; Guduric-Fuchs, J.; Stitt, A.W.; Medina, R.J. The Vasoreparative Potential of Endothelial Colony Forming Cells: A Journey Through Pre-clinical Studies. *Front. Med.* **2018**, *5*, 273. [CrossRef]

252. Faris, P.; Negri, S.; Perna, A.; Rosti, V.; Guerra, G.; Moccia, F. Therapeutic Potential of Endothelial Colony-Forming Cells in Ischemic Disease: Strategies to Improve their Regenerative Efficacy. *Int. J. Mol. Sci.* **2020**, *21*, 7406. [CrossRef] [PubMed]
253. Ingram, D.A.; Mead, L.E.; Tanaka, H.; Meade, V.; Fenoglio, A.; Mortell, K.; Pollok, K.; Ferkowicz, M.J.; Gilley, D.; Yoder, M.C. Identification of a novel hierarchy of endothelial progenitor cells using human peripheral and umbilical cord blood. *Blood* **2004**, *104*, 2752–2760. [CrossRef] [PubMed]
254. Paschalaki, K.E.; Randi, A.M. Recent Advances in Endothelial Colony Forming Cells Toward Their Use in Clinical Translation. *Front. Med.* **2018**, *5*, 295. [CrossRef] [PubMed]
255. Fadini, G.P.; Boscaro, E.; de Kreutzenberg, S.; Agostini, C.; Seeger, F.; Dimmeler, S.; Zeiher, A.; Tiengo, A.; Avogaro, A. Time course and mechanisms of circulating progenitor cell reduction in the natural history of type 2 diabetes. *Diabetes Care* **2010**, *33*, 1097–1102. [CrossRef]
256. Hortenhuber, T.; Rami-Mehar, B.; Satler, M.; Nagl, K.; Hobaus, C.; Hollerl, F.; Koppensteiner, R.; Schernthaner, G.; Schober, E.; Schernthaner, G.H. Endothelial progenitor cells are related to glycemic control in children with type 1 diabetes over time. *Diabetes Care* **2013**, *36*, 1647–1653. [CrossRef]
257. Zhang, Q.; Cannavicci, A.; Kutryk, M.J.B. Exploring Endothelial Colony-Forming Cells to Better Understand the Pathophysiology of Disease: An Updated Review. *Stem Cells Int.* **2022**, *2022*, 4460041. [CrossRef]
258. Altabas, V.; Marinkovic Radosevic, J.; Spoljarec, L.; Uremovic, S.; Bulum, T. The Impact of Modern Anti-Diabetic Treatment on Endothelial Progenitor Cells. *Biomedicines* **2023**, *11*, 3051. [CrossRef]
259. Muller-Ehmsen, J.; Braun, D.; Schneider, T.; Pfister, R.; Worm, N.; Wielckens, K.; Scheid, C.; Frommolt, P.; Flesch, M. Decreased number of circulating progenitor cells in obesity: Beneficial effects of weight reduction. *Eur. Heart J.* **2008**, *29*, 1560–1568. [CrossRef]
260. Tobler, K.; Freudenthaler, A.; Baumgartner-Parzer, S.M.; Wolzt, M.; Ludvik, B.; Nansalmaa, E.; Nowotny, P.J.; Seidinger, D.; Steiner, S.; Luger, A.; et al. Reduction of both number and proliferative activity of human endothelial progenitor cells in obesity. *Int. J. Obes.* **2010**, *34*, 687–700. [CrossRef]
261. Cedar, H.; Bergman, Y. Programming of DNA methylation patterns. *Annu. Rev. Biochem.* **2012**, *81*, 97–117. [CrossRef]
262. Smith, N.; Shirazi, S.; Cakouros, D.; Gronthos, S. Impact of Environmental and Epigenetic Changes on Mesenchymal Stem Cells during Aging. *Int. J. Mol. Sci.* **2023**, *24*, 6499. [CrossRef] [PubMed]
263. Tan, D.Q.; Suda, T. Reactive Oxygen Species and Mitochondrial Homeostasis as Regulators of Stem Cell Fate and Function. *Antioxid. Redox Signal.* **2018**, *29*, 149–168. [CrossRef] [PubMed]
264. Hahm, J.Y.; Park, J.; Jang, E.S.; Chi, S.W. 8-Oxoguanine: From oxidative damage to epigenetic and epitranscriptional modification. *Exp. Mol. Med.* **2022**, *54*, 1626–1642. [CrossRef]
265. Moreno-Luna, R.; Munoz-Hernandez, R.; Lin, R.Z.; Miranda, M.L.; Vallejo-Vaz, A.J.; Stiefel, P.; Praena-Fernandez, J.M.; Bernal-Bermejo, J.; Jimenez-Jimenez, L.M.; Villar, J.; et al. Maternal body-mass index and cord blood circulating endothelial colony-forming cells. *J. Pediatr.* **2014**, *164*, 566–571. [CrossRef]
266. Weiss, E.; Leopold-Posch, B.; Schrufer, A.; Cvitic, S.; Hiden, U. Fetal sex and maternal fasting glucose affect neonatal cord blood-derived endothelial progenitor cells. *Pediatr. Res.* **2022**, *92*, 1590–1597. [CrossRef] [PubMed]
267. Gumina, D.L.; Su, E.J. Endothelial Progenitor Cells of the Human Placenta and Fetoplacental Circulation: A Potential Link to Fetal, Neonatal, and Long-term Health. *Front. Pediatr.* **2017**, *5*, 41. [CrossRef]
268. Ingram, D.A.; Lien, I.Z.; Mead, L.E.; Estes, M.; Prater, D.N.; Derr-Yellin, E.; DiMeglio, L.A.; Haneline, L.S. In vitro hyperglycemia or a diabetic intrauterine environment reduces neonatal endothelial colony-forming cell numbers and function. *Diabetes* **2008**, *57*, 724–731. [CrossRef]
269. Blue, E.K.; DiGiuseppe, R.; Derr-Yellin, E.; Acosta, J.C.; Pay, S.L.; Hanenberg, H.; Schellinger, M.M.; Quinney, S.K.; Mund, J.A.; Case, J.; et al. Gestational diabetes induces alterations in the function of neonatal endothelial colony-forming cells. *Pediatr. Res.* **2014**, *75*, 266–272. [CrossRef]
270. Apatiga-Perez, R.; Soto-Rojas, L.O.; Campa-Cordoba, B.B.; Luna-Viramontes, N.I.; Cuevas, E.; Villanueva-Fierro, I.; Ontiveros-Torres, M.A.; Bravo-Munoz, M.; Flores-Rodriguez, P.; Garces-Ramirez, L.; et al. Neurovascular dysfunction and vascular amyloid accumulation as early events in Alzheimer's disease. *Metab. Brain Dis.* **2022**, *37*, 39–50. [CrossRef]
271. Hussain, B.; Fang, C.; Chang, J. Blood-Brain Barrier Breakdown: An Emerging Biomarker of Cognitive Impairment in Normal Aging and Dementia. *Front. Neurosci.* **2021**, *15*, 688090. [CrossRef]
272. Safar, M.M.; Arab, H.H.; Rizk, S.M.; El-Maraghy, S.A. Bone Marrow-Derived Endothelial Progenitor Cells Protect Against Scopolamine-Induced Alzheimer-Like Pathological Aberrations. *Mol. Neurobiol.* **2016**, *53*, 1403–1418. [CrossRef] [PubMed]
273. Zhang, S.; Zhi, Y.; Li, F.; Huang, S.; Gao, H.; Han, Z.; Ge, X.; Li, D.; Chen, F.; Kong, X.; et al. Transplantation of in vitro cultured endothelial progenitor cells repairs the blood-brain barrier and improves cognitive function of APP/PS1 transgenic AD mice. *J. Neurol. Sci.* **2018**, *387*, 6–15. [CrossRef] [PubMed]
274. Bigalke, B.; Schreitmuller, B.; Sopova, K.; Paul, A.; Stransky, E.; Gawaz, M.; Stellos, K.; Laske, C. Adipocytokines and CD34 progenitor cells in Alzheimer's disease. *PLoS ONE* **2011**, *6*, e20286. [CrossRef] [PubMed]
275. Breining, A.; Silvestre, J.S.; Dieudonne, B.; Vilar, J.; Faucounau, V.; Verny, M.; Neri, C.; Boulanger, C.M.; Boddaert, J. Biomarkers of vascular dysfunction and cognitive decline in patients with Alzheimer's disease: No evidence for association in elderly subjects. *Aging Clin. Exp. Res.* **2016**, *28*, 1133–1141. [CrossRef] [PubMed]

276. Lee, S.T.; Chu, K.; Jung, K.H.; Park, H.K.; Kim, D.H.; Bahn, J.J.; Kim, J.H.; Oh, M.J.; Lee, S.K.; Kim, M.; et al. Reduced circulating angiogenic cells in Alzheimer disease. *Neurology* **2009**, *72*, 1858–1863. [CrossRef]
277. Kong, X.D.; Zhang, Y.; Liu, L.; Sun, N.; Zhang, M.Y.; Zhang, J.N. Endothelial progenitor cells with Alzheimer's disease. *Chin. Med. J.* **2011**, *124*, 901–906.
278. Maler, J.M.; Spitzer, P.; Lewczuk, P.; Kornhuber, J.; Herrmann, M.; Wiltfang, J. Decreased circulating CD34$^+$ stem cells in early Alzheimer's disease: Evidence for a deficient hematopoietic brain support? *Mol. Psychiatry* **2006**, *11*, 1113–1115. [CrossRef]
279. Wang, Y.; Huang, J.; Ang, T.F.A.; Zhu, Y.; Tao, Q.; Mez, J.; Alosco, M.; Denis, G.V.; Belkina, A.; Gurnani, A.; et al. Circulating Endothelial Progenitor Cells Reduce the Risk of Alzheimer's Disease. *medRxiv* **2023**. [CrossRef]
280. Ferreira, N.V.; Goncalves, N.G.; Szlejf, C.; Goulart, A.C.; de Souza Santos, I.; Duncan, B.B.; Schmidt, M.I.; Barreto, S.M.; Caramelli, P.; Feter, N.; et al. Optimal cardiovascular health is associated with slower cognitive decline. *Eur. J. Neurol.* **2023**, *31*, e16139. [CrossRef]
281. Wang, H.H.; Wu, Y.J.; Tseng, Y.M.; Su, C.H.; Hsieh, C.L.; Yeh, H.I. Mitochondrial fission protein 1 up-regulation ameliorates senescence-related endothelial dysfunction of human endothelial progenitor cells. *Angiogenesis* **2019**, *22*, 569–582. [CrossRef] [PubMed]
282. Alvarado-Moreno, J.A.; Hernandez-Lopez, R.; Chavez-Gonzalez, A.; Yoder, M.C.; Rangel-Corona, R.; Isordia-Salas, I.; Hernandez-Juarez, J.; Cerbulo-Vazquez, A.; Gonzalez-Jimenez, M.A.; Majluf-Cruz, A. Endothelial colony-forming cells: Biological and functional abnormalities in patients with recurrent, unprovoked venous thromboembolic disease. *Thromb. Res.* **2016**, *137*, 157–168. [CrossRef] [PubMed]
283. Yu, B.B.; Zhi, H.; Zhang, X.Y.; Liang, J.W.; He, J.; Su, C.; Xia, W.H.; Zhang, G.X.; Tao, J. Mitochondrial dysfunction-mediated decline in angiogenic capacity of endothelial progenitor cells is associated with capillary rarefaction in patients with hypertension via downregulation of CXCR4/JAK2/SIRT5 signaling. *EBioMedicine* **2019**, *42*, 64–75. [CrossRef] [PubMed]
284. Yang, J.; Sun, M.; Cheng, R.; Tan, H.; Liu, C.; Chen, R.; Zhang, J.; Yang, Y.; Gao, X.; Huang, L. Pitavastatin activates mitophagy to protect EPC proliferation through a calcium-dependent CAMK1-PINK1 pathway in atherosclerotic mice. *Commun. Biol.* **2022**, *5*, 124. [CrossRef] [PubMed]
285. Besnier, M.; Finemore, M.; Yu, C.; Kott, K.A.; Vernon, S.T.; Seebacher, N.A.; Genetzakis, E.; Furman, A.; Tang, O.; Davis, R.L.; et al. Patient Endothelial Colony-Forming Cells to Model Coronary Artery Disease Susceptibility and Unravel the Role of Dysregulated Mitochondrial Redox Signalling. *Antioxidants* **2021**, *10*, 1547. [CrossRef] [PubMed]
286. Dai, X.; Wang, K.; Fan, J.; Liu, H.; Fan, X.; Lin, Q.; Chen, Y.; Chen, H.; Li, Y.; Liu, H.; et al. Nrf2 transcriptional upregulation of IDH2 to tune mitochondrial dynamics and rescue angiogenic function of diabetic EPCs. *Redox Biol.* **2022**, *56*, 102449. [CrossRef]
287. Shao, Y.; Chen, J.; Dong, L.J.; He, X.; Cheng, R.; Zhou, K.; Liu, J.; Qiu, F.; Li, X.R.; Ma, J.X. A Protective Effect of PPARα in Endothelial Progenitor Cells Through Regulating Metabolism. *Diabetes* **2019**, *68*, 2131–2142. [CrossRef]
288. Li, T.B.; Zhang, J.J.; Liu, B.; Luo, X.J.; Ma, Q.L.; Peng, J. Dysfunction of endothelial progenitor cells in hyperlipidemic rats involves the increase of NADPH oxidase derived reactive oxygen species production. *Can. J. Physiol. Pharmacol.* **2017**, *95*, 474–480. [CrossRef]
289. Li, T.B.; Zhang, Y.Z.; Liu, W.Q.; Zhang, J.J.; Peng, J.; Luo, X.J.; Ma, Q.L. Correlation between NADPH oxidase-mediated oxidative stress and dysfunction of endothelial progenitor cell in hyperlipidemic patients. *Korean J. Intern. Med.* **2018**, *33*, 313–322. [CrossRef]
290. Han, Y.; Yan, J.; Li, Z.Y.; Fan, Y.J.; Jiang, Z.L.; Shyy, J.Y.; Chien, S. Cyclic stretch promotes vascular homing of endothelial progenitor cells via Acsl1 regulation of mitochondrial fatty acid oxidation. *Proc. Natl. Acad. Sci. USA* **2023**, *120*, e2219630120. [CrossRef]
291. O'Neill, K.M.; Campbell, D.C.; Edgar, K.S.; Gill, E.K.; Moez, A.; McLoughlin, K.J.; O'Neill, C.L.; Dellett, M.; Hargey, C.J.; Abudalo, R.A.; et al. NOX4 is a major regulator of cord blood-derived endothelial colony-forming cells which promotes post-ischaemic revascularization. *Cardiovasc. Res.* **2020**, *116*, 393–405. [CrossRef] [PubMed]
292. Ren, R.; Guo, J.; Shi, J.; Tian, Y.; Li, M.; Kang, H. PKM2 regulates angiogenesis of VR-EPCs through modulating glycolysis, mitochondrial fission, and fusion. *J. Cell. Physiol.* **2020**, *235*, 6204–6217. [CrossRef] [PubMed]
293. Shao, Y.; Chen, J.; Freeman, W.; Dong, L.J.; Zhang, Z.H.; Xu, M.; Qiu, F.; Du, Y.; Liu, J.; Li, X.R.; et al. Canonical Wnt Signaling Promotes Neovascularization Through Determination of Endothelial Progenitor Cell Fate via Metabolic Profile Regulation. *Stem Cells.* **2019**, *37*, 1331–1343. [CrossRef] [PubMed]
294. Smith, R.A.; Murphy, M.P. Animal and human studies with the mitochondria-targeted antioxidant MitoQ. *Ann. N. Y Acad. Sci.* **2010**, *1201*, 96–103. [CrossRef] [PubMed]
295. Park, S.Y.; Pekas, E.J.; Headid, R.J., 3rd; Son, W.M.; Wooden, T.K.; Song, J.; Layec, G.; Yadav, S.K.; Mishra, P.K.; Pipinos, I.I. Acute mitochondrial antioxidant intake improves endothelial function, antioxidant enzyme activity, and exercise tolerance in patients with peripheral artery disease. *Am. J. Physiol. Heart Circ. Physiol.* **2020**, *319*, H456–H467. [CrossRef] [PubMed]
296. Rossman, M.J.; Santos-Parker, J.R.; Steward, C.A.C.; Bispham, N.Z.; Cuevas, L.M.; Rosenberg, H.L.; Woodward, K.A.; Chonchol, M.; Gioscia-Ryan, R.A.; Murphy, M.P.; et al. Chronic Supplementation with a Mitochondrial Antioxidant (MitoQ) Improves Vascular Function in Healthy Older Adults. *Hypertension* **2018**, *71*, 1056–1063. [CrossRef] [PubMed]
297. Shabalina, I.G.; Vyssokikh, M.Y.; Gibanova, N.; Csikasz, R.I.; Edgar, D.; Hallden-Waldemarson, A.; Rozhdestvenskaya, Z.; Bakeeva, L.E.; Vays, V.B.; Pustovidko, A.V.; et al. Improved health-span and lifespan in mtDNA mutator mice treated with the mitochondrially targeted antioxidant SkQ1. *Aging (Albany NY)* **2017**, *9*, 315–339. [CrossRef]

298. Sacks, B.; Onal, H.; Martorana, R.; Sehgal, A.; Harvey, A.; Wastella, C.; Ahmad, H.; Ross, E.; Pjetergjoka, A.; Prasad, S.; et al. Mitochondrial targeted antioxidants, mitoquinone and SKQ1, not vitamin C, mitigate doxorubicin-induced damage in H9c2 myoblast: Pretreatment vs. co-treatment. *BMC Pharmacol. Toxicol.* **2021**, *22*, 49. [CrossRef]
299. Anisimov, V.N.; Egorov, M.V.; Krasilshchikova, M.S.; Lyamzaev, K.G.; Manskikh, V.N.; Moshkin, M.P.; Novikov, E.A.; Popovich, I.G.; Rogovin, K.A.; Shabalina, I.G.; et al. Effects of the mitochondria-targeted antioxidant SkQ1 on lifespan of rodents. *Aging (Albany NY)* **2011**, *3*, 1110–1119. [CrossRef]
300. Lakomkin, V.L.; Abramov, A.A.; Kapel'ko, V.I. Mitochondrial antioxidant SkQl decreases intensity of ventricular arrhythmias caused by epinephrine. *Kardiologiia* **2011**, *51*, 60–64.
301. Ramil-Gomez, O.; Lopez-Pardo, M.; Fernandez-Rodriguez, J.A.; Rodriguez-Carmona, A.; Perez-Lopez, T.; Vaamonde-Garcia, C.; Perez-Fontan, M.; Lopez-Armada, M.J. Involvement of Mitochondrial Dysfunction in the Inflammatory Response in Human Mesothelial Cells from Peritoneal Dialysis Effluent. *Antioxidants* **2022**, *11*, 2184. [CrossRef] [PubMed]
302. Russo, S.; De Rasmo, D.; Signorile, A.; Corcelli, A.; Lobasso, S. Beneficial effects of SS-31 peptide on cardiac mitochondrial dysfunction in tafazzin knockdown mice. *Sci. Rep.* **2022**, *12*, 19847. [CrossRef] [PubMed]
303. Whitson, J.A.; Johnson, R.; Wang, L.; Bammler, T.K.; Imai, S.I.; Zhang, H.; Fredrickson, J.; Latorre-Esteves, E.; Bitto, A.; MacCoss, M.J.; et al. Age-related disruption of the proteome and acetylome in mouse hearts is associated with loss of function and attenuated by elamipretide (SS-31) and nicotinamide mononucleotide (NMN) treatment. *GeroScience* **2022**, *44*, 1621–1639. [CrossRef] [PubMed]
304. Deus, C.M.; Pereira, S.P.; Cunha-Oliveira, T.; Teixeira, J.; Simoes, R.F.; Cagide, F.; Benfeito, S.; Borges, F.; Raimundo, N.; Oliveira, P.J. A mitochondria-targeted caffeic acid derivative reverts cellular and mitochondrial defects in human skin fibroblasts from male sporadic Parkinson's disease patients. *Redox Biol.* **2021**, *45*, 102037. [CrossRef] [PubMed]
305. Amorim, R.; Cagide, F.; Tavares, L.C.; Simoes, R.F.; Soares, P.; Benfeito, S.; Baldeiras, I.; Jones, J.G.; Borges, F.; Oliveira, P.J.; et al. Mitochondriotropic antioxidant based on caffeic acid AntiOxCIN(4) activates Nrf2-dependent antioxidant defenses and quality control mechanisms to antagonize oxidative stress-induced cell damage. *Free Radic. Biol. Med.* **2022**, *179*, 119–132. [CrossRef] [PubMed]
306. Amorim, R.; Simoes, I.C.M.; Teixeira, J.; Cagide, F.; Potes, Y.; Soares, P.; Carvalho, A.; Tavares, L.C.; Benfeito, S.; Pereira, S.P.; et al. Mitochondria-targeted anti-oxidant AntiOxCIN(4) improved liver steatosis in Western diet-fed mice by preventing lipid accumulation due to upregulation of fatty acid oxidation, quality control mechanism and antioxidant defense systems. *Redox Biol.* **2022**, *55*, 102400. [CrossRef]
307. Xu, X.; Hua, Y.; Nair, S.; Bucala, R.; Ren, J. Macrophage migration inhibitory factor deletion exacerbates pressure overload-induced cardiac hypertrophy through mitigating autophagy. *Hypertension* **2014**, *63*, 490–499. [CrossRef]
308. Dutta, D.; Xu, J.; Kim, J.S.; Dunn, W.A., Jr.; Leeuwenburgh, C. Upregulated autophagy protects cardiomyocytes from oxidative stress-induced toxicity. *Autophagy* **2013**, *9*, 328–344. [CrossRef]
309. Huang, J.R.; Zhang, M.H.; Chen, Y.J.; Sun, Y.L.; Gao, Z.M.; Li, Z.J.; Zhang, G.P.; Qin, Y.; Dai, X.Y.; Yu, X.Y.; et al. Urolithin A ameliorates obesity-induced metabolic cardiomyopathy in mice via mitophagy activation. *Acta Pharmacol. Sin.* **2023**, *44*, 321–331. [CrossRef]
310. Li, Y.; Ma, Y.; Song, L.; Yu, L.; Zhang, L.; Zhang, Y.; Xing, Y.; Yin, Y.; Ma, H. SIRT3 deficiency exacerbates p53/Parkin-mediated mitophagy inhibition and promotes mitochondrial dysfunction: Implication for aged hearts. *Int. J. Mol. Med.* **2018**, *41*, 3517–3526. [CrossRef]
311. Agarwal, S.; Muqit, M.M.K. PTEN-induced kinase 1 (PINK1) and Parkin: Unlocking a mitochondrial quality control pathway linked to Parkinson's disease. *Curr. Opin. Neurobiol.* **2022**, *72*, 111–119. [CrossRef] [PubMed]
312. Price, N.L.; Gomes, A.P.; Ling, A.J.; Duarte, F.V.; Martin-Montalvo, A.; North, B.J.; Agarwal, B.; Ye, L.; Ramadori, G.; Teodoro, J.S.; et al. SIRT1 is required for AMPK activation and the beneficial effects of resveratrol on mitochondrial function. *Cell Metab.* **2012**, *15*, 675–690. [CrossRef] [PubMed]
313. Corona, J.C.; Duchen, M.R. PPARγ as a therapeutic target to rescue mitochondrial function in neurological disease. *Free Radic. Biol. Med.* **2016**, *100*, 153–163. [CrossRef] [PubMed]
314. Seabright, A.P.; Fine, N.H.F.; Barlow, J.P.; Lord, S.O.; Musa, I.; Gray, A.; Bryant, J.A.; Banzhaf, M.; Lavery, G.G.; Hardie, D.G.; et al. AMPK activation induces mitophagy and promotes mitochondrial fission while activating TBK1 in a PINK1-Parkin independent manner. *FASEB J.* **2020**, *34*, 6284–6301. [CrossRef] [PubMed]
315. Li, S.; Liu, M.; Chen, J.; Chen, Y.; Yin, M.; Zhou, Y.; Li, Q.; Xu, F.; Li, Y.; Yan, X.; et al. L-carnitine alleviates cardiac microvascular dysfunction in diabetic cardiomyopathy by enhancing PINK1-Parkin-dependent mitophagy through the CPT1a-PHB2-PARL pathways. *Acta Physiol.* **2023**, *238*, e13975. [CrossRef] [PubMed]
316. Memme, J.M.; Erlich, A.T.; Phukan, G.; Hood, D.A. Exercise and mitochondrial health. *J. Physiol.* **2021**, *599*, 803–817. [CrossRef]
317. Guedouari, H.; Daigle, T.; Scorrano, L.; Hebert-Chatelain, E. Sirtuin 5 protects mitochondria from fragmentation and degradation during starvation. *Biochim. Biophys. Acta (BBA) Mol. Cell Res.* **2017**, *1864*, 169–176. [CrossRef]
318. Um, J.H.; Lee, K.M.; Kim, Y.Y.; Lee, D.Y.; Kim, E.; Kim, D.H.; Yun, J. Berberine Induces Mitophagy through Adenosine Monophosphate-Activated Protein Kinase and Ameliorates Mitochondrial Dysfunction in PINK1 Knockout Mouse Embryonic Fibroblasts. *Int. J. Mol. Sci.* **2023**, *25*, 219. [CrossRef]
319. World Health Organization. 2023. Available online: https://www.who.int/news-room/fact-sheets/detail/cardiovascular-diseases-(cvds) (accessed on 18 January 2024).

320. Pereira, S.P.; Tavares, L.C.; Duarte, A.I.; Baldeiras, I.; Cunha-Oliveira, T.; Martins, J.D.; Santos, M.S.; Maloyan, A.; Moreno, A.J.; Cox, L.A.; et al. Sex-dependent vulnerability of fetal nonhuman primate cardiac mitochondria to moderate maternal nutrient reduction. *Clin. Sci.* **2021**, *135*, 1103–1126. [CrossRef]
321. Brislane, A.; Matenchuck, B.A.; Skow, R.J.; Steinback, C.D.; Davenport, M.H. Prenatal Exercise and Cardiovascular Health (PEACH) Study: Impact of pregnancy and exercise on rating of perceived exertion during non-weight-bearing exercise. *Appl. Physiol. Nutr. Metab.* **2022**, *47*, 804–809. [CrossRef]
322. Jevtovic, F.; Zheng, D.; Houmard, J.A.; Krassovskaia, P.M.; Lopez, C.A.; Wisseman, B.L.; Steen, D.M.; Broskey, N.T.; Isler, C.; DeVente, J.; et al. Effects of Maternal Exercise Modes on Glucose and Lipid Metabolism in Offspring Stem Cells. *J. Clin. Endocrinol. Metab.* **2023**, *108*, e360–e370. [CrossRef] [PubMed]
323. Chaves, A.; Weyrauch, L.A.; Zheng, D.; Biagioni, E.M.; Krassovskaia, P.M.; Davidson, B.L.; Broskey, N.T.; Boyle, K.E.; May, L.E.; Houmard, J.A. Influence of Maternal Exercise on Glucose and Lipid Metabolism in Offspring Stem Cells: ENHANCED by Mom. *J. Clin. Endocrinol. Metab.* **2022**, *107*, e3353–e3365. [CrossRef]
324. Boparai, R.; Skow, R.J.; Farooq, S.; Steinback, C.D.; Davenport, M.H. Prenatal exercise and cardiovascular health (PEACH) study: The remote effect of aerobic exercise training on conduit artery and resistance vessel function. *Appl. Physiol. Nutr. Metab.* **2021**, *46*, 1459–1468. [CrossRef]
325. May, L.E.; McDonald, S.; Forbes, L.; Jones, R.; Newton, E.; Strickland, D.; Isler, C.; Haven, K.; Steed, D.; Kelley, G.; et al. Influence of maternal aerobic exercise during pregnancy on fetal cardiac function and outflow. *Am. J. Obstet. Gynecol. MFM.* **2020**, *2*, 100095. [CrossRef] [PubMed]
326. Nyrnes, S.A.; Garnaes, K.K.; Salvesen, O.; Timilsina, A.S.; Moholdt, T.; Ingul, C.B. Cardiac function in newborns of obese women and the effect of exercise during pregnancy. A randomized controlled trial. *PLoS ONE* **2018**, *13*, e0197334. [CrossRef] [PubMed]
327. Yang, Y.; Xu, P.; Zhu, F.; Liao, J.; Wu, Y.; Hu, M.; Fu, H.; Qiao, J.; Lin, L.; Huang, B.; et al. The Potent Antioxidant MitoQ Protects Against Preeclampsia During Late Gestation but Increases the Risk of Preeclampsia When Administered in Early Pregnancy. *Antioxid. Redox Signal.* **2021**, *34*, 118–136. [CrossRef]
328. Sukjamnong, S.; Chan, Y.L.; Zakarya, R.; Nguyen, L.T.; Anwer, A.G.; Zaky, A.A.; Santiyanont, R.; Oliver, B.G.; Goldys, E.; Pollock, C.A.; et al. MitoQ supplementation prevent long-term impact of maternal smoking on renal development, oxidative stress and mitochondrial density in male mice offspring. *Sci. Rep.* **2018**, *8*, 6631. [CrossRef]
329. Aljunaidy, M.M.; Morton, J.S.; Kirschenman, R.; Phillips, T.; Case, C.P.; Cooke, C.M.; Davidge, S.T. Maternal treatment with a placental-targeted antioxidant (MitoQ) impacts offspring cardiovascular function in a rat model of prenatal hypoxia. *Pharmacol. Res.* **2018**, *134*, 332–342. [CrossRef]

biology

MDPI

Review

From Non-Alcoholic Fatty Liver to Hepatocellular Carcinoma: A Story of (Mal)Adapted Mitochondria

Ricardo Amorim [1,2,*], Carina C. Magalhães [1], Fernanda Borges [2], Paulo J. Oliveira [1] and José Teixeira [1,*]

[1] CNC—Center for Neuroscience and Cell Biology, CIBB—Centre for Innovative Biomedicine and Biotechnology, University of Coimbra, 3004-504 Coimbra, Portugal
[2] CIQUP-IMS/Department of Chemistry and Biochemistry, Faculty of Sciences, University of Porto, 4169-007 Porto, Portugal
* Correspondence: ramorim@cnc.uc.pt (R.A.); jteixeira@cnc.uc.pt (J.T.)

Simple Summary: Non-alcoholic fatty liver disease (NAFLD) is a global pandemic that affects 25% of the world's population and represents a serious health and economic concern worldwide resulting from unhealthy dietary habits combined with a sedentary lifestyle, although genetic contributions have been documented. Although the molecular mechanisms that cause the progression are not fully understood, metabolic-dysfunction-associated fatty liver disease is strong evidence that mitochondrial dysfunction plays a significant role in NAFLD. This review postulates that the regulation of hepatocytes' mitochondrial physiology to maintain hepatic mitochondrial mass, integrity, and function are differently altered during NAFLD progression. This review summarizes evidence linking mitochondrial (dys)function with NAFLD pathophysiology, discriminating it in different disease stages (simple steatosis, steatohepatitis, liver fibrosis, cirrhosis, and hepatocellular carcinoma). As mitochondrial dysfunction is considered a driving force in NAFLD progression, targeting hepatocytes' mitochondrial physiology could contribute to establishing an effective therapy for NAFLD. However, additional studies on distinct mitochondrial sub-populations roles in NAFLD, the impact of mitochondrial (mis)communication with other subcellular organelles (peroxisomes and lipid droplets), the impact of negligible pathways, such as fatty acid oxidation, de novo lipogenesis, and the pentose phosphate pathway in the hepatocytes' mitochondrial physiology in different stages of NAFLD are topics to explore.

Abstract: Non-alcoholic fatty liver disease (NAFLD) is a global pandemic affecting 25% of the world's population and is a serious health and economic concern worldwide. NAFLD is mainly the result of unhealthy dietary habits combined with sedentary lifestyle, although some genetic contributions to NAFLD have been documented. NAFLD is characterized by the excessive accumulation of triglycerides (TGs) in hepatocytes and encompasses a spectrum of chronic liver abnormalities, ranging from simple steatosis (NAFL) to steatohepatitis (NASH), significant liver fibrosis, cirrhosis, and hepatocellular carcinoma. Although the molecular mechanisms that cause the progression of steatosis to severe liver damage are not fully understood, metabolic-dysfunction-associated fatty liver disease is strong evidence that mitochondrial dysfunction plays a significant role in the development and progression of NAFLD. Mitochondria are highly dynamic organelles that undergo functional and structural adaptations to meet the metabolic requirements of the cell. Alterations in nutrient availability or cellular energy needs can modify mitochondria formation through biogenesis or the opposite processes of fission and fusion and fragmentation. In NAFL, simple steatosis can be seen as an adaptive response to storing lipotoxic free fatty acids (FFAs) as inert TGs due to chronic perturbation in lipid metabolism and lipotoxic insults. However, when liver hepatocytes' adaptive mechanisms are overburdened, lipotoxicity occurs, contributing to reactive oxygen species (ROS) formation, mitochondrial dysfunction, and endoplasmic reticulum (ER) stress. Impaired mitochondrial fatty acid oxidation, reduction in mitochondrial quality, and disrupted mitochondrial function are associated with a decrease in the energy levels and impaired redox balance and negatively affect mitochondria hepatocyte tolerance towards damaging hits. However, the sequence of events underlying mitochondrial failure from steatosis to hepatocarcinoma is still yet to be fully clarified.

This review provides an overview of our understanding of mitochondrial adaptation in initial NAFLD stages and highlights how hepatic mitochondrial dysfunction and heterogeneity contribute to disease pathophysiology progression, from steatosis to hepatocellular carcinoma. Improving our understanding of different aspects of hepatocytes' mitochondrial physiology in the context of disease development and progression is crucial to improving diagnosis, management, and therapy of NAFLD/NASH.

Keywords: non-alcoholic fatty liver disease (NAFLD); mitochondrial hepatic populations; mitochondrial adaptation; mitochondrial dysfunction

1. Introduction

Non-alcoholic fatty liver disease (NAFLD) is a spectrum of fatty liver phenotypes that do not result from alcohol consumption abuse (i.e., ≤30 g alcohol/day in men; ≤20 g alcohol/day in women), viral or autoimmune factors, or drug exposure. Global prevalence of NAFLD is around 25–29% and is closely associated with multiple metabolic disorders such as type 2 diabetes mellitus (T2M), obesity, hypertension, and hyperlipidemia, but a contribution of the hereditary component has also been demonstrated [1]. The diagnosis of this disease requires evidence of an excessive accumulation of TG in the hepatocytes while excluding other factors that also can lead to development of hepatic steatosis. NAFLD can range from NAFL or simple steatosis, a more benign stage, to NASH, which can progress to cirrhosis and hepatocellular carcinoma (HCC) [2,3]. The pathophysiology of NAFLD/NASH is multifactorial, and the progression to advanced forms remains unclear. Notwithstanding, two-hit or, more recently, the multiple-hit hypothesis is the most widely accepted explanation for NAFLD development. Accordingly, hepatic steatosis (first-hit) can progress to further stages due to several second hits (mitochondrial dysfunction, oxidative stress, proinflammatory cytokines, or gut-derived bacterial endotoxins).

Mitochondria play an important role in maintaining homeostasis in the liver and, consequently, are closely involved in the development of NAFLD disease. Although mitochondria counteract lipotoxic insults in the initial stage of the disease, prolonged uncontrolled stimulation of basal reactive oxygen species (ROS) production or failure of antioxidant defenses to neutralize them results in oxidative stress and hepatocyte injury [4]. Still, some aspects of hepatocytes' mitochondrial physiology in NAFLD remain unclear.

This review postulates that multiple pathways involved in regulating hepatocytes' mitochondrial physiology to maintain hepatic mitochondrial mass, integrity, and function are altered differently during NAFLD progression. This review summarizes the current evidence that links mitochondrial (dys)function with NAFLD pathophysiology, discriminating them in different disease stages. This knowledge of the mitochondrial physiology of hepatocytes and associated signaling pathways involved in disease development and progression will decisively impact diagnosis, management, and therapy of NAFLD/NASH.

2. NAFLD Disease

2.1. Epidemiology

The incidence and prevalence of NAFLD is increasing worldwide. Statistically, the global prevalence of NAFLD is around 25–29%, with the lowest rate in Africa (13%) and the highest in Southeast Asia (42%) [5]. In Europe, the prevalence of NAFLD is approximately 24%, with notoriously higher rates in Southern than Northern Europe [6,7]. Additionally, a time-dependent uptrend in NAFLD prevalence is documented (from 25% between 1999 and 2005, to 28% between 2006 and 2011, and 34% (32–36) between 2012 and 2017) [5]. NAFLD incidence is higher in men than in women (37% vs. 23% and more common in older populations (age ≥ 45 years) than in younger populations (age < 45 years; 32% vs. 27%) [5]. Although NAFLD is strongly associated with obesity episodes, lean NAFLD is also a health concern. From the NAFL patient population, 59% progress to NASH, of whom 41% develop fibrosis. Additionally, 40% of the patients with fibrosis become cirrhotic [8]. NASH has a global prevalence estimated between 3% to 5%. Still, NASH is responsible for 18% of all HCC cases in the USA, which corresponds to an 8-fold increase from 2002 to 2017 [9]. Concerningly, NAFLD is a rising cause of HCC worldwide.

2.2. Risk Factors

NAFLD is mainly the result of unhealthy dietary habits such as high caloric intake and fructose consumption combined with sedentary lifestyle [9]. A meta-analysis showed that 51% of patients with NAFLD were obese, 23% had type 2 diabetes mellitus (T2DM), 69% had hyperlipidemia, 39% had hypertension, and 42% had metabolic syndrome [5]. Obesity, defined by the World Health Organization (WHO) as a body mass index (BMI) higher or equal to 30, is proportional to the rising prevalence of NAFLD [10]. T2DM is another critical risk factor for NAFLD and NASH. The manifestation of NAFLD among people with diabetes is 56%, whereas the overall prevalence of NASH in people who have diabetes type II (T2DM) is around 37% [7]. Likewise, dyslipidemia is a risk factor that is characterized by exacerbated triglycerides (TGs) and low-density lipoprotein cholesterol (LDL-C) levels and by diminished high-density lipoprotein cholesterol (HDL-C) concentrations. Hypertension is also recognized as a major (cardio)metabolic risk for NAFLD, since 50% of hypertensive patients have the disease [11–13].

In addition, some genetic contributions to NAFLD have been documented, accounting for between 20–70% of NAFLD development (Table 1). Although five major variants in genes associated exclusively with NAFLD, such as patatin-like phospholipase domain-containing 3 (*PNPLA3*), transmembrane 6 superfamily member 2 (*TM6SF2*), glucokinase regulator (*GCKR*), membrane-bound O-acyltransferase domain-containing 7 (*MBOAT7*), and hydroxysteroid 17-beta dehydrogenase 13 (*HSD17B13*), have been described, rare variants were also reported in NAFLD patients [14]. *PNPLA3* gene, responsible for encoding adiponutrin (ADPN) protein and located on the lipid droplets of hepatocytes, acts as a hydrolase towards to TGs and transacylase at polyunsaturated fatty acids (PUFAs) in phospholipids. The replacement of glutamic acid with lysine at position 434 (PNPLA3 148M, rs2294918) impairs ubiquitylation and proteasomal degradation, resulting in lipid droplet accumulation and NAFLD development [15]. TM6SF2, highly abundant in the liver and small intestine, is mainly localized in the endoplasmic reticulum (ER) and the ER–Golgi intermediate compartment (ERGIC) and plays a regulatory function in liver fat metabolism, orchestrating triglyceride secretion and hepatic lipid droplet content. A nonsynonymous mutation in TM6SF2 (TM6SF2 E167K, rs58542926) leads to a substitution of a glutamine by a lysine at residue 167 that promotes protein degradation [16]. TM6SF2 E167K variant can contribute to liver steatosis due to abnormal TG synthesis or low secretion of VLDL-TG or a combination of both as it impairs the second stage of lipidation of VLDLs, affecting the incorporation of PUFAs into serum TGs and liver phosphocholines (PCs) [17]. The *GCKR gene* encodes glucokinase regulatory protein (GCKRP), which plays a huge role in preserving plasma glucose homeostasis and metabolic traits. A common missense variant (rs1260326) resulting from a proline-to-leucine substitution at position 446 (P446L) showed impaired regulation of fructose-6-phosphate levels that turned out to increase GCK activity [18] continually. In fact, augmented liver GCK activity is known to stimulate glycolytic flux, which promotes hepatic glucose metabolism and increased concentrations of malonyl-CoA, leading to hepatic fat storage due to β-oxidation blocking ability of malonyl-Coa [19]. *HSD17B13* gene expression is confined to the liver, in particular hepatocytes. It is a lipid droplet (LD)-associated protein involved in the insulin-regulated lipogenic transcription factor steroid-responsive element-binding protein 1c (SREBP1c) and upregulated in human NAFLD livers [20,21]. Additionally, it catalyzes multiple substrates such as steroids, lipids including leukotriene B4 and 12(R)-hydroxyeicosatetraenoic acid, and retinol. A protein-truncating variant of HSD17B13 (rs72613567) resulted in lower risks of developing chronic hepatic inflammation and ballooning as well as fibrosis [22]. Notably, this variant did not prevent steatosis, and its protective effect may be determined by the co-existence of other genetic variants such as PNPLA3 rs2294918 and TM6SF2 rs58542926 [21]. The *MBOAT7 gene* is highly expressed in circulating monocytes and lymphocytes codifying the MBOAT7 enzyme that participate in the phospholipid acyl-chain remodeling of the membranes. MBOAT7 catalyzes a desaturation of the second acyl-chain of phospholipids by transferring a PUFA in the form of acyl-CoA to lysophosphatidylinositol (LPI) and other lysophospholipids. Since it uses arachidonoyl-CoA as a substrate, MBOAT7 can regulate the levels of free arachidonic acid and consequently eicosanoids that are potent triggers for hepatic inflammation and fibrosis. The MBOAT7 variant (rs641738 C>T MBOAT7/TMC4) reduces the levels of the MBOAT7 protein in the liver and predisposes to advance forms of NAFLD, mainly by modifying the hepatic levels of phosphatidylinositol (PI) and LPI and stimulating hyperinsulinemia and hepatic IR [23,24]. Many other rare genetic variants related to NAFLD have been described. Among them, protein phosphatase 1 regulatory subunit 3B (*PPP1R3B*, rs4240624), autophagy-related 7 (*ATG7*, rs143545741), immunity-related GTPase M (*IRGM*, rs10065172), lipin 1 (*Lpin1*, rs13412852), uncoupling protein 2 (*UCP2*, rs695366), mitochondrial amidoxime reducing component 1 (*MARC1*, rs2642438), interferon-l4 (*IFNL4*, rs368234815), MER proto-oncogene, tyrosine kinase (*MERTK*, rs4374383), superoxide dismutase 2 (*SOD2*, rs4880), and Kruppel-like factor 6 (*KFL6*, rs3750861) were reported in NAFLD patients [25].

Table 1. Expression patterns and function of genes associated with NAFLD risk.

Gene	Function	Variant	Outcomes in NAFLD
PNPLA3	Lipid remodeling; Lipogenesis	rs738409	Decreased lipolysis, phospholipase and retinyl-plamitate lipase activity; [26] Increased hepatic fat content, elevated liver enzymes, hepatic fibrosis, and cirrhosis [27]
GCKR	Glucose uptake; Lipogenesis	rs1260326	Inhibition of glucokinase; [28] Increased glycolytic flux and malonyl-CoA levels; [29] Increased hepatic fat storage and decreased β-oxidation [30]
TM6SF2	VLDL secretion	rs58542926	Increased hepatic TG content and higher risk of advanced fibrosis in NAFLD; [31] Lower concentration of hepatic-derived TG-rich lipoproteins; [32] Impaired incorporation of polyunsaturated fatty acids into hepatic TGs, phospholipids, and cholesterol ester [20]
HSD17B13	Lipid droplet remodeling; Retinol metabolism	rs72613567	Decreased risk of chronic liver damage in NAFLD patients; [33] Increased hepatic phospholipids and downregulation of inflammation-related genes [21]
MBOAT7	Remodeling of PI	rs641738	Increased liver damage; [24] Decreased PI species with arachidonoyl side chains; [23] Increased PI species with monounsaturated fatty acids; [23] Elevated plasma levels of LPI [24]

In summary, rare genetic variants can contribute to NAFLD development, but the lack of information on the role of rare variants, as well as structural variation, gene-by-gene-interaction, and gene-by-environment interaction emphasize the need to improve our understanding as they likely contribute to the disease development and may impact NAFLD clinical diagnosis.

2.3. *Pathophysiology*

NAFLD pathophysiology is characterized by excessive fat in the liver, specifically when at least 5% of hepatocytes exhibit lipid droplets (LDs) that surpass 5–10% of total liver weight in patients. The histological hallmark of NAFLD is steatosis, the accumulation of hepatic TGs, which relies on the acinar architecture and is classified according to the percentage of liver parenchyma containing steatotic hepatocytes: 0–33%, 33–66%, or >66% [34]. The increasing FFA flux into the liver from lipolysis (the hydrolysis of FFAs and glycerol from triglyceride) within adipose tissue, dietary sources, and de novo lipogenesis (DNL), combined with an imbalance in its oxidation or secretion, leads to hepatic steatosis [35]. Once in the liver, FFAs are metabolized either through β-oxidation or re-esterification to TGs and storage as LD or wrapped and exported as very low-density lipoproteins (VLDLs). In NAFLD patients, 60% of liver TG content is derived from nonesterified fatty acid pool (NEFA), 26% from DNL, and 15% from the diet, while in healthy individuals DNL only contributes to <5% of hepatic TG formation [36].

Classically, progressive liver steatosis, if not treated, may advance to NASH and fibrosis. The NASH histological diagnostic criteria include steatosis, hepatocellular injury, and lobular inflammation, with or without fibrosis. As the subsequent impairment of insulin signaling in the adipose tissue results in the suppression of lipolysis and inflammation, and the adaptive mechanisms in the liver are overburdened, lipotoxicity occurs, a process that can contribute to ROS formation, mitochondrial dysfunction, and ER stress. Elevated proinflammatory adipocytokines such as TNF-α, IL-6, and IL-1β produced by adipose tissue activate the immune system in the liver and act as precursors to the development of insulin resistance and compensatory hyperinsulinemia [37]. The cellular damage caused by the combination of these insults leads to the transition from NASH to fibrosis [38]. Once fibrosis progresses, hepatic architectural remodeling occurs, and hepatocellular injury occurs in the form of ballooning, the formation of apoptotic bodies, and lytic necrosis. Hepatocyte ballooning describes the presence of enlarged, swollen hepatocytes, with rarefied cytoplasm that may have a reticulated appearance or contain Mallory–Denk bodies. The need to replace dead cells leads to the activation of liver regeneration and fibrogenesis, extracellular matrix (ECM) production, and augmenting collagen, promoting liver fibrosis [39]. Approximately 25% of NAFL-diagnosed patients develop advanced fibrosis during a relatively short follow-up period (median: 6.7 years; mean: 3.3 years), which reflects an active disease predisposing denominator to both liver- and non-liver related morbidity and mortality. Advanced fibrosis increases the likelihood of cirrhosis and, ultimately, may develop into hepatocellular cancer and liver failure due to impaired liver regeneration brought on by unsuccessful attempts to restore healthy liver architecture [39–41].

3. Two-Hit or Multiple-Hit Hypothesis

The full understanding of the mechanisms underlying the development of NAFLD is of extreme importance, although the pathophysiology is complex and incompletely understood. The 'two-hit' hypothesis is now obsolete, as it is inadequate to explain the several molecular and metabolic changes that take place in NAFLD. The "multiple-hit" hypothesis considers multiple insults acting together on genetically predisposed subjects to induce NAFLD and provides a more accurate explanation of NAFLD pathogenesis. According to this hypothesis, the first hit consists of hepatic fat accumulation that occurs in response to increased fat synthesis and delivery, decreased fat export, and/or diminished fat oxidation [42].

Hepatic steatosis can progress to further stages due to "second hits" such as mitochondrial dysfunction, proinflammatory cytokines (IL-1β, TNF-α, and IL-6) and adipokines (adiponectin and IL-37), ER stress, and gut-derived bacterial endotoxins [43–47]. The theory evolved as new evidence showed that NAFLD may be a consequence of parallel "multi-hits" [48]. In this context, insulin resistance leads to enhanced lipogenesis and increased uptake of FFAs into the liver, which predispose the liver to injury by "multiple parallel hits" (oxidative damage, activation of fibrogenic pathways, activation of hepatic stellate cells (HSCs), altered expression of adipokines) leading to NASH and fibrosis. Mitochondrial dysfunction has been described as a crucial driving force in NAFLD progression. In the sections below, the role of mitochondria in NAFLD progression will be discussed.

4. Mitochondrial (Dys)Function in NAFLD

4.1. Hepatic Mitochondrial Populations: Implications for NAFLD

The number and type of mitochondrial structures diverge from tissue to tissue, depending on their metabolic state. However mitochondrial heterogeneity can occur even within the same tissue, including liver. Experimental data using intact livers and isolated liver mitochondria revealed an increment in mitochondrial oxidative function induced by simple steatosis [49], even though in primary hepatocytes and human hepatoma cell lines subjected to lipotoxicity insults opposing effects were observed [50,51]. In a study in brown adipose tissue (BAT), two segregated populations of mitochondria, the peridroplet mitochondria (PDM) and the cytosolic mitochondria (CM), were detected [52]. Mitochondria bound to lipid droplets (LDs), namely PDM, can stimulate TG synthesis and expand LDs in a process involving protein perilipin 5 (PLIN5) [52]. Similarly, hepatic PLIN5 retains the dietary excess of FAs in LDs and blocks lipolysis, which protect hepatic from IR damage induced by HFD feeding [53]. Likewise, it was proposed that hepatocytes possess segregated mitochondria, which would be dedicated to sustaining dietary FA esterification into TGs but also to producing new FAs and assembling lipoproteins in the ER (Figure 1). As TG, cholesterol, and phospholipids can be carried inside of this type of lipoprotein, which allows their efflux from hepatocytes to plasma, a new segregated mitochondrial population, ER-anchored mitochondria, were suggested [54]. In this scenario, ER-anchored mitochondria showed inhibited CPT-1 activity and are probably responsible for lipoprotein assembly and de novo FA synthesis. Peridroplet mitochondria (PDM) have a limited capacity to execute FAO. On other hand, cytosolic mitochondria (CM) are proposed to be more involved in oxidizing FAs. Since hyperinsulinemia stimulates lipogenesis, it is possible that the increase in ER–mitochondria contacts with IR and that simple steatosis is a consequence of hyperinsulinemia [54]. Notably, overexpression of PLIN5 and consequently PDM do not augment de novo lipogenesis or the assembly of lipoproteins in the ER, as observed by the unchanged VLDL export and plasma lipid levels [55]. Furthermore, diacylglycerol o-acyltransferase 2 (DGAT2) and not PLIN5 appears to be the mediator in mitochondria segregation and ER-anchored lipogenic mitochondria generation [56], as demonstrated by the reduction on steatosis and hypertriglyceridemia upon DGAT2 ablation [57]. Functionally, DGAT2 catalyzes the last step of TG synthesis and is found in mitochondria-associated membranes (MAMs).

These segregated subpopulations of mitochondria can be independent and have diverse oxidative functions, which may explain why the tricarboxylic acid (TCA) cycle fluxes and mitochondrial fatty acid β-oxidation (FAO) rates increase in NAFLD (in animal models). This process is not always observed in isolated liver mitochondria by the inability to access in ex vivo experiments full mitochondrial oxidative function. Although studies on distinct mitochondrial sub-populations roles in NAFLD are still scarce, and their role in metabolic dysregulation remains poorly understood, the idea that liver ER-anchored mitochondria and PDM are functionally disconnected from cytosolic mitochondria can explain the mitochondria oxidative function heterogeneity in NAFLD.

4.2. Adaptation (Hormesis) vs. Maladaptation (Dysfunction)

Multiple pathways can be involved in the regulation of hepatocytes' mitochondrial physiology in order to maintain hepatic mitochondrial mass, integrity, and function. Alterations in mitochondria-associated signaling pathways decisively impact development and progression of NAFLD/NASH. Hormesis, a "biphasic dose response" [58], is defined as a beneficial or stimulatory effect caused by exposure to low doses of an agent capable of stimulating adaptive responses in cells and organisms to preserve homeostasis, promoting health and longevity. More recently, the "mitohormesis" concept was introduced as the hormetic response that promotes health and vitality upon sublethal mitochondrial stress [59]. Activation of ROS-mediated (mainly H_2O_2) cell signaling pathways is crucial for mitohormesis regulation [60,61].

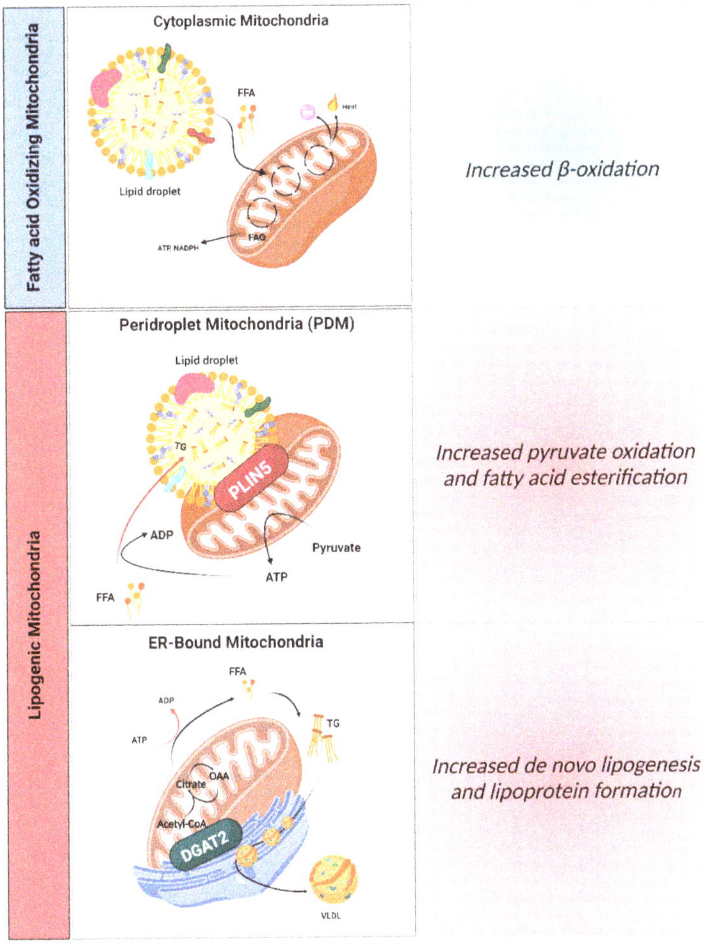

Figure 1. Distinct mitochondrial populations in hepatocytes. Mitochondria attached to different organelles can have distinct roles, reinforcing the hypothesis that not all mitochondria in the same cell are homogeneous. This concept supports the assumption that some mitochondria in hepatocytes can be specialized in synthesizing lipids, while other mitochondria can oxidize lipids. The functional segregation of mitochondria can be determined by their anchorage to specific organelles, which prevents motility and thus fusion between the different subpopulations. In this context, it is believed that three mitochondrial populations exist in hepatocytes: (1) cytosolic mitochondria, which are responsible for fatty acid oxidation, production of ketone bodies, and ureagenesis to support glucose production; (2) mitochondria attached to lipid droplets, namely peridroplet mitochondria (PDM), which promote the esterification of fatty acids into triglycerides; and (3) ER-anchored mitochondria, responsible for fatty acid synthesis, lipoprotein assembly, and excretion. VLDL, very low-density lipoprotein; PLIN5, perilipin 5; DGAT2, diacylglycerol O-acyltransferase 2; ER, endoplasmic reticulum; OAA, oxaloacetate. Created with BioRender.com (accessed on 5 February 2023).

NAFLD patients showed increased serum levels of antioxidant enzymes such as SOD, GPx, and GSH in an initial stage of NAFLD [62], indicating a possible adaptation mechanism to mild increase in oxidative stress (Figure 2). Activation of the SIRT1-PGC-1α pathway, either by an alteration in AMP/ATP ratio or AMPK activation and fluctuation in NAD^+ levels, can upregulate mitochondrial energy metabolism and biogenesis [63].

In mouse models, it was observed that SIRT1 overexpression attenuated HFD-induced liver steatosis and inflammation by inhibiting CD36 expression and the NF-κB signaling pathway [64].

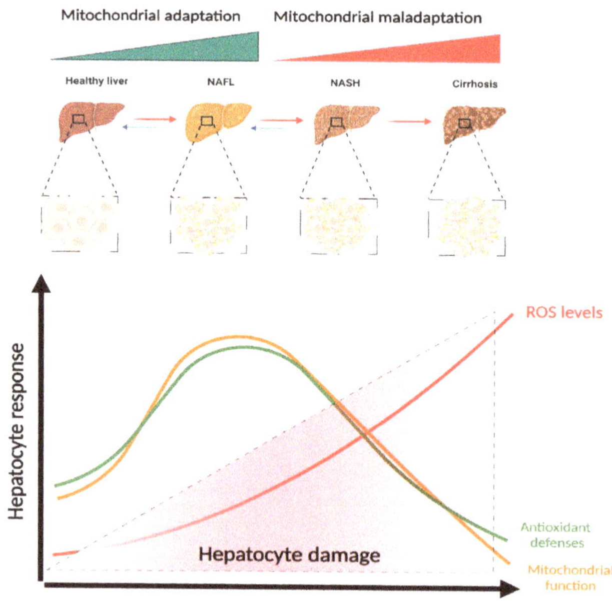

Figure 2. Mitochondrial adaptation and maladaptation in NAFLD progression. Different stages of Non-alcoholic fatty liver disease (NAFLD), comprising non-alcoholic fatty liver (NAFL), non-alcoholic steatohepatitis (NASH), cirrhosis, and hepatocellular carcinoma (HCC). During NAFLD progression, mitochondria increase their function in order to counteract lipotoxic insults. However, uncontrolled stimulation of basal ROS production or failure of antioxidant defenses to neutralize ROS results in exacerbated ROS levels that lead to oxidative stress and culminate in hepatocyte injury. ROS, reactive oxygen species. Created with BioRender.com (accessed on 5 February 2023).

Proteotoxic signals, such as mitochondrial unfolded protein response (UPR^{mt}), are also involved in hormetic processes. UPR^{mt} alteration was observed in mouse studies and obese humans [65–67], constituting a stimulus that may trigger UPRer, UPRmt, or both. Moreover, the downregulation of the TOR signaling pathway led to an early increase in mtROS levels [68]. In liver tumors, mTOR activation has been associated with NASH in both mouse models and humans [69]. The nuclear factor erythroid-derived 2-like 2 (Nrf2, NFE2L2) also contributes to hormetic induction of increased stress resistance [70]. Specific overexpression of hepatic Nrf2 in HFD-fed mice protects against OxS induced by prolonged methionine- and choline-deficient (MCD) exposure [71], while Nrf2 deletion results in progression from simple steatosis to NASH [72]. Interestingly, liver macrophages showed diminished levels of Nrf2 [73].

Mitochondrial homeostasis is assured by the successful removal of physiological ROS through endogenous antioxidant mechanisms as well as by assisting metabolic adaptations that prevent substrate supply to the TCA cycle. However, amplified and chronic mitochondrial ROS production and redox processes that damage mitochondria can be part of a deleterious cycle as mitochondria can continuously produce more ROS (Figure 2) [74]. While mitochondria are the preferential site of ROS production, particularly under pathological conditions, other mitochondrial enzymes such as glycerol 3-phosphate dehydrogenase and 2-oxoglutarate dehydrogenase can also contribute to a decay of mitochondrial homeostasis [75] and induce a stress signaling response and mitochondrial dysfunction. Liver tissues from patients with NASH exhibited high levels of mtROS and mtDNA damage [76]. mtDNA depletion and augmented levels of 8-hydroxy-20-deoxyguanosine (8-OHdG), an oxidized form deoxyguanosine, were reported in NAFLD [77]. Critical regulators of mitochondrial metabolism and biogenesis such as TFAM, Nrf2, and PGC-1α showed reduced expression levels in NAFLD [75]. Due to the high FA hepatic influx, patients with NAFLD have elevated mitochondrial FAO and TCA cycle turnover, which result in a consistent high source of reducing equivalents to the ETC. Although increased mitochondrial FAO characterizes NAFLD, in NAFLD patients and high-fat-fed mice, the upregulation proliferator-activated receptor-α (PPAR-α) and ACOX genes and higher levels of peroxisomal-related proteins in livers were detected [78,79]. The increased content of oxidized cardiolipin (CL), a phospholipid present in the inner mitochondrial membrane, contributes to mitochondria dysfunction by decreasing ETC complex activity and promoting the mPTP opening [80]. This process seems to involve ALCAT1, a lyso-CL acyltransferase.

Ceramides are crucial cell membranes components that can act as signaling molecules coordinating various cellular processes such as proliferation and apoptosis. In response to HFD feeding of mice, ceramide synthesis can be exacerbated, leading to the decrease in mitochondrial respiration and contributing to NASH. Sphingolipid ceramide 16:0 directly decreases mitochondrial FAO in hepatocytes from steatotic mice, accompanied by reduced hepatic insulin signaling and hyperglycemia [81]. Notably, the data from cohorts of NASH patients presented a strong correlation between serum and liver ceramide levels [82]. Exacerbated hepatic ceramide content is linked to diminished mitochondrial oxidative capacity [83]. Ceramides accelerate the synthesis of ganglioside GD3 at the ER, promoting its translocation to mitochondria, where it enhances OxS by stimulating superoxide anion production at complex III [84]. Steatotic livers from ob/ob mice also showed exacerbated levels of TNF-α and FFAs [4,85], together with decreased ETC coupling, as demonstrated by the higher proton leak and subsequent decrease in ATP synthesis [86].

The activation of pathways involving mitogen-activated protein kinases (MAPKs) play a critical role in the development of liver diseases and injuries, such as steatosis, NASH, fibrosis and hepatocarcinoma [87]. Oxidative stress prompts a progressive and irreversible escalation of oxidative damage that markedly influences critical aspects of mitochondrial physiology (oxygen consumption, ATP and ROS production, FAO, autophagy, among others), which might contribute to NAFLD disease progression. However, the mitochondrial capacity breaking point, i.e., the sequence by which signaling pathways transform functional mitochondria into dysfunctional mitochondria, is unknown.

5. Mitochondrial (Dys)Function in NAFLD Progression

5.1. Mitochondrial Function in Simples Steatosis

In simple steatosis, the dysregulation of lipid and glucose metabolism occurs mainly in the presence of a high intake of high-caloric fat diets, which results in accumulation of TGs and FFAs in the liver. The overall process contributes to modifying the mitochondrial proteome [88]. In response to fat overload, hepatocytes increase fatty acid oxidation (FAO) processes, followed by increasing the TCA cycle and OXPHOS to avoid hepatic lipid burden. AMPK triggers catabolic pathways (e.g., fatty acid and glucose oxidation pathways) by inducing the activation of PGC-1α (Figure 3) [89]. When PGC-1α is activated, it powerfully coordinates gene expression that stimulates mitochondrial fatty oxidation. Through interaction with PPAR-α, PGC-1α induces the expression of several enzymes involved in fatty acid-metabolism, including carnitine palmitoyltransferase-1 (CPT-1) and acyl-CoA dehydrogenases [76]. The carnitine palmitoyltransferase system is an essential step in the β-oxidation of long chain fatty acids, as CPT-1 catalyzes the import of FFAs into the mitochondria. Clinically, CPT-1 activation can increase NAFLD biomarkers in patients, as demonstrated by the decrease in serum levels of AST, ALT, bilirubin, and mtDNA [90]. Moreover, the observed alterations in the mitochondrial composition may reflect the adaptation to the chronic rise in gluconeogenesis and intrahepatic lipid management induced by NAFLD, leading to accumulation of mitochondrial ATP and TCA cycle intermediates.

Studies in the fatty liver of human and mice demonstrated that mitochondrial pyruvate oxidation and TCA cycle flux are elevated in the fasted stage and that ketogenesis does not follow the same tendency [91]. The mismatch of mitochondria between high TCA fluxes and decreased OXPHOS activity alongside high rates of FAO could be the key pathogenic mechanism in NAFLD. In fact, impaired ketosis can raise TCA flux in NAFLD, which increases acetyl-CoA available to the TCA cycle. Notably, in HFD mice, the deletion of the mitochondrial pyruvate carrier 1 (MPC1), which decreases TCA fluxes, led to diminished hepatic glucose production and inflammation [92,93].

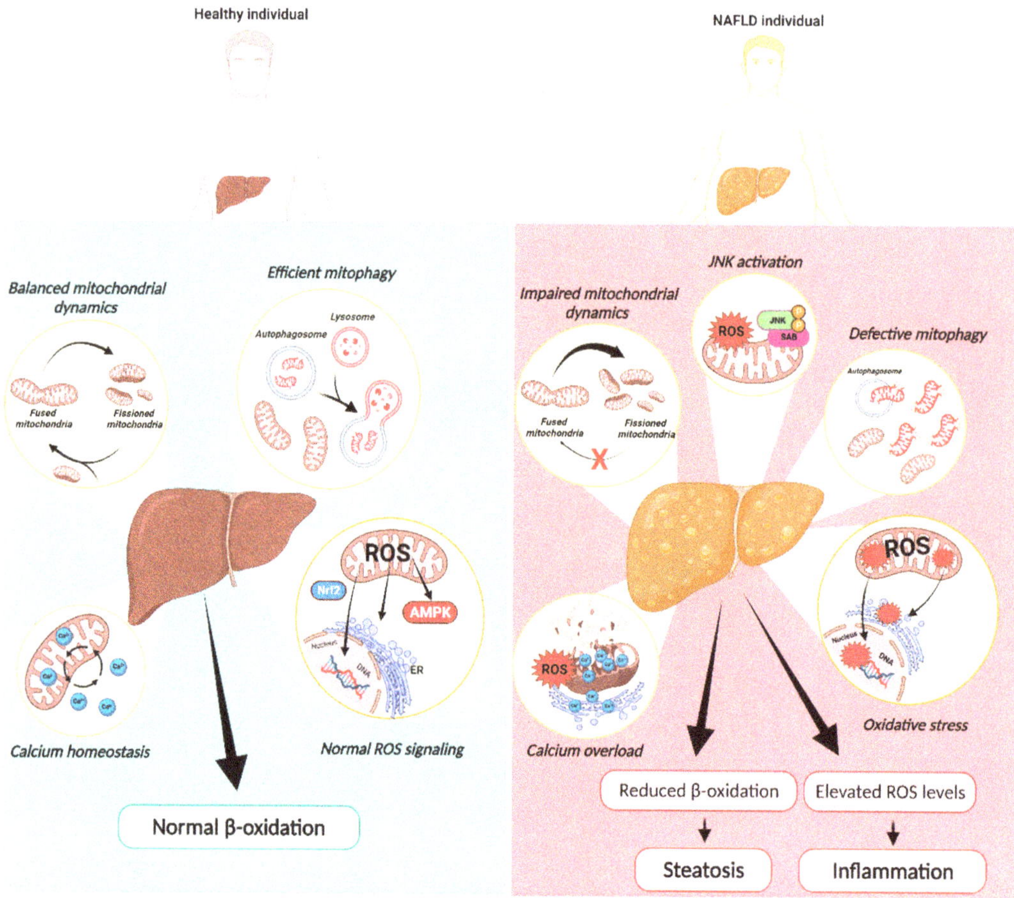

Figure 3. Mitochondrial dysfunction in NAFLD progression. Mitochondria rely on diverse mechanisms to preserve their function including dynamics, redox signaling, mitophagy, and calcium homeostasis. In contrast to a healthy liver, mitochondria in NAFLD were reported to be fragmented and overloaded with calcium, with decreased oxidative capacity and increased ROS production, which cause JNK activation. JNK activation itself can induce these same defects in mitochondrial function, constituting a feed-forward cycle of mitochondrial dysfunction. Mitochondrial dysfunction in NAFLD was also explained by defective mitophagy. The decrease in fatty acid oxidation (FAO) caused by this compromise in mitochondrial function may induce FA accumulation in hepatocytes while impairing insulin signaling. ER, endoplasmic reticulum; JNK, c-Jun NH2-terminal kinase; SAB, SH3 homology associated BTK-binding protein; ROS, reactive oxygen species. Created with BioRender.com (accessed on 5 February 2023).

Several in vitro studies mimicking NAFLD conditions as well as mice subjected to HFD showed impaired mitophagy, culminating in increased fat accumulation, elevated OxS, and inflammation [94,95] (Figure 3). HFD-fed mice presented exacerbated expression levels of ALCAT1 and defective mitophagy in isolated hepatocytes, which were restored after genetic ablation of ALCAT1, strengthening the importance of maintaining mitochondrial morphology and mtDNA integrity [96]. Knockout mouse studies showed that BNIP3, an important regulator of hepatic lipid metabolism, led to augmented lipid synthesis, mainly by reducing AMPK activity and increasing expression of lipogenic genes. In addition, decreased β-oxidation was reported [97]. Finally, it was found that peroxiredoxin 6 (PRDX6), an antioxidant PRDX family member, can translocate to dysfunctional mitochondria upon increased ROS production, where it plays a crucial role in the initial stage of mitophagy by controlling ROS homeostasis. Moreover, PRDX6 antagonizes the positive feedback loop between lipid accumulation and ROS production through the regulation of mitochondrial antioxidant function and β-oxidation to maintain mitochondrial integrity [98]. Although OxS is clearly documented as a trigger of NAFLD progression, the role of mitochondria ROS in severity transition remains controversial. In fact, several authors showed no alterations in ROS levels of isolated liver mitochondria from mice with the NAFL phenotype [99,100] Peroxisomes are important organelles in fat metabolism, also being responsible for ROS generation. The knowledge of how these two organelles communicate is very limited. Further studies on contact sites between mitochondria and peroxisomes and the sub-localization of ROS in steatosis are still needed.

5.2. Mitochondrial Function in NASH and Non-Alcoholic Fibrosis (NAF)

In liver biopsies of NASH patients, mitochondria presented ultrastructural abnormalities [101]. In NAFLD, the sequential events of increased FFAs and de novo lipogenesis (DNL) and accumulation of TGs induce adaptations of mitochondrial oxidative metabolism. However, even a dynamic organelle such as mitochondria cannot infinitely protect cells against lipotoxicity with the excessive deposition of FFAs.

NAFLD progression is amplified by inhibition of CPT-1, diminished mitochondrial FAO, and continuing ATP depletion, which is promoted by increased hepatic expression of uncoupling protein-2 (UCP2) [102]. Subsequently, increased ROS levels also contribute to TNF synthesis and several other cytokines, which can cause apoptosis and necroptosis. DNA-enriched mitochondria-derived danger-associated molecular patterns (DAMPs) (Figure 4) produced by damaged hepatocyte mitochondria, activate NOD-like receptor family pyrin domain-containing 3 (NLRP3) and other innate immune system inflammasomes through pattern recognition receptors such as toll-like receptors (TLRs) (Figure 4) [103–105]. Moreover, OxS and lipid peroxidation participate in inflammatory response by activating NF-κB and the production of proinflammatory cytokines (TNF-α, IL-1β, Il-6, and IL-8), which culminate in apoptosis and necrosis in hepatocytes [106,107]. The combination of events comprising ROS-associated lipid peroxidation, mitochondrial DAMPs, and activation of caspases promote chronic liver injury via intrusion of inflammatory cells [106,108]. Studies in HFD-fed mice showed that mtDNA released by injured hepatocytes activate TLR9 on Kupffer cells (KCs) and HSCs, stimulating the innate immune as well as fibrogenic responses [108]. Transition from steatosis to NASH is accelerated by mitochondrial cholesterol deposition, as it causes alterations in mitochondrial membrane permeability and impairs protein transport from mitochondria to cytosol and vice versa [109]. In fact, mPTP opening episodes appear critical in hepatocyte cell death [110]. This process seems to be correlated with overexpression of StARD1, a mitochondrial cholesterol-transporting polypeptide involved in the trafficking of cholesterol to IMM [109]. Although the impact of autophagic dysregulation in NAFL progression to NASH is still under debate, several mechanisms of autophagy impairment have been described in NAFLD. Decreased in ATG7 expression levels and increased activation of proteases, such as calpain-2, which can diminish autophagy proteins levels, namely ATG3, ATG5, Beclin1, and ATG7, were found to reduce autophagy flux in NAFLD [111]. Moreover, accumulation of LC3-II and p62 were detected in NASH patients, and their increase positively correlates with disease severity [112]. Silencing of macrophage stimulating 1 (MST1), a cell survival regulator, stimulated PINK1/Parkin-mediated mitophagy and counteracted HFD-induced liver injury [113]. Moreover, impairment of MFN2 activity induced by JNK activation during inflammation could trigger mitophagy defects, as MFN2 supports the formation of autophagosomes [114]. OPA1 ablation in the liver led to the recovery of mitochondrial homeostasis and reduced the accumulation of mitophagy intermediates, which could contribute to alleviation of MCD diet-induced liver damage in mice [115]. Patients diagnosed with NASH showed a negative correlation between cholesterol content and mitochondrial GSH levels [116], probably resulting from an impairment in the mitochondrial GSH transport system. Finally, the high levels of cholesterol in obese mice also seem to stimulate TNF-α and Fas-induced apoptosis in hepatocytes, contributing to mitochondrial GSH ablation [117]. Nutritional and genetic NASH mouse models exhibited an increased expression in the levels of SOD2, paralleled by a significant impairment in its activity, which may reflect sensitivity to OxS in the later NAFLD stages [118]. Interestingly, hepatocyte-specific deletion of GPx1 resulted in diminished hepatic lymphocytic infiltration, inflammation, and liver fibrosis in mice with the NASH phenotype [119]. As result of GPx1 ablation, H_2O_2 signaling led to protein-tyrosine phosphatase 1B (PTP1B) inactivation. Hyperactivation of PTP1B promotes IR and steatosis by dephosphorylating the insulin receptor and increasing SREBP-1c activity [120]. Moreover, heme oxygenase 1 (HMOX1) deletion in hepatocytes increased H_2O_2-mediated PTP1B inactivation, protecting mice from NAFLD and hyperglycemia [121].

Summing up, the transition from NAFL to NASH is accompanied by a decrease in mitochondrial plasticity, resulting in decline in ketogenesis, TCA turnover, OXPHOS capacity, and ATP production. As mitochondria are important immune-cell mediators, at this stage, the release of mitochondrial danger signals by damaged mitochondria impacts inflammation and leads to the recruitment and activation of KCs. Several mitochondrial damage-associated molecular patterns (DAMPs) containing intact mitochondria and high levels of mitochondrial oxidized DNA enclosed in microparticles of hepatocyte origin were already identified in plasma from patients with NASH [122]. However, it remains unclear whether DAMPs play a role in the development of extra-hepatic complications associated with NAFL/NASH.

5.3. Mitochondria Function in Hepatocellular Carcinoma (HCC)

The last stage of liver disease progression can be hepatocellular carcinoma (HCC). An increase in the prevalence of HCC was observed in NAFLD patients, in which tumor development occurred in non-cirrhotic livers, indicating that HCC can still develop in the NASH stage [123]. Lipotoxicity, inflammation, OxS, mitochondrial dysfunction, and ER stress are factors that produce an ideal environment for tumor promotion. Lipid-induced alterations in intracellular Ca^{2+} homeostasis play a crucial role in the progression of the disease. In fact, ob/ob mice fed with a high-fat diet exacerbated lipid accumulation causing ER stress and impaired ER–mitochondria connections in steatotic hepatocytes [124]. Moreover, changes in Ca^{2+} channels and transporters promote decreased Ca2+ concentration in the ER and increased Ca^{2+} concentration in the cytoplasm and in the mitochondrial matrix. As a consequence of the increase in ROS levels and subsequent mitochondrial damage, oxidative damage and mutations of both nDNA and mtDNA induce aberrant activation of proliferative pathways and inhibition of oncosuppressors [124]. Moreover, increased ROS levels induced by dysregulation of Ca^{2+} homeostasis can activate Nrf2 signaling pathways. Although Nrf2 is a transcription factor essential to protecting the liver from OxS in the initial stage of NAFLD, it is also considered a promotor of HCC [125]. In fact, activation of Nrf2 was found to contribute to the progression of the preneoplastic lesion to malignancy, which was confirmed by in vivo detection of the inhibition of the Nrf2 pathway that accompanied the regression of cytokeratin 19-positive [125]. In addition,

Nrf2 was found to take part in the protection processes of HCC cells by facilitating the survival response of FGF19 to endoplasmic reticulum stress [126].

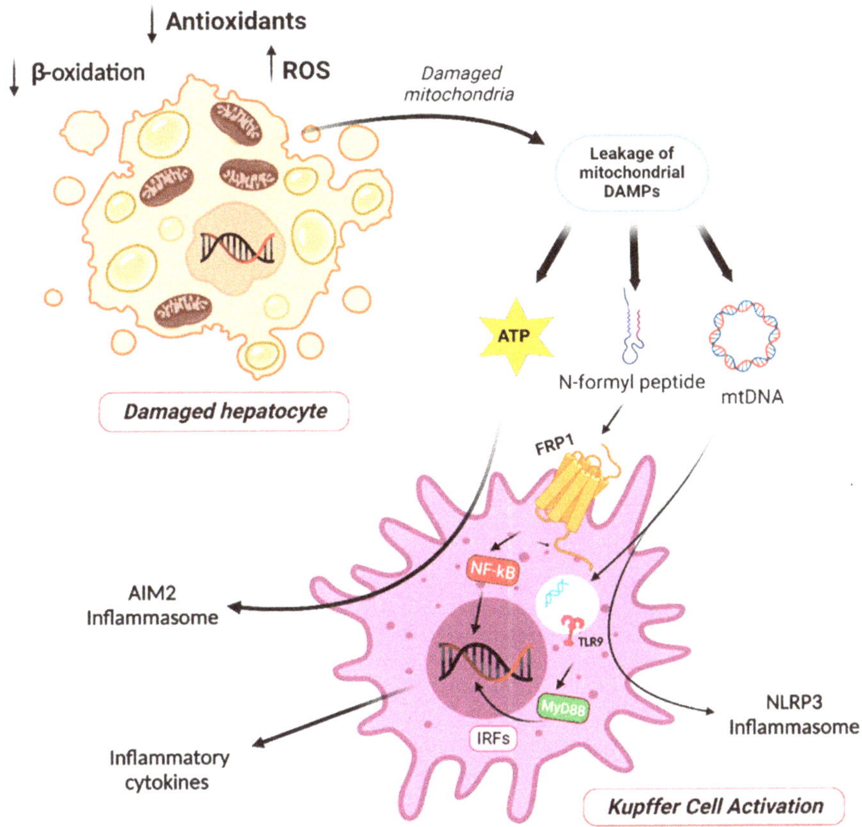

Figure 4. Mitochondria involvement in NAFL progression to steatohepatitis and fibrosis. The augmented accumulation of damaged/dysfunctional mitochondria within hepatocytes results in cell necrosis and induces the leakage of mitochondrial DAMPs, such as mtDNA, N-formyl peptides, and ATP. Further, these signals trigger the activation of toll-like receptor 9 (TLR9) and formyl peptide receptor 1 (FPR1), which in turn activates the IRFs and NF-kB and thereby the production of inflammatory cytokines. mtDNA and ATP also activate the inflammasomes NLRP3 and AIM2, respectively. Multiple inflammatory cytokines and the activation of inflammasomes provide a chronic inflammatory milieu, which contributes to the development of steatohepatitis and fibrosis. Created with BioRender.com (accessed on 5 February 2023).

One of the main hallmarks of cancer pathogenesis is metabolic reprogramming. In fact, HCC cells present a high DNL rate and survive in a highly rich lipid environment [127,128]. Thus, inhibition of lipogenesis might be a possible therapeutic target to counteract HCC progression. PGC-1β is the master regulator of oxidative metabolism, mitochondria biogenesis, and antioxidant response in the liver. However, in both genetic hepatic-specific PGC-1β-overexpressing (LivPGC-1β) and diethylnitrosamine (DEN)-induced HCC mouse models, PGC-1β plays an important role in HCC development, sustaining metabolic reprogramming through the induction of lipogenic enzymes and promoting tumor growth [128].

High levels of PGC-1β can boost reactive oxygen species (ROS) scavenger expression, therefore limiting the detrimental ROS accumulation and, consequently, apoptosis. Moreover, it supports tumor anabolism, enhancing gene expression in fatty acid and triglyceride synthesis. By contrast, the knockout of PGC-1β protects mice from developing HCC [128].

Mitochondrial dynamics have been also associated with cancer progression [129]. High metastatic HCC (MHCC-LM3, MHCC97-H, and MHCC97-L) cell lines appear to have more fragmented mitochondria due to the imbalance toward mitochondrial fission [130,131]. Z. Zhang et al. demonstrated that MFN1 overexpression, through the increase in mitochondrial fusion and expression of the epithelial marker E-cadherin, and reduction in expression of mesenchymal markers including N-cadherin inhibited tumor proliferation and subsequent metastatic potential [131]. MFN1 seems to also modulate metabolic reprogramming in HCC cells. Increased mitochondrial fusion by overexpression of MFN1 induced the expression of the main enzymes involved in OXPHOS and mediated metabolic shift from aerobic glycolysis to OXPHOS [131].

In summary, unbalanced mitochondrial dynamics alongside damaged mitochondria accumulation prompts metabolic reprogramming of hepatocytes, marked by the switch towards the Warburg effect, mutagenesis, epithelial–mesenchymal transition (EMT), and apoptosis escape, stimulating compensatory proliferation and HCC onset. Although mitochondrial metabolic reprogramming and mechanotransduction have been investigated in carcinogenesis, the crosstalk between the extracellular matrix and mitochondrial metabolism remains underexplored in NAFLD-driven HCC.

6. Conclusions

The prevalence of NAFLD is increasing at an impressive rate, and it is becoming the most common liver disease worldwide. The increase in NAFLD prevalence has led to an urgent need to develop better diagnostic and therapeutic approaches. In liver hepatocytes, multiple adaptive mechanisms are triggered to reduce liver fat accumulation and reestablish homeostasis. The failure of the adaptive mechanisms leads to OxS, ER stress, mitochondrial dysfunction, and inflammation, contributing to NAFLD progression. Indeed, mitochondria play a critical role in the advancement of NAFLD to NASH by decreasing mitochondrial FAO and continuing ATP depletion due to the loss of capacity to catabolize the excessive FFAs. During the development of NASH to HCC, the decreased FAO contributes to cancer cells adapting to the lipid-rich environment, and mitochondrial damage can also promote the activation of proliferative pathways. As mitochondrial dysfunction is considered a driving force in NAFLD progression, targeting these intracellular organelles and/or the pathways that can modulate their structure, function, and dynamics could contribute to establishing an effective therapy for NAFLD. However, a clear understanding of disease pathophysiology in its different stages is crucial but still not fully understood.

7. Future Perspectives

Regulation of different aspects of hepatocytes' mitochondrial physiology decisively impacts the development and progression of NAFLD/NASH. Nevertheless, studies on distinct mitochondrial sub-population roles in NAFLD are still scarce, and their role in metabolic dysregulation remains poorly understood. Moreover, the impact of mitochondrial (mis)communication with other subcellular organelles (peroxisomes, lipid droplets, etc.) is unclear in NAFLD. Additionally, the impact of negligible pathways, such as fatty acid oxidation, DNL, and PPP, in the hepatocytes' mitochondrial physiology in different stages of NAFLD is a topic to explore. As mitochondria are involved in the different stages of the disease, several molecular markers involved in mitochondrial metabolism, dynamics, and quality control mechanisms change differently across the disease spectrum; therefore, the study of these alterations may facilitate diagnosis. Finally, the impact of hepatocytes' mitochondrial physiology in NAFLD-associated HCC remains unclear. Thus, there is a well-justified need to improve our understanding of different aspects of hepatocytes' mitochondrial physiology in the context of NAFLD.

Author Contributions: R.A., C.C.M. and J.T. wrote the manuscript. J.T., P.J.O. and F.B. revised the manuscript. All authors have read and agreed to the published version of the manuscript.

Funding: This work was financed by the European Regional Development Fund (ERDF), through the Centro 2020 Regional Operational Programme and through the COMPETE 2020—Operational Programme for Competitiveness and Internationalisation and Portuguese national funds via FCT, under projects: EXPL/BIA-BQM/1361/2021, CENTRO-01-0246-FEDER-000010 (Multidisciplinary Institute of Ageing in Coimbra), UIDB/00081/2020 (CIQUP); LA/P/0056/2020 (IMS), UIDP/04539/2020, and LA/P/0058/2020 and Mitoboost v2.0—Prova de Conceito para o Uso de Polifenóis Dirigidos à Mitocôndria para Tratar a Doença do Fígado Gordo Não Alcoólico" (CENTRO-01-0145-FEDER-181226).

Institutional Review Board Statement: Not applicable.

Informed Consent Statement: Not applicable.

Data Availability Statement: Not applicable.

Acknowledgments: R. Amorim (SFRH/BD/131070/2017), J. Teixeira (2020.01560.CEECIND), and C.C. Magalhães (CENTRO-01-0145-FEDER-181226) acknowledge FCT, I.P. for the research contract.

Conflicts of Interest: The authors declare no conflict of interest.

Abbreviation

8-OHdG 8-Hydroxy-20-deoxyguanosine; **ACOX1** Peroxisomal acyl-coenzyme A oxidase 1; **ALCAT1** Acyl-CoA:lysocardiolipin acyltransferase-1; **ALT** Alanine transaminase; **AMP** Adenosine monophosphate; **AMPK** 5′ Adenosine monophosphate-activated protein kinase; **AST** Aspartate transaminase; **ATF6** Transcription factor 6; **ATG7** Autophagy-related protein 3; **ATG5** Autophagy-related protein 5; **ATG7** Autophagy-related protein 7; **BAT** Brown adipose tissue; **BMI** Body mass index; **BNIP3** BCL2/adenovirus E1B 19 kDa protein-interacting protein 3; **CAT** Catalase; **CHOP** C/EBP homologous protein; **CL** Cardiolipin; **CM** Cytosolic mitochondria; **CPT-1** Carnitine palmitoyltransferase-1; **CR** Caloric restriction; **DALYs** Disability-adjusted life years; **DAMPs** Danger-associated molecular patterns; **DEN** Diethylnitrosamine; **DGAT2** Diacylglycerol o-acyltransferase 2; **DNL** de novo lipogenesis; **ECM** Extracellular matrix; **ER** Endoplasmic reticulum; **ETC** Electron transport chain; **FAO** Mitochondrial fatty acid β-oxidation; **FFA** Free fatty acids; **GCKR** Glucokinase regulator; **GPAT1** Glycerol phosphate acyltransferase 1; **GPx** Glutathione peroxidase; **GSH** Glutathione; **H_2O_2** Hydrogen peroxide; **HCC** Hepatocellular carcinoma; **HDL-C** High-density lipoprotein cholesterol; **HFD** High-fat diet; **HMOX1** Heme oxygenase 1; **HSC** Hepatic stellate cells; **HSD17B13** hydroxysteroid 17-beta dehydrogenase 13; **IL-1β** Interleukin-1 beta; **IL-6** Interleukin-6; **IL-8** Interleukin-8; **INSR** Insulin receptor; **IR** Insulin resistance; **LC3** Microtubule-associated protein 1A/1B-light chain 3; **LDL-C** Low-density lipoprotein cholesterol; **LDs** lipid droplets; **LPI** Lysophosphatidylinositol; **MAFLD** Metabolic (dysfunction)-associated fatty liver disease; **MAM** Mitochondria-associated membranes; **MAPKs** Mitogen-activated protein kinases; **MBOAT7** Membrane-bound O-acyltransferase domain-containing 7; **MCD Methionine- and choline-deficient**; **MFN** Mitofusin; **MPC1** Mitochondrial pyruvate carrier 1; **mPTP** Mitochondrial permeability transition pore; **MST1** Macrophage stimulating 1; **mtROS** mitochondrial reactive oxygen species; **NADH** Nicotinamide adenine dinucleotide reduced form; **NAF** Non-alcoholic fibrosis; **NAFL** Non-alcoholic fatty liver; **NAFLD** Non-alcoholic fatty liver disease; **NASH** Non-alcoholic steatohepatitis; **NEFA** Nonesterified fatty acid; **NF-κB** Nuclear factor k-light-chain-enhancer of activated B cells; **NLRP3** NOD-like receptor family pyrin domain-containing 3; **Nrf2, NFE2L2** Nuclear factor erythroid-derived 2-like 2; **OPA1** Optic athrophy protein 1; **OXPHOS** Oxidative phosphorylation; **OxS** Oxidative stress; **PDM** Peridroplet mitochondria; **PGC-1** Peroxisome proliferator-activated receptor-gamma coactivator; **PI** Phosphatidylinositol; **PLIN5** Protein perilipin 5; ***PNPLA3*** Patatin-like phospholipase domain-containing 3; **PP2A** Protein phosphatase 2; **PPAR-α** Proliferator-activated receptor-α; **PPP** Pentose phosphate pathway; **PRDX6** Peroxiredoxin 6; **PTP1B** Protein-tyrosine phosphatase 1B; **ROS** Reactive oxygen species; **Sirt1** Sirtuin 1; **sn-1,2-DAGs** *sn*-1,2-diacylglycerols; **SOD** Superoxide dismutase; **SREBP1** Sterol regulatory element-binding protein 1; **StARD1** Steroidogenic acute regulatory protein; **T2DM** Type 2 diabetes mellitus; **TCA** Tricarboxylic acid; **TFAM** Mitochondrial transcription factor A; **TG** Triglycerides; **TLRs** Toll-like receptors; **TM6SF2** Transmembrane 6 superfamily member 2;

TNF-α Tumor necrosis factor α; **UCP2** Uncoupling protein-2; **UPR** Unfolded protein response; **VLDL** Very low-density lipoprotein; **WHO** World Health Organization; **XBP1** Xbox-binding protein.

References

1. Godoy-Matos, A.F.; Silva Júnior, W.S.; Valerio, C.M. NAFLD as a continuum: From obesity to metabolic syndrome and diabetes. *Diabetol. Metab. Syndr.* **2020**, *12*, 60. [CrossRef] [PubMed]
2. Adams, L.A.; Lymp, J.F.; St Sauver, J.; Sanderson, S.O.; Lindor, K.D.; Feldstein, A.; Angulo, P. The natural history of non-alcoholic fatty liver disease: A population-based cohort study. *Gastroenterology* **2005**, *129*, 113–121. [CrossRef] [PubMed]
3. White, D.L.; Kanwal, F.; El-Serag, H.B. Association between non-alcoholic fatty liver disease and risk for hepatocellular cancer, based on systematic review. *Clin. Gastroenterol. Hepatol.* **2012**, *10*, 1342–1359.e2. [CrossRef] [PubMed]
4. Begriche, K.; Massart, J.; Robin, M.-A.; Bonnet, F.; Fromenty, B. Mitochondrial adaptations and dysfunctions in non-alcoholic fatty liver disease. *Hepatology* **2013**, *58*, 1497–1507. [CrossRef] [PubMed]
5. Ye, Q.; Zou, B.; Yeo, Y.H.; Li, J.; Huang, D.Q.; Wu, Y.; Yang, H.; Liu, C.; Kam, L.Y.; Tan, X.X.E.; et al. Global prevalence, incidence, and outcomes of non-obese or lean non-alcoholic fatty liver disease: A systematic review and meta-analysis. *Lancet Gastroenterol. Hepatol.* **2020**, *5*, 739–752. [CrossRef]
6. Sayiner, M.; Koenig, A.; Henry, L.; Younossi, Z.M. Epidemiology of Non-alcoholic Fatty Liver Disease and Non-alcoholic Steatohepatitis in the United States and the Rest of the World. *Clin. Liver Dis.* **2016**, *20*, 205–214. [CrossRef]
7. Paik, J.M.; Golabi, P.; Younossi, Y.; Srishord, M.; Mishra, A.; Younossi, Z.M. The Growing Burden of Disability Related to Non-alcoholic Fatty Liver Disease: Data from the Global Burden of Disease 2007–2017. *Hepatol. Commun.* **2020**, *4*, 1769–1780. [CrossRef]
8. Singh, S.; Allen, A.M.; Wang, Z.; Prokop, L.J.; Murad, M.H.; Loomba, R. Fibrosis progression in non-alcoholic fatty liver vs non-alcoholic steatohepatitis: A systematic review and meta-analysis of paired-biopsy studies. *Clin. Gastroenterol. Hepatol.* **2015**, *13*, 640–643. [CrossRef]
9. Younossi, Z.; Tacke, F.; Arrese, M.; Chander Sharma, B.; Mostafa, I.; Bugianesi, E.; Wai-Sun Wong, V.; Yilmaz, Y.; George, J.; Fan, J.; et al. Global Perspectives on Non-alcoholic Fatty Liver Disease and Non-alcoholic Steatohepatitis. *Hepatology* **2019**, *69*, 2672–2682. [CrossRef]
10. Camhi, S.M.; Bray, G.A.; Bouchard, C.; Greenway, F.L.; Johnson, W.D.; Newton, R.L.; Ravussin, E.; Ryan, D.H.; Smith, S.R.; Katzmarzyk, P.T. The relationship of waist circumference and BMI to visceral, subcutaneous, and total body fat: Sex and race differences. *Obesity* **2011**, *19*, 402–408. [CrossRef]
11. Zhao, Y.-C.; Zhao, G.-J.; Chen, Z.; She, Z.G.; Cai, J.; Li, H. Non-alcoholic Fatty Liver Disease: An Emerging Driver of Hypertension. *Hypertension* **2020**, *75*, 275–284. [CrossRef] [PubMed]
12. López-Suárez, A.; Guerrero, J.M.R.; Elvira-González, J.; Beltrán-Robles, M.; Cañas-Hormigo, F.; Bascuñana-Quirell, A. Non-alcoholic fatty liver disease is associated with blood pressure in hypertensive and nonhypertensive individuals from the general population with normal levels of alanine aminotransferase. *Eur. J. Gastroenterol. Hepatol.* **2011**, *23*, 1011–1017. [CrossRef] [PubMed]
13. Zhou, D.; Xi, B.; Zhao, M.; Wang, L.; Veeranki, S.P. Uncontrolled hypertension increases risk of all-cause and cardiovascular disease mortality in US adults: The NHANES III Linked Mortality Study. *Sci. Rep.* **2018**, *8*, 9418. [CrossRef] [PubMed]
14. Jonas, W.; Schürmann, A. Genetic and epigenetic factors determining NAFLD risk. *Mol. Metab.* **2021**, *50*, 101111. [CrossRef]
15. BasuRay, S.; Smagris, E.; Cohen, J.C.; Hobbs, H.H. The PNPLA3 variant associated with fatty liver disease (I148M) accumulates on lipid droplets by evading ubiquitylation. *Hepatology* **2017**, *66*, 1111–1124. [CrossRef]
16. Luo, F.; Oldoni, F.; Das, A. TM6SF2: A Novel Genetic Player in Non-alcoholic Fatty Liver and Cardiovascular Disease. *Hepatol. Commun.* **2022**, *6*, 448–460. [CrossRef]
17. Borén, J.; Adiels, M.; Björnson, E.; Matikainen, N.; Söderlund, S.; Rämö, J.; Ståhlman, M.; Ripatti, P.; Ripatti, S.; Palotie, A.; et al. Effects of TM6SF2 E167K on hepatic lipid and very low-density lipoprotein metabolism in humans. *JCI Insight*, **2020**, *Epub ahead of print*. [CrossRef]
18. Santoro, N.; Zhang, C.K.; Zhao, H.; Pakstis, A.J.; Kim, G.; Kursawe, R.; Dykas, D.J.; Bale, A.E.; Giannini, C.; Pierpont, B.; et al. Variant in the glucokinase regulatory protein (GCKR) gene is associated with fatty liver in obese children and adolescents. *Hepatology* **2012**, *55*, 781–789. [CrossRef]
19. Nissim, I.; Horyn, O.; Nissim, I.; Daikhin, Y.; Wehrli, S.L.; Yudkoff, M.; Matschinsky, F.M. Effects of a glucokinase activator on hepatic intermediary metabolism: Study with 13C-isotopomer-based metabolomics. *Biochem. J.* **2012**, *444*, 537–551. [CrossRef]
20. Luukkonen, P.K.; Zhou, Y.; Nidhina Haridas, P.A.; Dwivedi, O.P.; Hyötyläinen, T.; Ali, A.; Juuti, A.; Leivonen, M.; Tukiainen, T.; Ahonen, L.; et al. Impaired hepatic lipid synthesis from polyunsaturated fatty acids in TM6SF2 E167K variant carriers with NAFLD. *J. Hepatol.* **2017**, *67*, 128–136. [CrossRef]
21. Luukkonen, P.K.; Tukiainen, T.; Juuti, A.; Sammalkorpi, H.; Haridas, P.N.; Niemelä, O.; Arola, J.; Orho-Melander, M.; Hakkarainen, A.; Kovanen, P.T.; et al. Hydroxysteroid 17-β dehydrogenase 13 variant increases phospholipids and protects against fibrosis in non-alcoholic fatty liver disease. *JCI Insight*, **2020**, *Epub ahead of print*. [CrossRef]

22. Abul-Husn, N.S.; Cheng, X.; Li, A.H.; Xin, Y.; Schurmann, C.; Stevis, P.; Liu, Y.; Kozlitina, J.; Stender, S.; Wood, G.C.; et al. A Protein-Truncating HSD17B13 Variant and Protection from Chronic Liver Disease. *N. Engl. J. Med.* **2018**, *378*, 1096–1106. [CrossRef]
23. Mancina, R.M.; Dongiovanni, P.; Petta, S.; Pingitore, P.; Meroni, M.; Rametta, R.; Borén, J.; Montalcini, T.; Pujia, A.; Wiklund, O.; et al. The MBOAT7-TMC4 Variant rs641738 Increases Risk of Nonalcoholic Fatty Liver Disease in Individuals of European Descent. *Gastroenterology* **2016**, *150*, 1219–1230.e6. [CrossRef] [PubMed]
24. Helsley, R.N.; Varadharajan, V.; Brown, A.L.; Gromovsky, A.D.; Schugar, R.C.; Ramachandiran, I.; Fung, K.; Kabbany, M.N.; Banerjee, R.; Neumann, C.K.; et al. Obesity-linked suppression of membrane-bound O-acyltransferase 7 (MBOAT7) drives non-alcoholic fatty liver disease. *eLife*, 2019; *Epub ahead of print*. [CrossRef]
25. Trépo, E.; Valenti, L. Update on NAFLD genetics: From new variants to the clinic. *J. Hepatol.* **2020**, *72*, 1196–1209. [CrossRef]
26. Pirazzi, C.; Valenti, L.; Motta, B.M.; Pingitore, P.; Hedfalk, K.; Mancina, R.M.; Burza, M.A.; Indiveri, C.; Ferro, Y.; Montalcini, T.; et al. PNPLA3 has retinyl-palmitate lipase activity in human hepatic stellate cells. *Hum. Mol. Genet.* **2014**, *23*, 4077–4085. [CrossRef]
27. Sookoian, S.; Pirola, C.J. Meta-analysis of the influence of I148M variant of patatin-like phospholipase domain containing 3 gene (PNPLA3) on the susceptibility and histological severity of non-alcoholic fatty liver disease. *Hepatology* **2011**, *53*, 1883–1894. [CrossRef]
28. Zain, S.M.; Mohamed, Z.; Mohamed, R. Common variant in the glucokinase regulatory gene rs780094 and risk of non-alcoholic fatty liver disease: A meta-analysis. *J. Gastroenterol. Hepatol.* **2015**, *30*, 21–27. [CrossRef] [PubMed]
29. Beer, N.L.; Tribble, N.D.; McCulloch, L.J.; Roos, C.; Johnson, P.R.; Orho-Melander, M.; Gloyn, A.L. The P446L variant in GCKR associated with fasting plasma glucose and triglyceride levels exerts its effect through increased glucokinase activity in liver. *Hum. Mol. Genet.* **2009**, *18*, 4081–4088. [CrossRef] [PubMed]
30. Sparsø, T.; Andersen, G.; Nielsen, T.; Burgdorf, K.S.; Gjesing, A.P.; Nielsen, A.L.; Albrechtsen, A.; Rasmussen, S.S.; Jørgensen, T.; Borch-Johnsen, K.; et al. The GCKR rs780094 polymorphism is associated with elevated fasting serum triacylglycerol, reduced fasting and OGTT-related insulinaemia, and reduced risk of type 2 diabetes. *Diabetologia* **2008**, *51*, 70–75. [CrossRef] [PubMed]
31. Liu, Y.-L.; Reeves, H.L.; Burt, A.D.; Tiniakos, D.; McPherson, S.; Leathart, J.B.S.; Allison, M.E.D.; Alexander, G.J.; Piguet, A.-C.; Anty, R.; et al. TM6SF2 rs58542926 influences hepatic fibrosis progression in patients with non-alcoholic fatty liver disease. *Nat. Commun.* **2014**, *5*, 4309. [CrossRef] [PubMed]
32. Mahdessian, H.; Taxiarchis, A.; Popov, S.; Silveira, A.; Franco-Cereceda, A.; Hamsten, A.; Eriksson, P.; Hooft, F.V. TM6SF2 is a regulator of liver fat metabolism influencing triglyceride secretion and hepatic lipid droplet content. *Proc. Natl. Acad. Sci. USA* **2014**, *111*, 8913–8918. [CrossRef] [PubMed]
33. Pirola, C.J.; Garaycoechea, M.; Flichman, D.; Arrese, M.; Martino, J.S.; Gazzi, C.; Castaño, G.O.; Sookoian, S. Splice variant rs72613567 prevents worst histologic outcomes in patients with non-alcoholic fatty liver disease. *J. Lipid Res.* **2019**, *60*, 176–185. [CrossRef]
34. Takahashi, Y.; Fukusato, T. Histopathology of non-alcoholic fatty liver disease/non-alcoholic steatohepatitis. *World J. Gastroenterol.* **2014**, *20*, 15539–15548. [CrossRef] [PubMed]
35. Postic, C.; Girard, J. Contribution of de novo fatty acid synthesis to hepatic steatosis and insulin resistance: Lessons from genetically engineered mice. *J. Clin. Investig.* **2008**, *118*, 829–838. [CrossRef] [PubMed]
36. Donnelly, K.L.; Smith, C.I.; Schwarzenberg, S.J.; Jessurun, J.; Boldt, M.D.; Parks, E.J. Sources of fatty acids stored in liver and secreted via lipoproteins in patients with non-alcoholic fatty liver disease. *J. Clin. Investig.* **2005**, *115*, 1343–1351. [CrossRef] [PubMed]
37. Hardy, T.; Oakley, F.; Anstee, Q.M.; Day, C.P. Non-alcoholic Fatty Liver Disease: Pathogenesis and Disease Spectrum. *Annu. Rev. Pathol.* **2016**, *11*, 451–496. [CrossRef] [PubMed]
38. Haas, J.T.; Francque, S.; Staels, B. Pathophysiology and Mechanisms of Non-alcoholic Fatty Liver Disease. *Annu. Rev. Physiol.* **2016**, *78*, 181–205. [CrossRef] [PubMed]
39. Diehl, A.M.; Day, C. Cause, Pathogenesis, and Treatment of Non-alcoholic Steatohepatitis. *N. Engl. J. Med.* **2017**, *377*, 2063–2072. [CrossRef]
40. Kumar, S.; Duan, Q.; Wu, R.; Harris, E.N.; Su, Q. Pathophysiological communication between hepatocytes and non-parenchymal cells in liver injury from NAFLD to liver fibrosis. *Adv. Drug Deliv. Rev.* **2021**, *176*, 113869. [CrossRef]
41. Tiniakos, D.G.; Vos, M.B.; Brunt, E.M. Non-alcoholic fatty liver disease: Pathology and pathogenesis. *Annu. Rev. Pathol.* **2010**, *5*, 145–171. [CrossRef]
42. Ipsen, D.H.; Lykkesfeldt, J.; Tveden-Nyborg, P. Molecular mechanisms of hepatic lipid accumulation in non-alcoholic fatty liver disease. *Cell. Mol. Life Sci.* **2018**, *75*, 3313–3327. [CrossRef]
43. Kessoku, T.; Kobayashi, T.; Imajo, K.; Tanaka, K.; Yamamoto, A.; Takahashi, K.; Kasai, Y.; Ozaki, A.; Iwaki, M.; Nogami, A.; et al. Endotoxins and Non-Alcoholic Fatty Liver Disease. *Front. Endocrinol.* **2021**, *12*, 770986. [CrossRef]
44. Adolph, T.E.; Grander, C.; Grabherr, F.; Tilg, H. Adipokines and Non-Alcoholic Fatty Liver Disease: Multiple Interactions. *Int. J. Mol. Sci.* **2017**, *148*, 1649. [CrossRef] [PubMed]
45. Fei, N.; Bruneau, A.; Zhang, X.; Wang, R.; Wang, J.; Rabot, S.; Gérard, P.; Zhao, L. Endotoxin Producers Overgrowing in Human Gut Microbiota as the Causative Agents for Non-alcoholic Fatty Liver Disease. *MBio* **2020**, *11*, e03263-19. [CrossRef] [PubMed]
46. Lebeaupin, C.; Vallée, D.; Hazari, Y.; Hetz, C.; Chevet, E.; Bailly-Maitre, B. Endoplasmic reticulum stress signalling and the pathogenesis of non-alcoholic fatty liver disease. *J. Hepatol.* **2018**, *69*, 927–947. [CrossRef] [PubMed]

47. Fontes-Cal, T.C.M.; Mattos, R.T.; Medeiros, N.I.; Pinto, B.F.; Belchior-Bezerra, M.; Roque-Souza, B.; Dutra, W.O.; Ferrari, T.C.; Vidigal, P.V.; Faria, L.C.; et al. Crosstalk Between Plasma Cytokines, Inflammation, and Liver Damage as a New Strategy to Monitoring NAFLD Progression. *Front. Immunol.* **2021**, *12*, 708959. [CrossRef]
48. Buzzetti, E.; Pinzani, M.; Tsochatzis, E.A. The multiple-hit pathogenesis of non-alcoholic fatty liver disease (NAFLD). *Metabolism* **2016**, *65*, 1038–1048. [CrossRef]
49. Brady, L.J.; Brady, P.S.; Romsos, D.R.; Hoppel, C.L. Elevated hepatic mitochondrial and peroxisomal oxidative capacities in fed and starved adult obese (ob/ob) mice. *Biochem. J.* **1985**, *231*, 439–444. [CrossRef]
50. Moravcová, A.; Červinková, Z.; Kučera, O.; Mezera, V.; Rychtrmoc, D.; Lotkova, H. The effect of oleic and palmitic acid on induction of steatosis and cytotoxicity on rat hepatocytes in primary culture. *Physiol. Res.* **2015**, *64*, S627–S636. [CrossRef]
51. Amorim, R.; Simões, I.C.M.; Veloso, C.; Carvalho, A.; Simões, R.F.; Pereira, F.B.; Thiel, T.; Normann, A.; Morais, C.; Jurado, A.S.; et al. Exploratory Data Analysis of Cell and Mitochondrial High-Fat, High-Sugar Toxicity on Human HepG2 Cells. *Nutrients* **2021**, *13*, 1723. [CrossRef]
52. Benador, I.Y.; Veliova, M.; Mahdaviani, K.; Petcherski, A.; Wikstrom, J.D.; Assali, E.A.; Acín-Pérez, R.; Shum, M.; Oliveira, M.F.; Cinti, S.; et al. Mitochondria Bound to Lipid Droplets Have Unique Bioenergetics, Composition, and Dynamics that Support Lipid Droplet Expansion. *Cell Metab.* **2018**, *27*, 869–885.e6. [CrossRef]
53. Wang, C.; Zhao, Y.; Gao, X.; Li, L.; Yuan, Y.; Liu, F.; Zhang, L.; Wu, J.; Hu, P.; Zhang, X.; et al. Perilipin 5 improves hepatic lipotoxicity by inhibiting lipolysis. *Hepatology* **2015**, *61*, 870–882. [CrossRef]
54. Shum, M.; Ngo, J.; Shirihai, O.S.; Liesa, M. Mitochondrial oxidative function in NAFLD: Friend or foe? *Mol. Metab.* **2021**, *50*, 101134. [CrossRef] [PubMed]
55. Trevino, M.B.; Mazur-Hart, D.; Machida, Y.; King, T.; Nadler, J.; Galkina, E.V.; Poddar, A.; Dutta, S.; Imai, Y. Liver Perilipin 5 Expression Worsens Hepatosteatosis but Not Insulin Resistance in High Fat-Fed Mice. *Mol. Endocrinol.* **2015**, *29*, 1414–1425. [CrossRef] [PubMed]
56. Stone, S.J.; Levin, M.C.; Zhou, P.; Han, J.; Walther, T.C.; Farese, R.V. The endoplasmic reticulum enzyme DGAT2 is found in mitochondria-associated membranes and has a mitochondrial targeting signal that promotes its association with mitochondria. *J. Biol. Chem.* **2009**, *284*, 5352–5361. [CrossRef] [PubMed]
57. Gluchowski, N.L.; Gabriel, K.R.; Chitraju, C.; Bronson, R.T.; Mejhert, N.; Boland, S.; Wang, K.; Lai, Z.W.; Farese, R.V.; Walther, T.C. Hepatocyte Deletion of Triglyceride-Synthesis Enzyme Acyl CoA: Diacylglycerol Acyltransferase 2 Reduces Steatosis without Increasing Inflammation or Fibrosis in Mice. *Hepatology* **2019**, *70*, 1972–1985. [CrossRef] [PubMed]
58. Tapia, P.C. Sublethal mitochondrial stress with an attendant stoichiometric augmentation of reactive oxygen species may precipitate many of the beneficial alterations in cellular physiology produced by caloric restriction, intermittent fasting, exercise and dietary p. *Med. Hypotheses* **2006**, *66*, 832–843. [CrossRef] [PubMed]
59. Hoppins, S.; Lackner, L.; Nunnari, J. The machines that divide and fuse mitochondria. *Annu. Rev. Biochem.* **2007**, *76*, 751–780. [CrossRef] [PubMed]
60. Palmeira, C.M.; Teodoro, J.S.; Amorim, J.A.; Steegborn, C.; Sinclair, D.A.; Rolo, A.P. Mitohormesis and metabolic health: The interplay between ROS, cAMP and sirtuins. *Free Radic. Biol. Med.* **2019**, *141*, 483–491. [CrossRef]
61. Finkel, T. Signal transduction by mitochondrial oxidants. *J. Biol. Chem.* **2012**, *287*, 4434–4440. [CrossRef]
62. Perlemuter, G.; Davit-Spraul, A.; Cosson, C.; Conti, M.; Bigorgne, A.; Paradis, V.; Corre, M.P.; Prat, L.; Kuoch, V.; Basdevant, A.; et al. Increase in liver antioxidant enzyme activities in non-alcoholic fatty liver disease. *Liver Int.* **2005**, *25*, 946–953. [CrossRef]
63. Fang, E.F.; Lautrup, S.; Hou, Y.; Demarest, T.G.; Croteau, D.L.; Mattson, M.P.; Bohr, V.A. NAD(+) in Aging: Molecular Mechanisms and Translational Implications. *Trends Mol. Med.* **2017**, *23*, 899–916. [CrossRef]
64. Niu, B.; He, K.; Li, P.; Gong, J.; Zhu, X.; Ye, S.; Ou, Z.; Ren, G. SIRT1 upregulation protects against liver injury induced by a HFD through inhibiting CD36 and the NF-κB pathway in mouse kupffer cells. *Mol. Med. Rep.* **2018**, *18*, 1609–1615. [CrossRef] [PubMed]
65. Yi, H.S. Implications of Mitochondrial Unfolded Protein Response and Mitokines: A Perspective on Fatty Liver Diseases. *Endocrinol. Metab.* **2019**, *34*, 39–46. [CrossRef] [PubMed]
66. Gariani, K.; Menzies, K.J.; Ryu, D.; Wegner, C.J.; Wang, X.; Ropelle, E.R.; Moullan, N.; Zhang, H.; Perino, A.; Lemos, V.; et al. Eliciting the mitochondrial unfolded protein response by nicotinamide adenine dinucleotide repletion reverses fatty liver disease in mice. *Hepatology* **2016**, *63*, 1190–1204. [CrossRef] [PubMed]
67. Chung, H.K.; Kim, J.T.; Kim, H.-W.; Kwon, M.; Kim, S.Y.; Shong, M.; Kim, K.S.; Yi, H.S. GDF15 deficiency exacerbates chronic alcohol- and carbon tetrachloride-induced liver injury. *Sci. Rep.* **2017**, *7*, 17238. [CrossRef]
68. Bonawitz, N.D.; Chatenay-Lapointe, M.; Pan, Y.; Shadel, G.S. Reduced TOR signaling extends chronological life span via increased respiration and upregulation of mitochondrial gene expression. *Cell Metab.* **2007**, *5*, 265–277. [CrossRef]
69. Ferrín, G.; Guerrero, M.; Amado, V.; Rodríguez-Perálvarez, M.; De la Mata, M. Activation of mTOR Signaling Pathway in Hepatocellular Carcinoma. *Int. J. Mol. Sci.* **2020**, *21*, 1266. [CrossRef]
70. Bárcena, C.; Mayoral, P.; Quirós, P.M. Mitohormesis, an Antiaging Paradigm. *Int. Rev. Cell Mol. Biol.* **2018**, *340*, 35–77.
71. Lee, L.-Y.; Köhler, U.A.; Zhang, L.; Roenneburg, D.; Werner, S.; Johnson, J.A.; Foley, D.P. Activation of the Nrf2-ARE pathway in hepatocytes protects against steatosis in nutritionally induced non-alcoholic steatohepatitis in mice. *Toxicol. Sci.* **2014**, *142*, 361–374. [CrossRef]

72. Wang, C.; Cui, Y.; Li, C.; Zhang, Y.; Xu, S.; Li, X.; Li, H.; Zhang, X. Nrf2 deletion causes 'benign' simple steatosis to develop into non-alcoholic steatohepatitis in mice fed a high-fat diet. *Lipids Health Dis.* **2013**, *12*, 165. [CrossRef]
73. Wang, P.; Ni, M.; Tian, Y.; Wang, H.; Qiu, J.; You, W.; Wei, S.; Shi, Y.; Zhou, J.; Cheng, F.; et al. Myeloid Nrf2 deficiency aggravates non-alcoholic steatohepatitis progression by regulating YAP-mediated NLRP3 inflammasome signaling. *iScience* **2021**, *24*, 102427. [CrossRef]
74. Mantena, S.K.; Vaughn, D.P.; Andringa, K.K.; Eccleston, H.B.; King, A.L.; Abrams, G.A.; Doeller, J.E.; Kraus, D.W.; Darley-Usmar, V.M.; Bailey, S.M. High fat diet induces dysregulation of hepatic oxygen gradients and mitochondrial function in vivo. *Biochem. J.* **2009**, *417*, 183–193. [CrossRef] [PubMed]
75. Aharoni-Simon, M.; Hann-Obercyger, M.; Pen, S.; Madar, Z.; Tirosh, O. Fatty liver is associated with impaired activity of PPARγ-coactivator 1α (PGC1α) and mitochondrial biogenesis in mice. *Lab. Investig.* **2011**, *91*, 1018–1028. [CrossRef] [PubMed]
76. Pessayre, D. Role of mitochondria in non-alcoholic fatty liver disease. *J. Gastroenterol. Hepatol.* **2007**, *22* (Suppl. S1), S20–S27. [CrossRef]
77. Tanaka, S.; Miyanishi, K.; Kobune, M.; Kawano, Y.; Hoki, T.; Kubo, T.; Hayashi, T.; Sato, T.; Sato, Y.; Takimoto, R.; et al. Increased hepatic oxidative DNA damage in patients with non-alcoholic steatohepatitis who develop hepatocellular carcinoma. *J. Gastroenterol.* **2013**, *48*, 1249–1258. [CrossRef]
78. Matsuzawa-Nagata, N.; Takamura, T.; Ando, H.; Nakamura, S.; Kurita, S.; Misu, H.; Ota, T.; Yokoyama, M.; Honda, M.; Miyamoto, K.-I.; et al. Increased oxidative stress precedes the onset of high-fat diet-induced insulin resistance and obesity. *Metabolism* **2008**, *57*, 1071–1077. [CrossRef]
79. Knebel, B.; Hartwig, S.; Haas, J.; Lehr, S.; Goeddeke, S.; Susanto, F.; Bohne, L.; Jacob, S.; Koellmer, C.; Nitzgen, U.; et al. Peroxisomes compensate hepatic lipid overflow in mice with fatty liver. *Biochim. Biophys. Acta* **2015**, *1851*, 965–976. [CrossRef] [PubMed]
80. Li, J.; Romestaing, C.; Han, X.; Li, Y.; Hao, X.; Wu, Y.; Sun, C.; Liu, X.; Jefferson, L.S.; Xiong, J.; et al. Cardiolipin remodeling by ALCAT1 links oxidative stress and mitochondrial dysfunction to obesity. *Cell. Metab.* **2010**, *12*, 154–165. [CrossRef]
81. Turpin, S.M.; Nicholls, H.T.; Willmes, D.M.; Mourier, A.; Brodesser, S.; Wunderlich, C.M.; Mauer, J.; Xu, E.; Hammerschmidt, P.; Brönneke, H.S.; et al. Obesity-induced CerS6-dependent C16:0 ceramide production promotes weight gain and glucose intolerance. *Cell. Metab.* **2014**, *20*, 678–686. [CrossRef]
82. Zhu, C.; Huai, Q.; Zhang, X.; Dai, H.; Li, X.; Wang, H. Insights into the roles and pathomechanisms of ceramide and sphigosine-1-phosphate in non-alcoholic fatty liver disease. *Int. J. Biol. Sci.* **2023**, *19*, 311–330. [CrossRef]
83. Apostolopoulou, M.; Gordillo, R.; Koliaki, C.; Gancheva, S.; Jelenik, T.; De Filippo, E.; Herder, C.; Markgraf, D.; Jankowiak, F.; Esposito, I.; et al. Specific Hepatic Sphingolipids Relate to Insulin Resistance, Oxidative Stress, and Inflammation in Non-alcoholic Steatohepatitis. *Diabetes Care* **2018**, *41*, 1235–1243. [CrossRef]
84. Reiniers, M.J.; van Golen, R.F.; van Gulik, T.M.; Heger, M. Reactive oxygen and nitrogen species in steatotic hepatocytes: A molecular perspective on the pathophysiology of ischemia-reperfusion injury in the fatty liver. *Antioxid. Redox Signal.* **2014**, *21*, 1119–1142. [CrossRef] [PubMed]
85. Marette, A. Molecular mechanisms of inflammation in obesity-linked insulin resistance. *Int. J. Obes. Relat. Metab. Disord. J. Int. Assoc. Study Obes.* **2003**, *27* (Suppl. S3), S46–S48. [CrossRef] [PubMed]
86. Begriche, K.; Massart, J.; Fromenty, B. Effects of β-aminoisobutyric acid on leptin production and lipid homeostasis: Mechanisms and possible relevance for the prevention of obesity. *Fundam. Clin. Pharmacol.* **2010**, *24*, 269–282. [CrossRef] [PubMed]
87. Tilg, H.; Moschen, A.R. Evolution of inflammation in non-alcoholic fatty liver disease: The multiple parallel hits hypothesis. *Hepatology* **2010**, *52*, 1836–1846. [CrossRef] [PubMed]
88. Eccleston, H.B.; Andringa, K.K.; Betancourt, A.M.; King, A.L.; Mantena, S.K.; Swain, T.M.; Tinsley, H.N.; Nolte, R.N.; Nagy, T.R.; Abrams, G.A.; et al. Chronic exposure to a high-fat diet induces hepatic steatosis, impairs nitric oxide bioavailability, and modifies the mitochondrial proteome in mice. *Antioxid. Redox Signal.* **2011**, *15*, 447–459. [CrossRef]
89. Herzig, S.; Shaw, R.J. AMPK: Guardian of metabolism and mitochondrial homeostasis. *Nat. Rev. Mol. Cell. Biol.* **2018**, *19*, 121–135. [CrossRef]
90. Lim, C.Y.; Jun, D.W.; Jang, S.S.; Cho, W.K.; Chae, J.D.; Jun, J.H. Effects of carnitine on peripheral blood mitochondrial DNA copy number and liver function in non-alcoholic fatty liver disease. *Korean J. Gastroenterol.* **2010**, *55*, 384–389. [CrossRef]
91. Sunny, N.E.; Parks, E.J.; Browning, J.D.; Burgess, S.C. Excessive hepatic mitochondrial TCA cycle and gluconeogenesis in humans with non-alcoholic fatty liver disease. *Cell. Metab.* **2011**, *14*, 804–810. [CrossRef]
92. Gray, L.R.; Sultana, M.R.; Rauckhorst, A.J.; Oonthonpan, L.; Tompkins, S.C.; Sharma, A.; Fu, X.; Miao, R.; Pewa, A.D.; Brown, K.S.; et al. Hepatic Mitochondrial Pyruvate Carrier 1 Is Required for Efficient Regulation of Gluconeogenesis and Whole-Body Glucose Homeostasis. *Cell. Metab.* **2015**, *22*, 669–681. [CrossRef]
93. Rauckhorst, A.J.; Gray, L.R.; Sheldon, R.D.; Fu, X.; Pewa, A.D.; Feddersen, C.R.; Dupuy, A.J.; Gibson-Corley, K.N.; Cox, J.E.; Burgess, S.C.; et al. The mitochondrial pyruvate carrier mediates high fat diet-induced increases in hepatic TCA cycle capacity. *Mol. Metab.* **2017**, *6*, 1468–1479. [CrossRef]
94. Ma, X.; McKeen, T.; Zhang, J.; Ding, W.-X. Role and Mechanisms of Mitophagy in Liver Diseases. *Cells* **2020**, *9*, 837. [CrossRef] [PubMed]

95. Li, J.; Zou, B.; Yeo, Y.H.; Feng, Y.; Xie, X.; Lee, D.H.; Fujii, H.; Wu, Y.; Kam, L.Y.; Ji, F.; et al. Prevalence, incidence, and outcome of non-alcoholic fatty liver disease in Asia, 1999–2019: A systematic review and meta-analysis. *Lancet Gastroenterol. Hepatol.* **2019**, *4*, 389–398. [CrossRef] [PubMed]
96. Edmunds, L.R.; Xie, B.; Mills, A.M.; Huckestein, B.R.; Undamatla, R.; Murali, A.; Pangburn, M.M.; Martin, J.; Sipula, I.; Kaufman, B.A. Liver-specific Prkn knockout mice are more susceptible to diet-induced hepatic steatosis and insulin resistance. *Mol. Metab.* **2020**, *41*, 101051. [CrossRef]
97. Glick, D.; Zhang, W.; Beaton, M.; Marsboom, G.; Gruber, M.; Simon, M.C.; Hart, J.; Dorn, G.W.; Brady, M.J.; Macleod, K.F. BNip3 regulates mitochondrial function and lipid metabolism in the liver. *Mol. Cell. Biol.* **2012**, *32*, 2570–2584. [CrossRef]
98. Lee, D.H.; Jung, Y.Y.; Park, M.H.; Jo, M.R.; Han, S.B.; Yoon, D.Y.; Roh, Y.S.; Hong, J.T. Peroxiredoxin 6 Confers Protection Against Non-alcoholic Fatty Liver Disease Through Maintaining Mitochondrial Function. *Antioxid. Redox Signal.* **2019**, *31*, 387–402. [CrossRef]
99. Simoes, I.C.M.; Karkucinska-Wieckowska, A.; Janikiewicz, J.; Szymanska, S.; Pronicki, M.; Dobrzyn, P.; Dabrowski, M.; Do-brzyn, A.; Oliveira, P.J.; Zischka, H.; et al. Western Diet Causes Obesity-Induced Nonalcoholic Fatty Liver Disease Development by Differentially Compromising the Autophagic Response. *Antioxidants* **2020**, *9*, 993. [CrossRef] [PubMed]
100. Gnaiger, E.; Gnaiger, E. Mitochondrial Pathways and Respiratory Control: An Introduction to OXPHOS Analysis Mitochondrial Pathways and Respiratory Control. In *An Introduction to OXPHOS Analysis*; OROBOROS MiPNet Publications: Innsbruck, Austria, 2012.
101. Sanyal, A.J.; Campbell-Sargent, C.; Mirshahi, F.; Rizzo, W.B.; Contos, M.J.; Sterling, R.K.; Luketic, V.A.; Shiffman, M.L.; Clore, J.N. Non-alcoholic steatohepatitis: Association of insulin resistance and mitochondrial abnormalities. *Gastroenterology* **2001**, *120*, 1183–1192. [CrossRef]
102. Serviddio, G.; Bellanti, F.; Tamborra, R.; Rollo, T.; Capitanio, N.; Romano, A.D.; Sastre, J.; Vendemiale, G.; Altomare, E. Uncoupling protein-2 (UCP2) induces mitochondrial proton leak and increases susceptibility of non-alcoholic steatohepatitis (NASH) liver to ischaemia-reperfusion injury. *Gut* **2008**, *57*, 957–965. [CrossRef]
103. Elsheikh, A.; Lavergne, S.N.; Castrejon, J.L.; Farrell, J.; Wang, H.; Sathish, J.; Pichler, W.J.; Park, B.K.; Naisbitt, D.J. Drug antigenicity, immunogenicity, and costimulatory signaling: Evidence for formation of a functional antigen through immune cell metabolism. *J. Immunol.* **2010**, *185*, 6448–6460. [CrossRef]
104. Marques, P.E.; Oliveira, A.G.; Pereira, R.V.; David, B.A.; Gomides, L.F.; Saraiva, A.M.; Pires, D.A.; Novaes, J.T.; Patricio, D.O.; Cisalpino, D.; et al. Hepatic DNA deposition drives drug-induced liver injury and inflammation in mice. *Hepatology* **2015**, *61*, 348–360. [CrossRef]
105. Lee, J.; Park, J.-S.; Roh, Y.S. Molecular insights into the role of mitochondria in non-alcoholic fatty liver disease. *Arch. Pharm. Res.* **2019**, *42*, 935–946. [CrossRef] [PubMed]
106. Pessayre, D.; Mansouri, A.; Fromenty, B. Non-alcoholic steatosis and steatohepatitis. V. Mitochondrial dysfunction in steatohepatitis. *Am. J. Physiol. Gastrointest. Liver Physiol.* **2002**, *282*, G193–G199. [CrossRef] [PubMed]
107. Carter-Kent, C.; Zein, N.N.; Feldstein, A.E. Cytokines in the pathogenesis of fatty liver and disease progression to steatohepatitis: Implications for treatment. *Am. J. Gastroenterol.* **2008**, *103*, 1036–1042. [CrossRef] [PubMed]
108. Garcia-Martinez, I.; Santoro, N.; Chen, Y.; Hoque, R.; Ouyang, X.; Caprio, S.; Shlomchik, M.J.; Coffman, R.L.; Candia, A.; Mehal, W.Z. Hepatocyte mitochondrial DNA drives non-alcoholic steatohepatitis by activation of TLR9. *J. Clin. Investig.* **2016**, *126*, 859–864. [CrossRef] [PubMed]
109. Caballero, F.; Fernández, A.; De Lacy, A.M.; Fernández-Checa, J.C.; Caballería, J.; García-Ruiz, C. Enhanced free cholesterol, SREBP-2 and StAR expression in human NASH. *J. Hepatol.* **2009**, *50*, 789–796. [CrossRef] [PubMed]
110. Chavin, K.D.; Yang, S.; Lin, H.Z.; Chatham, J.; Chacko, V.P.; Hoek, J.B.; Walajtys-Rode, E.; Rashid, A.; Chen, C.-H.; Huang, C.-C.; et al. Obesity induces expression of uncoupling protein-2 in hepatocytes and promotes liver ATP depletion. *J. Biol. Chem.* **1999**, *274*, 5692–5700. [CrossRef] [PubMed]
111. Zhao, Q.; Guo, Z.; Deng, W.; Fu, S.; Zhang, C.; Chen, M.; Ju, W.; Wang, D.; He, X. Calpain 2-mediated autophagy defect increases susceptibility of fatty livers to ischemia-reperfusion injury. *Cell. Death Dis.* **2016**, *7*, e2186. [CrossRef]
112. González-Rodríguez, A.; Mayoral, R.; Agra, N.; Valdecantos, M.P.; Pardo, V.; Miquilena-Colina, M.E.; Vargas-Castrillón, J.; Lo Iacono, O.; Corazzari, M.; Fimia, G.M.; et al. Impaired autophagic flux is associated with increased endoplasmic reticulum stress during the development of NAFLD. *Cell. Death Dis.* **2014**, *5*, e1179. [CrossRef]
113. Zhou, T.; Chang, L.; Luo, Y.; Zhou, Y.; Zhang, J. Mst1 inhibition attenuates non-alcoholic fatty liver disease via reversing Parkin-related mitophagy. *Redox Biol.* **2019**, *21*, 101120. [CrossRef]
114. Sebastián, D.; Hernández-Alvarez, M.I.; Segalés, J.; Sorianello, E.; Muñoz, J.P.; Sala, D.; Waget, A.; Liesa, M.; Paz, J.C.; Gopalacharyulu, P.; et al. Mitofusin 2 (Mfn2) links mitochondrial and endoplasmic reticulum function with insulin signaling and is essential for normal glucose homeostasis. *Proc. Natl. Acad. Sci. USA* **2012**, *109*, 5523–5528. [CrossRef]
115. Yamada, T.; Murata, D.; Kleiner, D.E.; Anders, R.; Rosenberg, A.Z.; Kaplan, J.; Hamilton, J.P.; Aghajan, M.; Levi, M.; Wang, N.Y.; et al. Prevention and regression of megamitochondria and steatosis by blocking mitochondrial fusion in the liver. *iScience* **2022**, *25*, 103996. [CrossRef] [PubMed]
116. Gan, L.T.; Van Rooyen, D.M.; Koina, M.E.; McCuskey, R.S.; Teoh, N.C.; Farrell, G.C. Hepatocyte free cholesterol lipotoxicity results from JNK1-mediated mitochondrial injury and is HMGB1 and TLR4-dependent. *J. Hepatol.* **2014**, *61*, 1376–1384. [CrossRef] [PubMed]

117. Marí, M.; Caballero, F.; Colell, A.; Morales, A.; Caballeria, J.; Fernandez, A.; Enrich, C.; Fernandez-Checa, J.C.; García-Ruiz, C. Mitochondrial free cholesterol loading sensitizes to TNF- and Fas-mediated steatohepatitis. *Cell. Metab.* **2006**, *4*, 185–198. [CrossRef] [PubMed]
118. Von Montfort, C.; Matias, N.; Fernandez, A.; Fucho, R.; de la Rosa, L.C.; Martinez-Chantar, M.L.; Mato, J.M.; Machida, K.; Tsukamoto, H.; Murphy, M.P.; et al. Mitochondrial GSH determines the toxic or therapeutic potential of superoxide scavenging in steatohepatitis. *J. Hepatol.* **2012**, *57*, 852–859. [CrossRef]
119. Merry, T.L.; Tran, M.; Dodd, G.T.; Mangiafico, S.P.; Wiede, F.; Kaur, S.; McLean, C.L.; Andrikopoulos, S.; Tiganis, T. Hepatocyte glutathione peroxidase-1 deficiency improves hepatic glucose metabolism and decreases steatohepatitis in mice. *Diabetologia* **2016**, *59*, 2632–2644. [CrossRef]
120. Delibegovic, M.; Zimmer, D.; Kauffman, C.; Rak, K.; Hong, E.-G.; Cho, Y.-R.; Kim, J.K.; Kahn, B.B.; Neel, B.G.; Bence, K.K. Liver-specific deletion of protein-tyrosine phosphatase 1B (PTP1B) improves metabolic syndrome and attenuates diet-induced endoplasmic reticulum stress. *Diabetes* **2009**, *58*, 590–599. [CrossRef]
121. Jais, A.; Einwallner, E.; Sharif, O.; Gossens, K.; Lu, T.T.-H.; Soyal, S.M.; Medgyesi, D.; Neureiter, D.; Paier-Pourani, J.; Dalgaard, K.; et al. Heme oxygenase-1 drives metaflammation and insulin resistance in mouse and man. *Cell* **2014**, *158*, 25–40. [CrossRef]
122. Inzaugarat, M.E.; Wree, A.; Feldstein, A.E. Hepatocyte mitochondrial DNA released in microparticles and toll-like receptor 9 activation: A link between lipotoxicity and inflammation during non-alcoholic steatohepatitis. *Hepatology* **2016**, *64*, 669–671. [CrossRef]
123. Kawada, N.; Imanaka, K.; Kawaguchi, T.; Tamai, C.; Ishihara, R.; Matsunaga, T.; Gotoh, K.; Yamada, T.; Tomita, Y. Hepatocellular carcinoma arising from non-cirrhotic non-alcoholic steatohepatitis. *J. Gastroenterol.* **2009**, *44*, 1190–1194. [CrossRef]
124. Ali, E.S.; Rychkov, G.Y.; Barritt, G.J. Deranged hepatocyte intracellular Ca(2+) homeostasis and the progression of non-alcoholic fatty liver disease to hepatocellular carcinoma. *Cell. Calcium* **2019**, *82*, 102057. [CrossRef]
125. Xu, D.; Xu, M.; Jeong, S.; Qian, Y.; Wu, H.; Xia, Q.; Kong, X. The Role of Nrf2 in Liver Disease: Novel Molecular Mechanisms and Therapeutic Approaches. *Front. Pharmacol.* **2019**, *9*, 1428. [CrossRef]
126. Teng, Y.; Zhao, H.; Gao, L.; Zhang, W.; Shull, A.Y.; Shay, C. FGF19 Protects Hepatocellular Carcinoma Cells against Endoplasmic Reticulum Stress via Activation of FGFR4-GSK3β-Nrf2 Signaling. *Cancer Res.* **2017**, *77*, 6215–6225. [CrossRef] [PubMed]
127. Calvisi, D.F.; Wang, C.; Ho, C.; Ladu, S.; Lee, S.A.; Mattu, S.; Destefanis, G.; Delogu, S.; Zimmermann, A.; Ericsson, J.; et al. Increased lipogenesis, induced by AKT-mTORC1-RPS6 signaling, promotes development of human hepatocellular carcinoma. *Gastroenterology* **2011**, *140*, 1071–1083. [CrossRef] [PubMed]
128. Piccinin, E.; Peres, C.; Bellafante, E.; Ducheix, S.; Pinto, C.; Villani, G.; Moschetta, A. Hepatic peroxisome proliferator-activated receptor γ coactivator 1β drives mitochondrial and anabolic signatures that contribute to hepatocellular carcinoma progression in mice. *Hepatology* **2018**, *67*, 884–898. [CrossRef] [PubMed]
129. Simula, L.; Nazio, F.; Campello, S. The mitochondrial dynamics in cancer and immune-surveillance. *Semin. Cancer Biol.* **2017**, *47*, 29–42. [CrossRef] [PubMed]
130. Sun, X.; Cao, H.; Zhan, L.; Yin, C.; Wang, G.; Liang, P.; Li, J.; Wang, Z.; Liu, B.; Huang, Q.; et al. Mitochondrial fission promotes cell migration by Ca(2+) /CaMKII/ERK/FAK pathway in hepatocellular carcinoma. *Liver Int.* **2018**, *38*, 1263–1272. [CrossRef]
131. Zhang, Z.; Li, T.-E.; Chen, M.; Xu, D.; Zhu, Y.; Hu, B.-Y.; Lin, Z.-F.; Pan, J.-J.; Wang, X.; Wu, C.; et al. MFN1-dependent alteration of mitochondrial dynamics drives hepatocellular carcinoma metastasis by glucose metabolic reprogramming. *Br. J. Cancer* **2020**, *122*, 209–220. [CrossRef]

biology

MDPI

Article

Phenotypic Characterization of Female Carrier Mice Heterozygous for Tafazzin Deletion

Michelle V. Tomczewski [1], John Z. Chan [1], Duaa M. Al-Majmaie [1], Ming Rong Liu [1], Alex D. Cocco [1], Ken D. Stark [1], Douglas Strathdee [2] and Robin E. Duncan [1,*]

[1] Department of Kinesiology and Health Sciences, Faculty of Health, University of Waterloo, 200 University Ave W., BMH1044, Waterloo, ON N2L 3G1, Canada; mvtomczewski@uwaterloo.ca (M.V.T.); l292zhan@uwaterloo.ca (J.Z.C.); almajmad@uoguelph.ca (D.M.A.-M.); mr2liu@uwaterloo.ca (M.R.L.); kstark@uwaterloo.ca (K.D.S.)

[2] Transgenic Technology Laboratory, Cancer Research UK Beatson Institute, Switchback Road, Glasgow G61 1BD, Scotland, UK; d.strathdee@beatson.gla.ac.uk

* Correspondence: reduncan@uwaterloo.ca; Tel.: +1-519-888-4567

Simple Summary: Barth syndrome (BTHS) is a disease that affects energy production. It results from mutations on the X chromosome, and thus it mainly affects males since they have only one copy (females have two X chromosomes). Although BTHS is rare, the consequences can be severe. BTHS affects the heart, immune system, and muscles, so boys and men with BTHS are at a high risk of heart attacks and death from infections, and they tire easily, which impacts quality of life. Women with one mutated X chromosome are typically thought to be asymptomatic, so they have not been studied very much. However, in other diseases caused by X chromosome mutations, females that were thought to be healthy developed symptoms after they got older. In this work, we studied female mice with one mutated X chromosome, which are models of female carriers of BTHS. We found that with advancing age, the carriers have some slowdown in their running speed, which is like that seen in male mice but less severe. They also weigh less and are better able to maintain their blood sugar, which could be beneficial. Our work shows that female carriers can have symptoms and supports further research in women.

Abstract: Barth syndrome (BTHS) is caused by mutations in tafazzin resulting in deficits in cardiolipin remodeling that alter major metabolic processes. The tafazzin gene is encoded on the X chromosome, and therefore BTHS primarily affects males. Female carriers are typically considered asymptomatic, but age-related changes have been reported in female carriers of other X-linked disorders. Therefore, we examined the phenotype of female mice heterozygous for deletion of the tafazzin gene (*Taz*-HET) at 3 and 12 months of age. Food intakes, body masses, lean tissue and adipose depot weights, daily activity levels, metabolic measures, and exercise capacity were assessed. Age-related changes in mice resulted in small but significant genotype-specific differences in *Taz*-HET mice compared with their female *Wt* littermates. By 12 months, *Taz*-HET mice weighed less than *Wt* controls and had smaller gonadal, retroperitoneal, and brown adipose depots and liver and brain masses, despite similar food consumption. Daily movement, respiratory exchange ratio, and total energy expenditure did not vary significantly between the age-matched genotypes. *Taz*-HET mice displayed improved glucose tolerance and insulin sensitivity at 12 months compared with their *Wt* littermates but had evidence of slightly reduced exercise capacity. Tafazzin mRNA levels were significantly reduced in the cardiac muscle of 12-month-old *Taz*-HET mice, which was associated with minor but significant alterations in the heart cardiolipin profile. This work is the first to report the characterization of a model of female carriers of heterozygous tafazzin deficiency and suggests that additional study, particularly with advancing age, is warranted.

Keywords: tafazzin; cardiolipin; Barth syndrome; mitochondria; energy metabolism; exercise capacity; mice; X-linked diseases; carriers; heterozygous

1. Introduction

Cardiolipin is a component of the inner mitochondrial membrane, constituting approximately 15–20% of the glycerolipids present [1]. The dimeric nature of cardiolipin makes it structurally unique among phospholipids, allowing for esterification of four fatty acyl chains rather than two [2]. While this permits, in theory, the generation of thousands of different possible molecular species of cardiolipin, lipidomic analyses indicate that only a handful of major species predominate [3]. In general, cardiolipin species in all tissues are enriched with 18-carbon fatty acyl chains, and while different tissues tend to have different cardiolipin molecular profiles, there is often conservation in these tissue profiles across organisms [2]. One molecular species, tetralinoleoyl (L4)-cardiolipin), which is comprised of four linoleic acid moieties, is particularly enriched in heart muscle from various organisms, ranging from approximately 80% of cardiolipin molecules in human hearts [4] to 1/3rd of cardiolipin molecules in mouse hearts [5].

Cardiolipin synthesis occurs initially in the Kennedy pathway [6]. However, the enzymes involved in de novo synthesis pathways lack the acyl-chain specificity needed to create the signature molecular profiles that are evident in various tissues [2]. To this end, at least five cardiolipin remodeling enzymes have been identified [7–12]. These enzymes function to re-esterify fatty acyl chains onto monolyso- or dilyso-cardiolipin produced from the action of various phospholipases on nascent cardiolipin, resulting in the generation of a mature form of this complex lipid [2]. Among these, the enzyme tafazzin has been extensively studied as a phosphatidylcholine:monolysocardiolipin transacylase that is critical for the generation of L4-cardiolipin [2].

Tafazzin is highly expressed in cardiac and skeletal muscle but is also expressed at variable levels in other tissues [2]. Mutations in tafazzin cause Barth syndrome (BTHS), a disease associated with L4-cardiolipin deficiency, resulting in variable clinical findings including cardiac and skeletal myopathies as well as immunological deficits and changes in cognition, taste, and sensory perception, among other symptoms [13]. BTHS is an X-linked recessive disorder, and therefore individuals with Barth Syndrome are almost entirely male [14]. The prevalence of the disease is low, affecting an estimated 1:300,000 to 1:400,000 live births [14]. The number of female carriers likely exceeds the number of clinically diagnosed males, however, since historically 70% of affected males perished in childhood due to the disease [15,16].

Female carriers of tafazzin mutations are typically considered clinically asymptomatic [14], but whether heterozygous tafazzin deficiency causes phenotypic changes at either younger or older ages in female carriers remains poorly understood. In other X-linked disorders of lipid metabolism, such as X-linked adrenoleukodystrophy, clinically relevant symptoms have been reported with advancing age [17]. We have therefore studied female mice heterozygous for tafazzin at ages 3 and 12 months.

2. Materials and Methods

2.1. Mice

The generation and maintenance of the *Taz*-KO mice were approved by a UK Home Office Licence (PP9886217). Animal procedures, including breeding and all experiments performed at the University of Waterloo (UW), were approved by the UW Animal Care Committee under AUPP#30055 (17-19), approved 25 July 2017; AUPP#41822, approved 27 August 2020; and AUPP#43431, approved 9 July 2021, and comply with Canadian Council on Animal Care guidelines and ARRIVE guidelines. Mice were housed in a temperature- and humidity-controlled environment on a 12:12 h light/dark cycle with enrichment materials and free access to standard rodent chow (Teklad 22/5 Rodent diet from Envigo, Haslett, MI, USA) and water, together with their sex-matched littermates.

Gene targeting was performed at the Beatson Institute (Cancer Research UK), resulting in the generation of mice with a germline deletion of exons 5–10 of tafazzin, and has been previously reported in detail [18,19]. Mice were backcrossed onto a C57BL/6J line >20 generations before use. Heterozygous females ($Taz^{\Delta/+}$ [*Taz*-HET]) and wildtype (*Wt*) littermate females ($Taz^{+/+}$) used in experiments were generated by mating male C57BL/6J mice (Jackson Labs, Bar Harbor, ME, USA) with $Taz^{\Delta/+}$ females. This also generated *Wt* male ($Taz^{+/Y}$) and hemizygous null ($Taz^{\Delta/Y}$ [*Taz*-KO]) male mice. Their phenotypic characterization has been reported separately [18,20].

Genotype was analyzed using an extract of genomic DNA isolated from ear punches, and the presence of the KO *Taz* allele was verified by generation of a 280 bp amplicon, visualized under ultraviolet light following gel electrophoresis using 1% TAE-agarose gels with ethidium bromide. The amplicon was produced by PCR using FastStart™ Master Mix (Roche Life Science, Mississauga, ON, Canada) and a Bio-Rad® T100 thermocycler (Mississauga, ON, Canada) under the following conditions: 95 °C for 4 min; 39 cycles of 95 °C for 30 s, 56 °C for 30 s, 72 °C for 1 min; and a final extension step of 72 °C for 7 min, with the KO-U1 (5′-CCAAGTTGCTAGCCCACAAG-3′) forward primer and WT-D1 (5′-CAGGCACATGGTCCTGTTTC-3′) reverse primer. Since the mating strategy could only produce *Wt* ($Taz^{+/+}$) or heterozygous ($Taz^{\Delta/+}$) females, detection of the null allele was sufficient to genotype mice as heterozygous, with those lacking the null allele designated as *Wt*.

2.2. Comprehensive Laboratory Animal Monitoring System Measures

Indirect calorimetry measures were analyzed in 3- and 12-month-old mice over a 24 h period, essentially as we have previously described [20]. Twenty-four hours prior to testing, mice were single-housed to allow for determination of food consumption and to assist them in adjusting to individual housing conditions prior to entering the Comprehensive Laboratory Animal Monitoring System (CLAMS, Columbus Instruments, Columbus, OH, USA). Mice were then placed in individual CLAMS chambers for an additional 2 h of acclimatization prior to the onset of data recording. Throughout the experiment, mice had unlimited access to chow and water and were maintained at room temperature (22–23 °C) with 12:12 h light/dark cycle (light 07:00–19:00 h, dark 19:00–07:00 h). Air flow in the chambers was exchanged at 0.5 L/min. Immediately prior to testing, gas sensors were calibrated with mixtures of standard gases (20.5% oxygen, 0.5% carbon dioxide, and nitrogen at balance), and oxygen consumption (VO_2; mL/kg/h) and carbon dioxide production (VCO_2; mL/kg/h) rates were analyzed at 28-min intervals. The respiratory exchange ratio (RER) was calculated from measures of VCO_2/VO_2 [21]. The Lusk equation [$(3.815 + 1.232 \times \text{RER}) \times VO_2$ (in liters)] was used to calculate total energy expenditure (TEE), which was normalized to individual body weights (kg) [22]. Infrared beam breaks were used to determine activity in three directions: x (locomotion), y (ambulation), and z (rearing) planes.

2.3. Glucose Tolerance Testing (GTT)

Mice at 12 months of age were tested for glucose tolerance, as we have previously described [20]. Food was withdrawn 6 h prior to testing at 15:00 h. Tail vein blood glucose levels were measured at baseline and 15, 30, 60, 90, and 120 min following *i.p.* injection of D-glucose (2.0 g/kg) using Freestyle Lite test strips and glucometer (Abbot Laboratories, Mississauga, ON, Canada). Area-under-the-curve (AUC) analysis was performed to allow for comparisons between overall test effects.

2.4. Insulin Tolerance Testing (ITT)

Twelve-month-old mice were tested for insulin sensitivity, essentially as we have previously described [20]. Following a 2 h fast (13:00–15:00 h), baseline glucose levels were measured using the Freestyle Lite glucose monitoring system, and then mice received an *i.p.* injection of insulin (0.5 U per kg body weight). Glucose levels were monitored in tail-vein blood at 15, 30, 60, 90, and 120 min and analyzed to determine AUC responses [23].

2.5. Treadmill Exercise Capacity Test

Mice at 3 and 12 months of age were subjected to an incremental treadmill exercise test using a five-lane motor-driven treadmill (Panlab; Harvard Apparatus, Barcelona, Spain) with a fixed slope of 5°, based on prior protocols [24,25], essentially as we have previously described [20]. Briefly, on the first 3 days of training, mice were placed on the treadmill in an immobile setting for 5 min, and then the treadmill was turned on to settings of 5 cm/s for a period of 5 min, followed by increases to 10 cm/s for 2 min, and then 15 cm/s for 3 min. On the third day, mice were placed on the static treadmill for 5 min, then it was set to speeds of 5 cm/s for a 3 min interval, 10 cm/s for 2 min, 15 cm/s for 2 min, and then 20 cm/s for 3 min. Mice rested on Day 4. An exhaustive exercise test was performed on Day 5 by placing mice on the treadmill for 5 min at a stationary setting, followed by an initial speed of 10 cm/s, which was increased by 3 cm/s every 2 min until a maximum speed of 70 cm/s was achieved. Running time and total distance ran until exhaustion were monitored. Sessions were performed from 16:00–19:00 h, which fell within the dark photoperiod for the mice since mice are normally most active nocturnally. Sessions were completed in a dark room, where illumination was provided using red lighting to prevent disruption to the dark cycle.

2.6. Tafazzin Gene Expression

Total RNA was extracted from mouse heart tissue using TRIzol® Reagent (Invitrogen, Waltham, MA, USA) according to the manufacturer's protocol after tissue was mechanically disrupted using a POLYTRON® PT 1200 E homogenizer (VWR, Radnor, PA, USA) set at maximum speed. Quantity of RNA was measured spectrophotometrically using a Nanodrop 2000 Spectrophotometer (ThermoFisher, Waltham, MA, USA), and 2 µg of RNA per 20 µL reaction was used to synthesize cDNA via random hexamer priming using a High-Capacity cDNA Reverse Transcription kit from Applied Biosystems (Waltham, MA, USA) according to the manufacturer's protocol. cDNA was diluted 1:5 in ddH_2O. The quantitative real-time (qRT)-PCR duplex reactions contained 7.5 µL PerfeCTa ToughMix qPCR MasterMix (Quantabio, Beverly, MA, USA), 0.75 µL each of the Taqman gene expression assays for FAM-labeled tafazzin (Mm04239390_g1), spanning exons 2/3, and VIC-labeled β-actin (Mm02619580_g1) (Applied Biosystems, Mississauga, ON, Canada), 5 µL of ddH_2O, and 1 µL of cDNA. Transcript levels were measured on a CFX-96 Connect Real Time qPCR Detection System (BioRad, Hercules, CA, USA). Thermal cycling conditions were 50 °C for 2 min, then 95 °C for 20 s, followed by 40 cycles at 95 °C for 3 s, then 60 °C for 30 s. All measurements were run in duplicate. Tafazzin expression was analyzed using the ΔΔCt method, with the Ct values normalized to β-actin.

2.7. Gas Chromatography Analysis of Cardiolipin

Mouse heart tissue was homogenized in phosphate-buffer saline (PBS) using a TissueLyser II for 2 min at a frequency of 25 Hz. Total lipids were extracted from the homogenate by the addition of 2:1 (*v*/*v*) chloroform:methanol with the antioxidant butylated hydroxytoluene (BHT) and overnight storage. The next day, phosphate buffered saline was added, the samples were vortexed, and then centrifugated at 3000 rpm for 5 min to separate the organic and aqueous phases. The organic phase was carefully collected and desiccated under a stream of nitrogen gas. To separate the individual phospholipid species, the organic phase was resuspended in chloroform and applied onto Silica Gel HF plates measuring 20 cm × 20 cm with a layer thickness of 250 µM (Analtech Inc., Cole-Parmer Canada, Montreal, QC, Canada), and resolved using thin-layer chromatography with a solvent system of chloroform:methanol:2-propanol:0.25% KCl:trimethylamine (30:9:25:6:18, *v*/*v*/*v*/*v*/*v*) [26]. Cardiolipin bands were detected using UV illumination after spraying with 0.1% 2,7-dichlorofuorescin in methanol (*w*/*v*) and scrapped in reference to known cardiolipin standards (Avanti Polar Lipids, Millipore Sigma, Mississauga, ON, Canada). To prepare for gas chromatography (GC) analysis, the fatty acyl species within cardiolipin underwent transesterification to fatty acyl methyl esters on a heating block for 1 h at 95 °C using 14% boron trifluoride in methanol and hexane (Thermo Scientific, Bellfonte, PA, USA), overlaid with nonadecanoic acid (19:0) as an internal standard (Nu-Chek Prep, Elysian, MN, USA). Following centrifugation at 3000 rpm for 5 min, the hexane layer was collected, transferred, desiccated under nitrogen gas, and resuspended in 65 µL of heptane. Subsequent analysis using gas chromatography with flame ionization detection was performed using a SCION 8300 GC (Scion Instruments Canada, Edmonton, AB, Canada) equipped with a DB-FFAP 15 m length × 0.10 mm inner diameter × 0.10 µm film thickness nitroterephthalic acid-modified polyethylene glycol capillary column (J&W Scientific/Agilent Technologies, Mississauga, ON, Canada) with hydrogen as the carrier gas. Specifically, 1 µL of samples were introduced by an Scion 8400Pro autosampler into the injector and heated to a temperature of 250 °C with a split ratio of 100:1. The initial temperature was set at 150 °C and maintained for 0.25 min, followed by a ramp of 35 °C/min to 200 °C, a 1 °C/min ramp to 211 °C, and an 80 °C/min ramp to 245 °C with a final hold of 4 min. The flame ionization detector temperature was maintained at 300 °C, while the make-up gas comprised air and nitrogen, flowing at rates of 300 and 30 mL/min, respectively. Sampling frequency was set at 50 Hz. The quantification of fatty acyl composition was expressed both in terms of concentrations (µg fatty acids per mg of tissue) and relative weight percentages, reflecting the proportion of each fatty acyl species within the total mass of fatty acids analyzed. Subsequently, the total content of cardiolipin was computed based on the cumulative mass of all cardiolipin fatty acyl species present within each sample.

2.8. Statistical Analyses

Comparisons between *Wt* and *Taz*-HET mice at 3 and 12 months of age were conducted using a two-way ANOVA to detect an interaction between genotype and age as main factors. Following identification of significant effects, Holm-Sidak's multiple comparison tests were used to identify significant differences in means within genotypes between ages and significant differences between age-matched animals with different genotypes.

Blood glucose levels across timepoints were compared between *Wt* and *Taz*-HET mice by repeated measures ANOVA. Area-under-the-curve (AUC) analyses were performed to determine the overall response of individual mice, and means from each group were compared using Student's t-test.

Differences between genotypes for tafazzin gene expression and cardiolipin measures were assessed by Student's t-test.

GraphPad Prism (version 9.0.0 for Mac, San Diego, CA, USA) was used to perform all statistical analyses. Data are presented as means ± standard error of the mean (SEM), and differences were considered significant when $p < 0.05$.

3. Results

3.1. Body, Organ, and Lean Tissue Weights

Mice of both genotypes grew from 3 to 12 months of age, as evidenced both by increases in absolute body weights (Figure 1A) and increases in tibial lengths within genotype groups (Figure 1B). At 3 months of age, there were no significant differences in body weights between *Taz*-HET and *Wt* mice (19.50 ± 1.13 g vs. 20.83 ± 1.10 g, respectively), but by 12 months, *Taz*-HET mice weighed 8% less than their *Wt* littermate controls (25.25 ± 3.24 g vs. 27.46 ± 2.90 g, respectively) (Figure 1A). Tibial lengths, however, did not differ between age-matched *Wt* and *Taz*-HET mice at either age examined, suggesting that differences in body weights at 12 months may reflect differences in body composition rather than absolute body stature per se.

Masses of hearts (Figure 1C), pancreas (Figure 1E), kidneys (Figure 1H), and gastrocnemius muscles (Figure 1K) increased with age in both genetic groups of mice but did not differ between age-matched genotypes. Masses of lungs (Figure 1D), spleens (Figure 1G), ovaries (Figure 1J), and soleus muscles (Figure 1L) did not differ significantly between genotypes at either age examined or between ages within a genotype group, indicating that maximal size for these organs and tissues was already attained by 3 months in all animals.

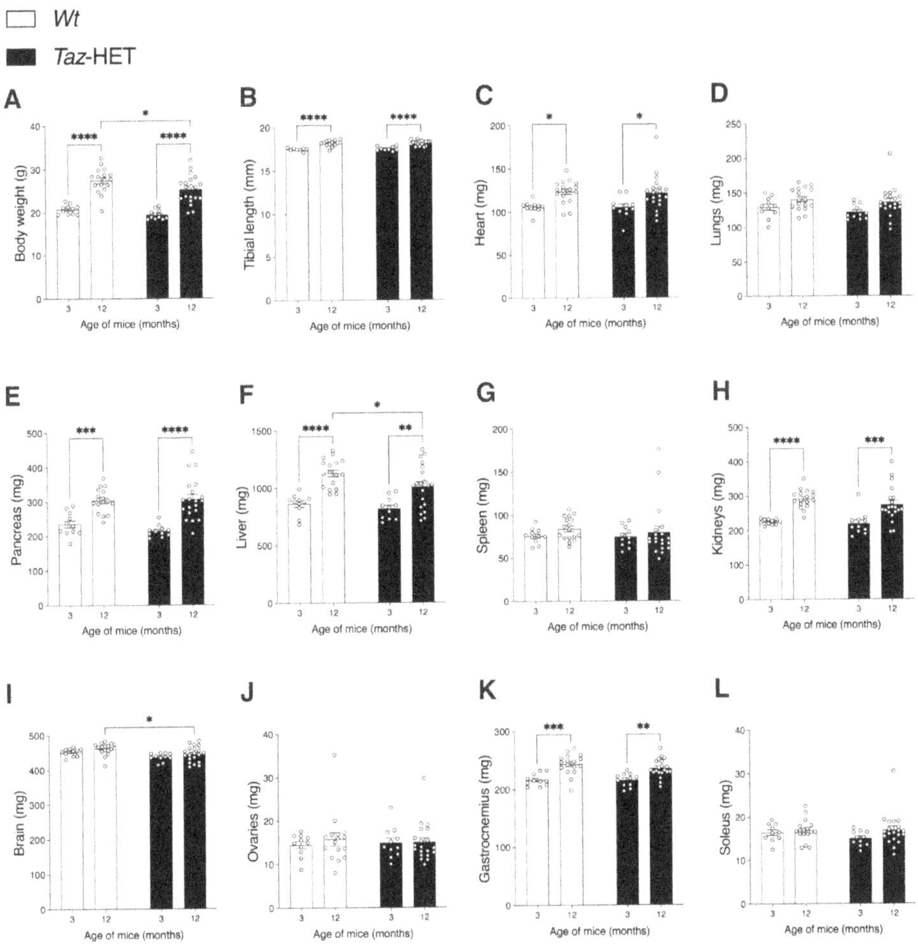

Figure 1. Body weights and lean tissue masses obtained by dissection of female *Wt* and *Taz*-HET mice at 3 and 12 months of age. Body weights (**A**) and tibial lengths (**B**), organ weights (**C**–**J**), and skeletal muscle masses (**K**,**L**) are shown according to genotype and age. Data are means ± SEM, with individual datapoints shown as circles, n = 11 per group at 3 months of age and n = 17–20 per genotype at 12 months of age. Comparisons between genotypes for age-matched mice, and comparisons between ages for mice within genotype groups are shown: * $p < 0.05$, ** $p < 0.01$, *** $p < 0.001$, **** $p < 0.0001$.

Only two organs differed in size between genotype groups, and significant differences were evident only at 12 months of age. Liver weights increased significantly from 3 to 12 months of age in both *Wt* and *Taz*-HET mice (Figure 1F). However, at 12 months of age, *Taz*-HET liver weights were ~11% lower than *Wt* liver weights.

Brain masses did not change significantly from 3 to 12 months of age in either the *Wt* or *Taz*-HET mouse groups. At both 3 and 12 months of age, brain masses were ~4% lower in *Taz*-HET mice compared with age-matched *Wt* mice, but this was only statistically significantly different at 12 months of age (Figure 1I), possibly due to the greater power associated with the larger sample size examined at this timepoint.

3.2. Adipose Tissue Masses

From 3 to 12 months of age, both *Wt* and *Taz*-HET mouse white adipose tissue (WAT) visceral (i.e., gonadal, perirenal, and retroperitoneal) and subcutaneous (i.e., inguinal) depots increased significantly in mass (Figure 2). At 3 months, there were no significant differences between *Wt* and *Taz*-HET mice in the mass of any individual WAT depot (Figure 2A–D). At 12 months, however, gonadal (Figure 2A) and retroperitoneal (Figure 2D) WAT depots were, respectively, 29% and 31% lower in mass in *Taz*-HET compared with *Wt* mice (Figure 2A,D).

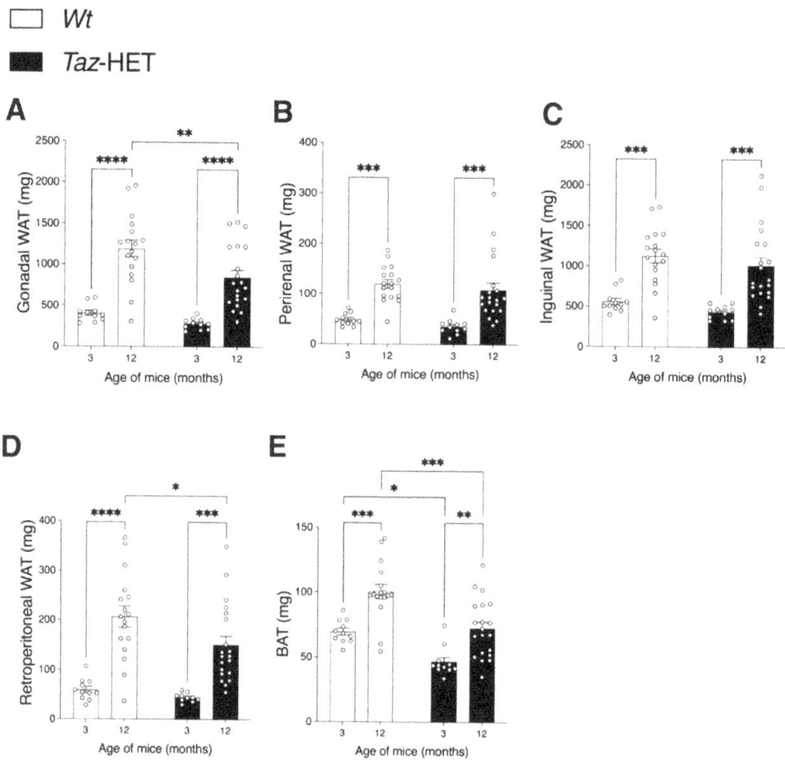

Figure 2. White (WAT) and brown adipose tissue (BAT) masses obtained by dissection from female *Wt* and *Taz*-HET mice at 3 and 12 months of age. WAT depots (**A–D**) and BAT depots (**E**) are shown according to genotype and age. Data are means ± SEM, with individual datapoints shown as circles, $n = 11$ per group at 3 months of age and $n = 17–20$ per genotype at 12 months of age. Differences were analyzed by 2-way ANOVA, and comparisons between genotypes for age-matched mice and between ages for mice within genotype groups are shown: * $p < 0.05$, ** $p < 0.01$, *** $p < 0.001$, **** $p < 0.0001$.

Interscapular brown adipose tissue (BAT) depots increased in mass from 3 to 12 months of age in both *Wt* and *Taz*-HET mice (Figure 2E). *Taz*-HET mice had 33% smaller BAT masses at 3 months and 28% smaller BAT masses at 12 months compared with their age-matched *Wt* littermates.

3.3. Food Intake

Using the CLAMS, a series of measures were performed. Mouse food intake was averaged over a 24 h period (Figure 3A) and also normalized to body weight (Figure 3B). At three months of age, absolute and weight-normalized food intake did not differ between genotypes. Total and weight-normalized food intakes decreased in *Wt* mice from 3 to

12 months. During this same period, total food intakes did not decrease significantly in *Taz*-HET mice, although there was a significant decline in weight-normalized measures. Food intake measured per gram of body weight at 12 months of age was higher in *Taz*-HET mice compared with their *Wt* littermates.

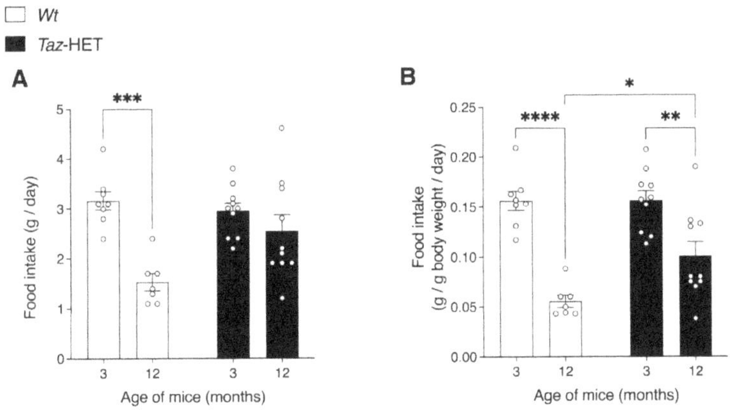

Figure 3. Total and weight-normalized daily food intakes of cohorts of 3- and 12-month-old mice. Twenty-four h absolute food intake (**A**) and food intake normalized to body weight (**B**) are shown. Data are means ± SEM, with individual datapoints shown (circles), $n = 7$–8 (*Wt*), $n = 10$ (*Taz*-HET), * $p < 0.05$, ** $p < 0.01$, *** $p < 0.001$, **** $p < 0.0001$.

3.4. Movement

Mice at 3 and 12 months of age were monitored in the CLAMS apparatus, with motion recorded over a 24 h period. Motion was detected through the monitoring of infrared beam breaks. The locomotion axis records breaks of the X-plane, which include all beam breaks due to combined repetitive activity such as feeding or grooming, in addition to activity from walking, and is termed locomotor activity. The Y-plane runs the length of the enclosure and records instances when a mouse breaks two different beams, indicating a traverse of the cage, which is termed ambulatory activity. Monitoring of the rearing axis only accounts for the infrared beam breaks in the Z-plane, such as when mice rear up on their hind legs (Figure 4).

Locomotor activity is shown in Figure 4 (upper panel), where line graphs show total beam breaks across the X-plane of the cage during each 28 min interval for 3-month-old (top, left) and 12-month-old (top, right) *Taz*-HET mice and their *Wt* littermates. Analysis of the average daily locomotor activity per 28 min interval indicated no significant differences between groups across ages and genotypes (bottom, left). *Wt* mice experienced an age-related significant decline in locomotor activity during the light phase, when mice are typically less active (bottom, middle), but otherwise there were no significant differences in average 28 min interval beam breaks across the X-plane in either the light or dark (bottom, right) cycles.

Line graphs of ambulatory activity (Figure 4, middle panel, top) indicate total values during 28 min intervals for beam breaks across the Y-plane of the cage recorded over a 24 h period, including both the light and dark cycles. Averages for these 28 min intervals are shown in this panel for the full 24 h period (bottom, left), the 12 h light phase (bottom, middle), and the 12 h dark phase (bottom, right). Similar to results seen for locomotor activity, ambulatory activity decreased significantly from 3 to 12 months of age in *Wt* mice during the light phase, specifically, but there were no significant differences between genotypes in age-matched mice and no other age-related differences within genotype groups.

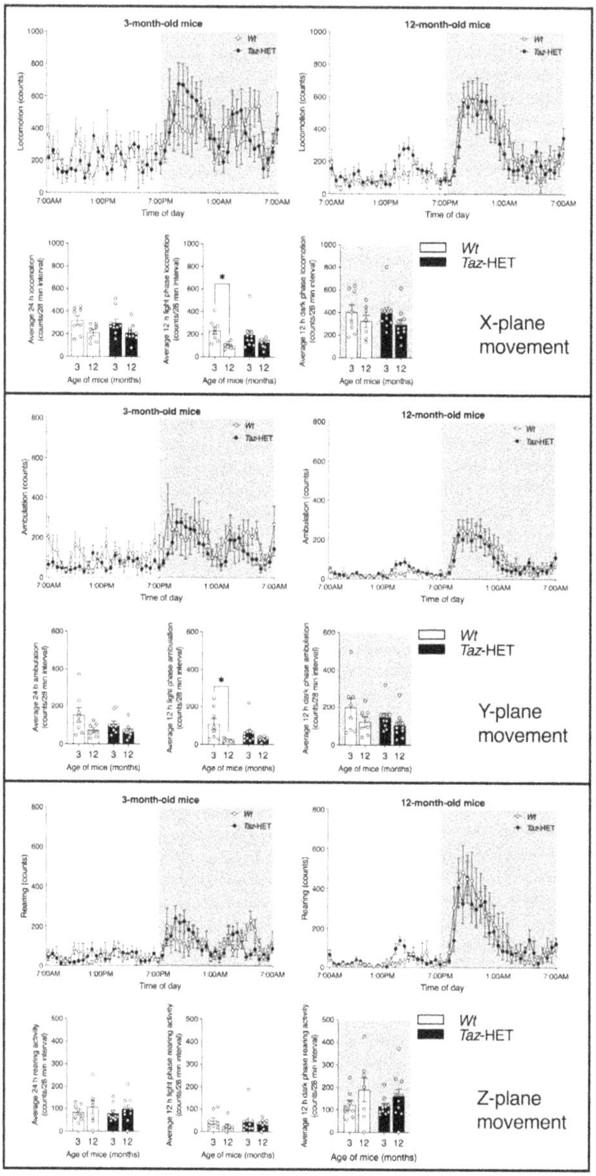

Figure 4. Movement of 3- and 12-month-old cohorts of mice over a period of 24 h housed in metabolic chambers equipped with infrared beams. Corresponding bar graphs of the daily and photoperiod average number of beam breaks per 28-min interval are shown. The movements of mice in the X (locomotor) plane (upper panel), Y (ambulatory) plane (middle panel), and Z (rearing) plane (lower panel) are shown. Shading indicates the duration of the dark cycle. Data are means ± SEM, with individual datapoints shown (circles), n = 7–10, * $p < 0.05$.

Rearing activity, denoted by activity in the Z-plane, was recorded during a 24 h period, and the total number of rearing events per 28 min interval is plotted according to genotype and age of mice (Figure 4, lower panel, top). Daily averages of these values (bottom, left) and averages during the light (bottom, middle) and dark (bottom, right) phases indicated no significant effects of age or genotype.

3.5. *Respiratory Exchange Ratio and Total Energy Expenditure*

Respiratory exchange ratios (RER) and total energy expenditures (TEE) were analyzed for 3- and 12-month-old *Wt* and *Taz*-HET mice and recorded every 28 min (Figure 5, top and bottom panels).

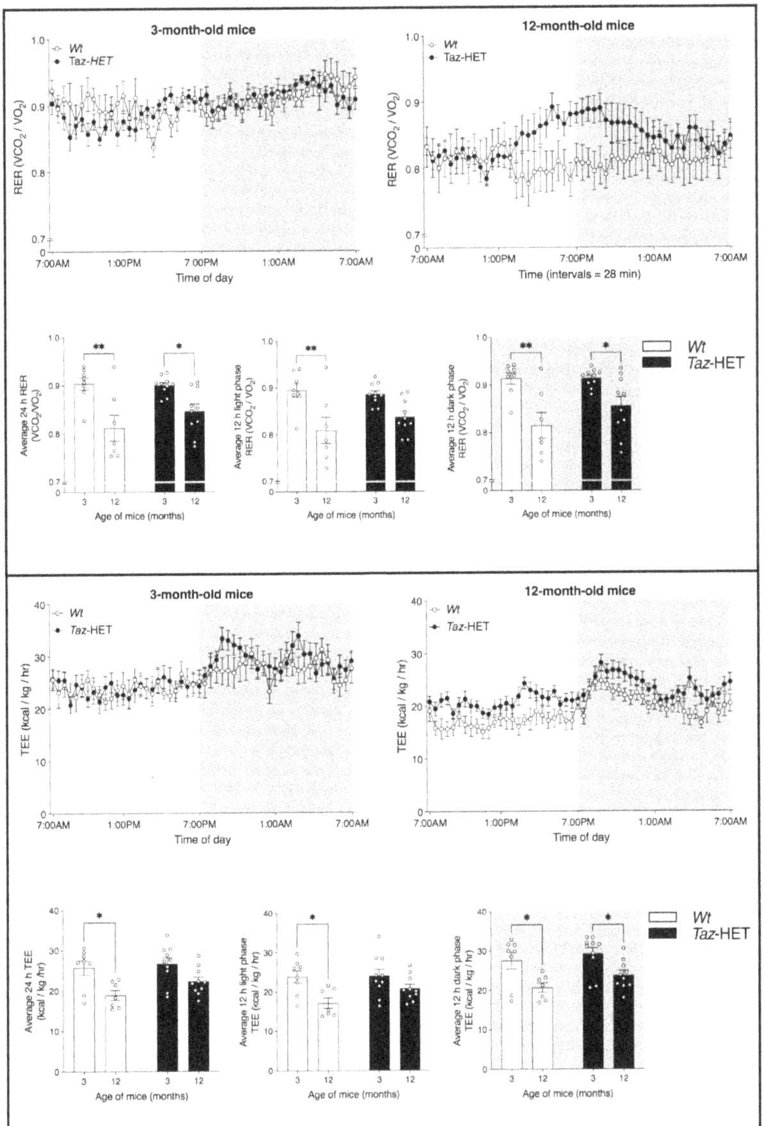

Figure 5. Respiratory exchange ratio (RER) and total energy expenditure (TEE). Cohorts of mice were monitored at 3 and 12 months of age for 24 h in the CLAMS apparatus, with measures taken every 28 min. Corresponding bar graphs of the daily and photoperiod average RER and TEE are shown. Data are means ± SEM, with individual datapoints shown (circles), n = 7–10, * $p < 0.05$, ** $p < 0.01$.

Line graphs show comparisons of RER measures taken every 28 min from *Wt* and *Taz*-HET mice at 3 months (Figure 5, upper panel, top right) and 12 months (top left) of age. Both *Wt* and *Taz*-HET mice underwent an age-related decrease in 24 h and dark phase RER (Figure 5, top panel, lower left and right). During the light phase, RER declined significantly from 3 to 12 months of age for *Wt* but not *Taz*-HET mice (Figure 5, top panel, middle). No significant differences were observed between age-matched *Wt* and *Taz*-HET mice in RER.

TEE measures are shown in Figure 5 (lower panel), with line graphs illustrating measures at 28 min intervals in 3-month-old (top, left) and 12-month-old (top, right) mice. Average TEE decreased significantly from 3 to 12 months of age in *Wt* mice during both the light and dark phases and also over the 24 h period measured overall (Figure 5, lower panel, bottom left, middle, and right). *Taz*-HET mice, however, only exhibited a statistically significant age-related decrease in TEE during the dark phase (bottom, right). Age-matched mice did not differ significantly in TEE measures by genotype.

3.6. *VO_2 and VCO_2*

Oxygen consumption rates (VO_2) were analyzed in 3- and 12-month-old *Wt* and *Taz*-HET mice. Line graphs depicting average VO_2 measures taken over 28 min intervals are shown (Figure 6, upper panel, top left and right). *Wt* mice exhibited a significant decrease in oxygen consumption with aging (upper panel, bottom left, middle, and right). Notably, this decrease in VO_2 was evident when averages over the entire 24 h period were considered, as well as when averages were compared during the less active light period and the more active dark period. In *Taz*-HET mice, however, oxygen consumption rates did not decline significantly from 3 to 12 months of age, suggesting greater resistance to age-related metabolic changes. In age-matched mice, however, there were no significant differences between *Wt* and *Taz*-HET littermates in measures of VO_2.

Carbon dioxide production rates (VCO_2) were also analyzed over a 24 h period in 3- and 12-month-old littermates. VCO_2 rates were graphed at 28 min intervals for 3-month-old (Figure 6, lower panel, top right) and 12-month-old (Figure 6, lower panel, top left) *Wt* and *Taz*-HET mice. Calculation and analysis of average rates of carbon dioxide production indicated significant age-related decreases in both *Wt* and *Taz*-HET mice from 3 to 12 months of age overall (Figure 6, lower panel, bottom left) and specifically during the 12 h dark period (bottom right). During the light period, an age-related decrease in VCO_2 was evident in *Wt* mice but not in *Taz*-HET mice (bottom middle). As with measures of VO_2, there were no significant differences between age-matched mice of different genotypes in VCO_2 overall or during either the light or dark periods.

3.7. *Glucose Tolerance and Insulin Sensitivity*

Genotype-specific differences in body weights and WAT masses were observed in older but not younger mice (Figures 1 and 2), although both genotypes undergo a decline in respiratory exchange ratio with age, suggesting changes in the relative use of major fuel types. Thus, tests of glucose tolerance (GTT) and insulin sensitivity (ITT) were performed in 12-month-old mice to determine if older animals exhibit genotype-specific differences.

There were no significant differences in baseline glucose measures between *Wt* and *Taz*-HET mice (Figure 7A). Following injection of mice with glucose, both genotypes demonstrated a rise in blood glucose by 15 min, although mean levels did not differ significantly between genotypes at that timepoint. Blood glucose levels were, on average, 2.41 mM lower in *Taz*-HET mice compared with their *Wt* littermates at 30 min post-injection and 2.74 mM lower at 60 min. Total blood glucose excursions were quantified by calculation of total AUC (Figure 7B) and were 16% lower in 12-month-old *Taz*-HET mice compared with *Wt* mice, indicating significantly better glucose disposal following an injected glucose challenge.

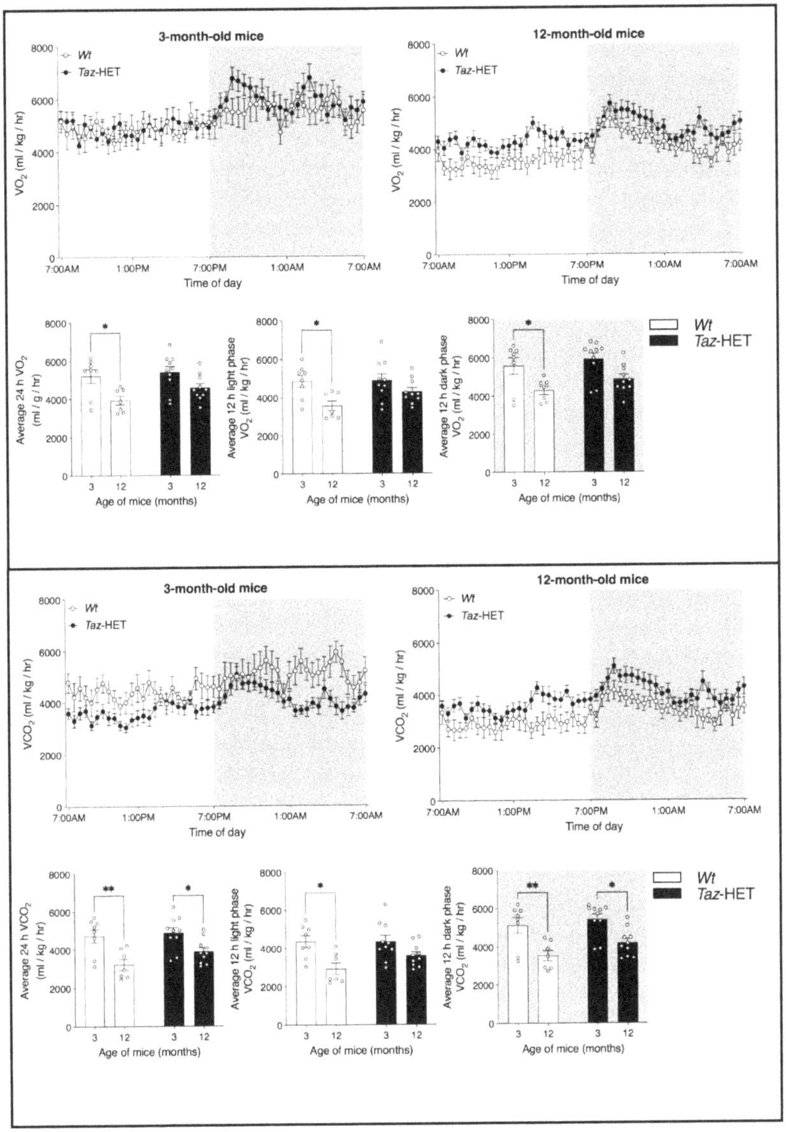

Figure 6. VO_2 and VCO_2 rates in 3- and 12-month-old cohorts of *Wt* and *Taz*-HET mice. Three- and twelve-month-old mice were monitored in the CLAMS apparatus, where measures of oxygen consumption rate and carbon dioxide production rate were calculated every 28 min. Corresponding bar graphs of the daily and photoperiod averages of VO_2 and VCO_2 are shown. Data are means ± SEM, with individual datapoints shown (circles), $n = 7$–10, * $p < 0.05$, ** $p < 0.01$.

Blood glucose concentrations at the start of the ITT protocol did not differ significantly between groups or at specific timepoints post-injection when analyzed by repeated measures ANOVA (Figure 7C). However, measures of total AUC indicated that blood glucose levels were suppressed to a greater overall extent in *Taz*-HET mice compared with their *Wt* littermates, indicating a greater response to insulin injection.

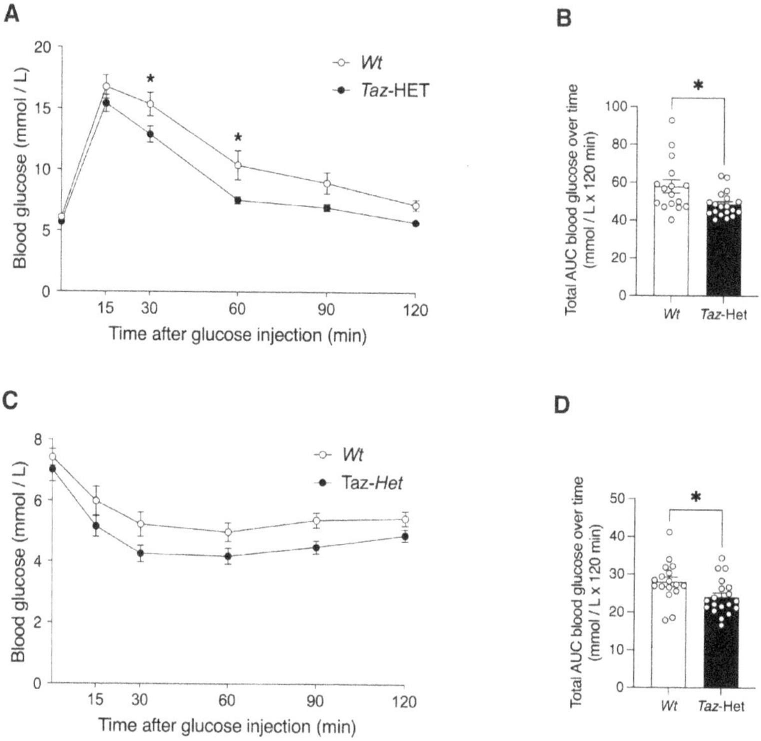

Figure 7. Blood glucose responses in 12-month-old female *Wt* and *Taz*-HET mice during GTT and ITT. Blood glucose responses immediately prior to *i.p.* injection with glucose and at 15, 30, 60, 90, and 120 min after injection were determined (**A**), and total glucose excursions were calculated by area-under-the-curve (AUC) analysis (**B**). Following *i.p.* insulin injection, blood glucose responses were monitored at the timepoints indicated (**C**), and total insulin-mediated glucose excursions were calculated by AUC analysis and mean AUC values during the experiment were compared (**D**). Data are means ± SEM, with individual datapoints shown (circles), n = 16–19, * $p < 0.05$, with differences indicated between mice of different genotypes at the same timepoint (**A**,**C**) or as indicated on the graph (**B**,**D**).

3.8. Exercise Endurance Capacity

The exercise capacity of mice was determined using an exhaustive treadmill running protocol after 3 days of training. Three measures of exercise performance were determined. The time to exhaustion declined significantly in both *Wt* and *Taz*-HET mice from 3 to 12 months of age (Figure 8A). However, there was no significant difference in time to exhaustion between the genotypes when mice were compared at the same ages. Furthermore, regardless of genotype, mice at 3 months of age were able to run over 1/3 longer than mice at 12 months of age.

Similar effects were observed for distance to exhaustion (Figure 8B). Twelve-month-old mice of either genotype achieved a total distance during the trial that was ~40–50% less than that of younger mice, regardless of genotype. In age-matched mice, there were no significant differences between distances achieved at exhaustion.

While measures of distance and time to exhaustion are continuous variables and therefore tend to have greater variation in outcomes, the maximal speed achieved is a discrete variable since it is increased in stepwise increments. When maximal speeds were analyzed, a difference between genotypes was observed. Mice at 12 months of age were able to achieve a significantly lower maximal speed than mice at 3 months of age, regardless of genotype, indicating an age-related decline in performance in both groups, which was similar to that observed for both time to exhaustion and distance to exhaustion measures. However, a small but significant difference between *Wt* and *Taz*-HET mice was observed specifically at 12 months of age. Since the treadmill speed was increased in 3 cm/s increments, the maximum speed achieved by *Wt* mice was, on average, 49 cm/s, while the maximum speed achieved by *Taz*-HET mice was, on average, 46 cm/s, indicating that the performance of *Taz*-HET females peaked at a level lower than that of the *Wt* females.

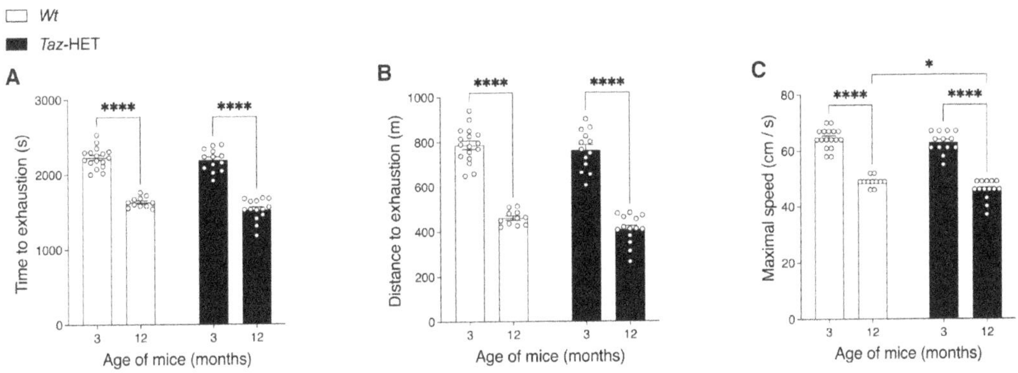

Figure 8. Treadmill exercise capacity testing. Three- and twelve-month-old cohorts of *Wt* and *Taz*-HET mice were trained for 3 days and then tested after one day of rest for maximal exercise capacity, measuring time to exhaustion (**A**), distance to exhaustion (**B**), and maximal speed achieved (**C**). Data are means ± SEM, with individual datapoints shown (circles), n = 11–17, * $p < 0.05$, **** $p < 0.0001$.

3.9. *Tafazzin Gene Expression and Cardiolipin Analysis*

Altered exercise performance in middle-aged *Taz*-HET females prompted us to investigate tafazzin expression and cardiolipin content in the hearts of mice at this timepoint. Tafazzin mRNA levels were ~36% lower in the hearts of *Taz*-HET females compared with *Wt* females (Figure 9A). Despite a lack of statistically significant differences in total cardiolipin content between *Taz*-HET and *Wt* females (Figure 9B), the total n-6 polyunsaturated fatty acid (PUFA) content was significantly lower in the 12-month-old *Taz*-HET females compared with age-matched *Wt* females (Figure 9C). Analysis of the abundance of specific fatty acyl species of cardiolipin revealed no differences in saturated fatty acids (SFA), monounsaturated fatty acids (MUFAs), and n-3 PUFAs (Figure 9C–E,G), although the n-6 PUFAs 18:2n-6 (linoleic acid) and 20:3n-6 (dihomo-γ-linolenic acid) were significantly lower by ~14% and ~18%, respectively, in the *Taz*-HET females (Figure 9F). Analysis of the relative abundance of fatty acyls in cardiac cardiolipin showed similar species-specific differences to those observed in absolute abundance comparisons and additionally showed a significant increase in MUFA content, particularly 18:1n-7 (vaccenic acid), in *Taz*-HET mice compared with *Wt* females (Supplementary Table S1).

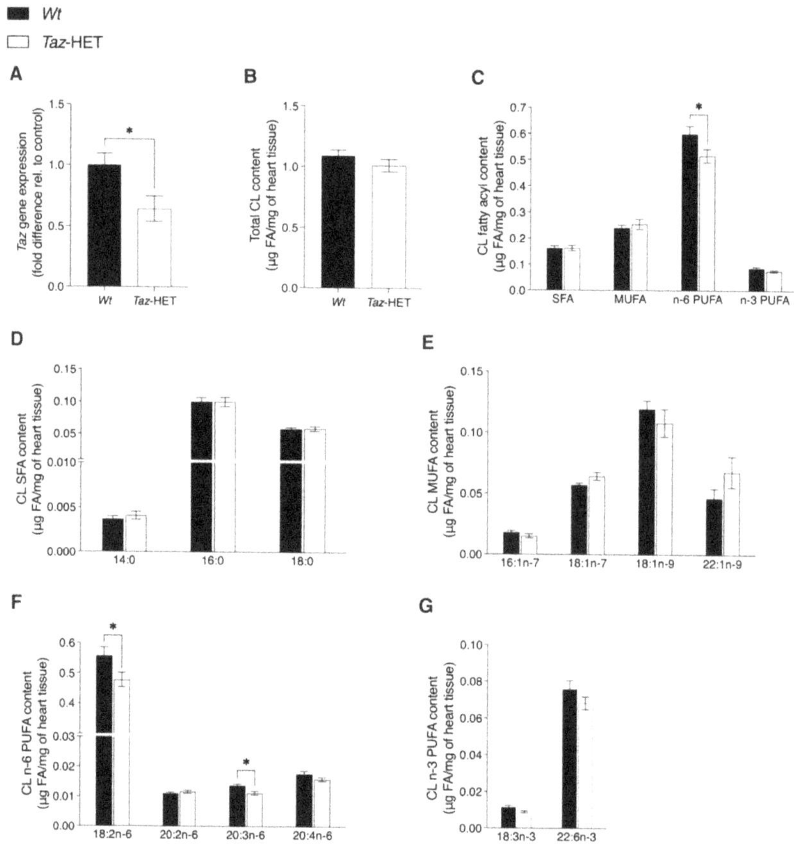

Figure 9. Tafazzin (*Taz*) gene expression and cardiolipin analysis in the cardiac tissue of 12-month-old mice. Tafazzin gene expression, normalized to β-actin, in the hearts of *Taz*-HET and control female mice (**A**). Total cardiolipin content (**B**), absolute content of major fatty acyl (FA) classes (i.e., saturates (SFA), monounsaturates (MUFA), n-6 polyunsaturated fatty acids (n-6 PUFAs), and n-3 PUFAs within cardiolipin (**C**), and cardiolipin absolute contents of specific FA species among SFA (**D**), MUFA (**E**), n-6 PUFA (**F**), and n-3 PUFA (**G**). Data are means ± SEM, n = 9–12, * $p < 0.05$.

4. Discussion

The molecular pathogenesis of BTHS involves cellular deficiencies in both L4-cardiolipin and total cardiolipin, together with an accumulation of monolysocardiolipin [14]. Female carriers are typically thought to be asymptomatic [14] and reportedly lack these hallmark biochemical abnormalities in tests of platelets and lymphocytes [27,28]. Additionally, carriers are also reported to lack perturbations in blood plasma measures of 3-methylglutaconic acid, cholesterol and cholesterol precursors, amino acids, and lactic acid that can occur in those with manifest disease [29–31]. Although a comprehensive clinical examination of carriers has not been performed, case reports also largely indicate an absence of female cardiac disease in the family history [32–34]. Moreover, assessment of cardiac function in mothers of BTHS patients typically reveals normal results through echocardiography [30,33,35,36] or electrocardiography [33].

We have recently published work reporting the characterization of male mice deficient in tafazzin (*Taz*-KO) [20]. In the present study, we assessed the characteristics of female mice that were heterozygous for a targeted disruption of the tafazzin gene. Whereas the male *Taz*-KO mice exhibited significant and sizeable reductions in body weights, major organ weights, adipose depot weights, and exercise capacity compared with male littermate control mice, the corresponding differences between *Taz*-HET female mice and their *Wt* female littermates were smaller. These results are largely consistent with the view that BTHS carriers are non-manifesting [14], since at both age points there were more similarities than differences between the two genotypes of female mice. Overall, changes that manifested with age in the *Taz*-HET females were subtle and unlikely to reach a threshold constituting clinically relevant pathology. Regardless, some differences were observed and are relevant for understanding the biological role of tafazzin in carriers.

Taz-HET mice were mostly indistinguishable from control littermates, as was expected based on reports from female carriers [14]. In instances where *Taz*-HET mice differed from their *Wt* counterparts, their phenotype recapitulated that of the *Taz*-KO males, but to a milder degree. Notable genotype-specific differences included lower body weights of 12-month-old *Taz*-HET mice compared with control females, in part due to lower weights of organs such as the brain and liver but more so due to smaller masses of select regional adipose depots. While the *Wt* mice had significantly reduced food intake with advancing age, this age-related change was lacking in the *Taz*-HET mice, despite their lower body weights. Systemic energy expenditure and basal substrate metabolism were comparable between the two groups at both age points and thus underwent similar age-related changes, while there were no notable differences in the movement or activity of the mice between genotypes at either age. Taken together, these data suggest some decreased efficiency of fuel use by female *Taz*-HET mice that may either manifest at an advanced age or compound as an accrued deficit over time.

Neither genotype was overtly glucose intolerant or insulin resistant at 12-months of age, since mean blood glucose measures in both groups returned to baseline 2 h following glucose injection and both groups exhibited significant declines in blood glucose levels following insulin injection [37]. Differences between genotypes, however, were evident. Aged *Taz*-HET females exhibited an enhanced ability to maintain glucose homeostasis in the face of a glucose challenge, with a lower overall response during GTT. *Taz*-HET mice also exhibited a better response to insulin over the course of the ITT. In theory, these metabolic changes could offer health benefits with aging and may contribute to a lower risk of diabetes and obesity development [38], although this has not been studied yet in humans.

In the treadmill exercise capacity test, the maximum speed achieved, total running distance, and running time before exhaustion were the same between the *Taz*-HET and *Wt* mice at 3-months of age. At 12-months of age, however, a phenotypic difference in their performance became discernible, as the maximum speed achieved before exhaustion was slightly but significantly lower in the *Taz*-HET females. This finding of a difference is particularly interesting given that mitochondrial insufficiency and exercise intolerance are hallmarks of BTHS. To the best of our knowledge, this is the first study to identify a difference, albeit minor, in exercise capacity associated with heterozygous loss of tafazzin in female carriers. The largely protected phenotype of *Taz*-HET females could potentially be attributed to a relatively high degree of haplosufficiency of tafazzin or to a skewed X chromosome inactivation (XCI).

Females have two X chromosomes, and, normally, one of the two is randomly chosen to be rendered transcriptionally inactive in each cell of the early embryo [39]. Throughout the cascading cell division that drives embryonic development, the inactivation of a specific X chromosome is permanent for all descendants of a cell [39]. Random XCI creates epigenetic cellular mosaicism in the tissues of females, which are composed of two populations of cells, with either the maternal or paternal chromosome as the active X [39]. In the framework of random XCI, one-half of the cells in a given tissue of *Taz*-HET mice should have the X chromosome with the mutant tafazzin gene active, and thus those cells should be deficient in the tafazzin protein.

Although we did not directly analyze XCI patterns in the current study, we found that twelve-month-old *Taz*-HET females showed an ~1/3 reduction in cardiac tafazzin expression, suggesting that the X chromosome possessing the recombined knock-out tafazzin locus, missing exons 5–10, is likely active in a subset of cardiomyocytes of the mice. Since tafazzin has a well-established role in incorporating, specifically, linoleic acid chains into cardiolipin in mammalian hearts [40], thereby completing the transformation of nascent cardiolipin into its mature form specific to this tissue, it is noteworthy that the subtle decrease in tafazzin expression that we observed was associated with a correspondingly minor but significant and specific decline in cardiolipin linoleic acid content in the hearts of *Taz*-HET mice. Indeed, in BTHS patients [40], male tafazzin knock-down mice [5,41], and cardiomyocyte-specific tafazzin knockout mice [42], notable and specific reductions in the linoleic acid content of cardiac cardiolipin are observed. This decline is hypothesized to be causative of the hallmark exercise intolerance of BTHS [43,44], due to the associated decreases in concentration of the proteins of oxidative phosphorylation at the mitochondrial inner membrane that are enriched in L4-cardiolipin [45]. In the current work, the decrease in tafazzin expression, alterations in cardiolipin composition, and resulting exercise deficits are collectively minor in the *Taz*-HET female mice. This aligns with the notion that the *Taz*-HET model shares similarities with reports from human female carriers, where skewed XCI has been reported [32], but future studies should investigate this directly.

Studies of XCI status in human BTHS carriers suggest that skewed XCI is responsible for their asymptomatic status [32]. Ørstavik et al. analyzed the XCI status of peripheral blood cells from 16 obligate carriers of BTHS, none with known cardiac disease, and 148 female controls [32]. The majority of carriers possessed an almost completely skewed XCI pattern (>=95:5), since six of the sixteen carriers (i.e., 38%) expressed the X chromosome with the normal tafazzin gene in 95% or more of their blood cells, with 5% or less of their blood cells using the mutated X chromosome as the active X. This degree of imbalance in parental X chromosome activation was absent in the 148 controls. Extremely skewed XCI status was found in carriers at both early life and senior ages and was confirmed in skin fibroblasts and granulocytes collected from two of the carriers. Interestingly, random XCI inactivation (defined as ratios between 50:50 and 65:35) was observed in 19% of carriers (three out of sixteen) and was significantly lower than the 55% incidence observed in the control group. Notably, carriers with an extremely skewed status and with a random status were found in the same families. The remainder of carriers studied displayed moderately skewed (defined as 65:35 to 80:20) or skewed (defined as 80:20 to 95:5) XCI, and, thus, 81% of BTHS carriers possessed discernible levels of skewed XCI, favoring the expression of the normal tafazzin gene [32].

Levels of skewness can be clinically relevant in some disorders [46,47] and have been associated with the development of overt pathology in BTHS since predominant expression of the mutant X chromosome has been found in the two known cases of females with manifestations of clinical disease. The first case of BTHS in a female was reported in 2012 [35]. The infant presented with severe heart failure at 1 month of age, and her clinical course was characterized by recurrent episodes of severe acute heart failure, progressive skeletal myopathy, and cyclic neutropenia until she succumbed to a fatal septic shock at 3 years of age. Cytogenetic analysis performed on lymphocytes and skin fibroblasts determined that the girl had inherited a mutated maternal X chromosome with a large intragenic deletion for exons 1–5 of the tafazzin gene that would preclude the synthesis of a functional enzyme. Her paternal X chromosome was either structurally abnormal, in a ring conformation and missing the whole Xq28 region, or completely absent in cells. In effect, the female patient, like affected males with BTHS, was deficient in functional tafazzin and hence presented with clinical disease [35].

The second female BTHS patient, reported in 2016, was mildly affected by hypertrophic left-ventricular noncompaction and hypotonia [48]. She received a diagnosis of BTHS only after her younger male sibling presented with the classical phenotype. Genetic investigation of her peripheral blood cells revealed that the manifesting carrier daughter and her asymptomatic carrier mother had similar degrees of XCI skewness, but in opposite directions, where the daughter had the X chromosome with the mutant tafazzin gene as the transcriptionally active one in 97% of her cells, while her mother exhibited predominant activation of the normal X chromosome in 93% of her cells. Notably, the daughter had a random XCI pattern in epithelial cells collected from a buccal swab and urine specimens. The daughter had a normal karyotype, and it is unknown why the mutant X chromosome was preferentially activated in her blood cells and presumably other mesoderm-derived tissues [48]. Although further study is warranted, this demonstrates support for the notion that XCI patterns are a determinant of clinical phenotype in carriers with BTHS, where most but not all carriers exhibit skewness towards inactivation of the mutant X chromosome in a majority of their cells [32].

Although XCI was not analyzed in the present study, the relatively small differences observed suggest that *Taz*-HET mice undergo similar patterns to humans of skewed XCI, with a majority of mutant X chromosomes inactivated. Our findings of heterogeneity in performance responses and outcomes within genotype-age categories also suggest that, as with human carriers, female *Taz*-HET mice may experience variation in the degree of mutant XCI between individuals. As many as 19% of BTHS carriers possess random XCI [32], but whether this plays a causal role in clinical symptoms is yet unknown. Case reports occasionally produce results showing a carrier displaying mild cardiac symptoms, although these reports lack accompanying XCI analysis. For example, a woman who was the carrier of a de novo tafazzin mutation and the mother of a BTHS patient had mild trabeculations of the left ventricle as revealed by echocardiography, but her total cardiac function and electrocardiogram were normal [49]. In a different case, examination of the pedigree of a boy with BTHS possessing a newly documented tafazzin mutation revealed a female relative that was diagnosed with Wolff-Parkinson-White syndrome and affected by dilated cardiomyopathy [50]. This woman lost her son to dilated cardiomyopathy, and the presence of a tafazzin mutation and BTHS diagnosis was suspected but never confirmed due to a lack of sample acquisition prior to death. Nonetheless, genetic sequencing confirmed the woman as a carrier of the novel tafazzin mutation. Additionally, neutropenia in a carrier has also been observed [30], although this is the single exception to the majority of carriers that do not present with neutropenia [30,51].

It is possible that subtle, subclinical differences may exist between unaffected carriers and controls at the molecular level, even when there is apparent haplosufficiency. A study by Kuijpers et al. on annexin-V-based apoptosis in neutrophils from BTHS patients, carriers, and controls uncovered differences between the three subject groups [51]. Neutrophils from BTHS patients demonstrated avid binding to annexin-V. Although the neutrophils from carriers displayed a wide range in binding levels, they fell into an intermediate range between BTHS patients and healthy controls. None of the carriers had neutropenia, although the biological significance of the increased annexin-V binding is unknown, especially since Kuijpers et al. noted an absence of apoptosis in BTHS neutrophils despite their binding to annexin-V. Likewise, the underlying cause for increased annexin-V binding remains unclear, although cardiolipin-independent modifications to the cellular membranes have been suggested [51]. Future work should incorporate XCI analysis in order to examine the relative association between clinical symptoms of carrier women and the degree of tafazzin insufficiency.

We studied the *Taz*-HET mouse model at two different age points, focusing on cohorts corresponding to young (3-month-old) and middle-aged (12-month-old) timepoints [52], since age-related manifestations of subclinical and clinical features have been reported in carriers of other X-linked disorders, such as Duchenne muscular dystrophy [53–55], glucose-6-phosphate dehydrogenase deficiency [56,57], and X-linked adrenoleukodystrophy [17,58]. The importance of studying X-linked disorders across the lifespan is highlighted by the experience of discovery in X-linked adrenoleukodystrophy, where carriers were originally considered to be asymptomatic [59,60], leading to misdiagnoses with multiple sclerosis, hereditary spastic paraparesis, or fibromyalgia [61–65]. Although reports of manifesting carriers began to accumulate over decades [58,61,66–69], it was not until the first systematic study in 2014 on disease manifestations in carriers that it was established that more than

80% of women experience symptoms at ages 60 years or older [17]. Notably, this provided a sharp increase from the 18% of symptomatic women aged 40 years or younger [17].

Interestingly, in X-ALD, the significance of the XCI pattern for the symptomatic status remains uncertain, despite studies [17,70–72]. The effects of age on clinical outcomes have not been formally investigated in BTHS carriers, although extreme XCI skewness away from expression of the mutant tafazzin allele predominates in both children and seniors [32]. Our findings suggest that the *Taz*-HET mouse model can be used to further explore expected interactions between age, XCI status, and symptom penetrance and severity in human female carriers.

5. Conclusions

Here, we have identified the development of subtle phenotypic differences between 12-month-old *Taz*-HET and *Wt* mice, which were nearly indistinguishable at 3 months of age. At 1 year of age, *Taz*-HET females have lower total body weights and enhanced glucose control compared with their *Wt* littermates. However, mild impairments in exercise capacity are also observed in the *Taz*-HET females at this age point, which are likely precipitated, in part, by lower tafazzin expression and linoleic acid content of cardiolipin in the hearts. While the subtle differences between the genotypes in this study corroborate the many reports of asymptomatic carriers of BTHS [27,29–36] and suggest that for the majority of BTHS carriers, abnormalities are likely to remain in a subclinical state, our findings of emergent differences at 12 months indicate that future work should examine later ages in both animals and humans. In particular, phenotypic differences may become more pronounced in model mice with advancing age, particularly at the threshold when aging progresses to senescence, which is typically observed around the 18-month milestone [52,73], and future studies should examine this directly.

Supplementary Materials: The following supporting information can be downloaded at: https://www.mdpi.com/article/10.3390/biology12091238/s1, Table S1: Relative mass percentage of fatty acid species and major fatty acid classes within cardiolipin in the hearts of 12-month-old Taz-HET mice and Wt female littermates.

Author Contributions: M.V.T. participated in conceptualization, investigation, methodology, formal analysis, writing—original draft, and writing—review and editing. J.Z.C. participated in investigation, methodology, formal analysis, and writing—review and editing. D.M.A.-M. participated in investigation, methodology, formal analysis, writing—review and editing. M.R.L. participated in investigation, methodology, formal analysis, writing—original draft, and writing—review and editing. A.D.C. participated in investigation, methodology, and writing—review and editing. K.D.S. participated in funding acquisition, supervision, formal analysis, methodology, and writing—review and editing. D.S. participated in methodology, resources, and writing—review and editing. R.E.D. participated in conceptualization, funding acquisition, supervision, formal analysis, methodology, and writing—original draft, and writing—review and editing. All authors have read and agreed to the published version of the manuscript.

Funding: This work was supported by Idea grants (2015 and 2019) from the Barth Syndrome Foundation, the Barth Syndrome Foundation of Canada, and the Barth Syndrome Foundation U.K., as well as the Canada Foundation for Innovation—Leader's Opportunity Fund and the Government of Ontario—Ontario Research Fund (Project No. 30259), the Government of Ontario Early Researcher Award (ERA)—Ministry of Research, Innovation and Science (ER16-12-162), and the Natural Sciences and Engineering Research Council of Canada (NSERC) #RGPIN-2019-05642, #RGPIN-2012-418213, and RGPAS-2019-00008 to R.E.D. J.Z.C was supported by a doctoral scholarship from NSERC (PGS-D). The generation of the Taz-KO mouse strain was supported by Cancer Research UK. Gas chromatography studies were supported by an NSERC Discovery grant #RGPIN-2018-04334 and an NSERC Research Tools and Instruments grant #RTI-2022-00006 to K.D.S. The funding agencies had no role in the study design, the collection, analysis, or interpretation of data, the writing of the report, or the decision to submit the article for publication.

Institutional Review Board Statement: All animal procedures were performed with the approval of the University of Waterloo Animal Care Committee (AUPP#30055 (17-19), approved 25 July 2017; AUPP# 41822, approved 27 August 2020; AUPP#43431, approved 9 July 2021) and comply with the guidelines of the Canadian Council on Animal Care. The generation and maintenance of the TazKO mice are covered by a UK Home Office Licence (PP9886217).

Informed Consent Statement: Not applicable.

Data Availability Statement: Data are available upon reasonable request to the authors.

Acknowledgments: The authors thank Jean Flanagan and Angela Wagler for expert assistance with mouse maintenance and care.

Conflicts of Interest: The authors declare no conflict of interest. The funders had no role in the design of the study; in the collection, analyses, or interpretation of data; in the writing of the manuscript; or in the decision to publish the results.

References

1. Pennington, E.R.; Funai, K.; Brown, D.A.; Shaikh, S.R. The role of cardiolipin concentration and acyl chain composition on mitochondrial inner membrane molecular organization and function. *Biochim. Biophys. Acta Mol. Cell Biol. Lipids* **2019**, *1864*, 1039–1052. [CrossRef] [PubMed]
2. Bradley, R.M.; Stark, K.D.; Duncan, R.E. Influence of tissue, diet, and enzymatic remodeling on cardiolipin fatty acyl profile. *Mol. Nutr. Food Res.* **2016**, *60*, 1804–1818. [CrossRef]
3. Han, X.; Yang, K.; Yang, J.; Cheng, H.; Gross, R.W. Shotgun lipidomics of cardiolipin molecular species in lipid extracts of biological samples. *J. Lipid Res.* **2006**, *47*, 864–879. [CrossRef] [PubMed]
4. Schlame, M.; Towbin, J.A.; Heerdt, P.M.; Jehle, R.; DiMauro, S.; Blanck, T.J. Deficiency of tetralinoleoyl-cardiolipin in Barth syndrome. *Ann. Neurol.* **2002**, *51*, 634–637. [CrossRef] [PubMed]
5. Acehan, D.; Vaz, F.; Houtkooper, R.H.; James, J.; Moore, V.; Tokunaga, C.; Kulik, W.; Wansapura, J.; Toth, M.J.; Strauss, A.; et al. Cardiac and skeletal muscle defects in a mouse model of human Barth syndrome. *J. Biol. Chem.* **2011**, *286*, 899–908. [CrossRef] [PubMed]
6. Kennedy, E.P.; Weiss, S.B. The function of cytidine coenzymes in the biosynthesis of phospholipides. *J. Biol. Chem.* **1956**, *222*, 193–214. [CrossRef]
7. Bione, S.; D'Adamo, P.; Maestrini, E.; Gedeon, A.K.; Bolhuis, P.A.; Toniolo, D. A novel X-linked gene, G4.5. is responsible for Barth syndrome. *Nat. Genet.* **1996**, *12*, 385–389. [CrossRef]
8. Bradley, R.M.; Hashemi, A.; Aristizabal-Henao, J.J.; Stark, K.D.; Duncan, R.E. PLAAT1 Exhibits Phosphatidylcholine: Monolysocardiolipin Transacylase Activity. *Int. J. Mol. Sci.* **2022**, *23*, 6714. [CrossRef]
9. Ma, B.J.; Taylor, W.A.; Dolinsky, V.W.; Hatch, G.M. Acylation of monolysocardiolipin in rat heart. *J. Lipid Res.* **1999**, *40*, 1837–1845. [CrossRef]
10. Taylor, W.A.; Hatch, G.M. Identification of the human mitochondrial linoleoyl-coenzyme A monolysocardiolipin acyltransferase (MLCL AT-1). *J. Biol. Chem.* **2009**, *284*, 30360–30371. [CrossRef]
11. Taylor, W.A.; Mejia, E.M.; Mitchell, R.W.; Choy, P.C.; Sparagna, G.C.; Hatch, G.M. Human trifunctional protein alpha links cardiolipin remodeling to beta-oxidation. *PLoS ONE* **2012**, *7*, e48628. [CrossRef]
12. Cao, J.; Liu, Y.; Lockwood, J.; Burn, P.; Shi, Y. A novel cardiolipin-remodeling pathway revealed by a gene encoding an endoplasmic reticulum-associated acyl-CoA:lysocardiolipin acyltransferase (ALCAT1) in mouse. *J. Biol. Chem.* **2004**, *279*, 31727–31734. [CrossRef] [PubMed]
13. Zegallai, H.M.; Hatch, G.M. Barth syndrome: Cardiolipin, cellular pathophysiology, management, and novel therapeutic targets. *Mol. Cell. Biochem.* **2021**, *476*, 1605–1629. [CrossRef]
14. Clarke, S.L.; Bowron, A.; Gonzalez, I.L.; Groves, S.J.; Newbury-Ecob, R.; Clayton, N.; Martin, R.P.; Tsai-Goodman, B.; Garratt, V.; Ashworth, M.; et al. Barth syndrome. *Orphanet J. Rare Dis.* **2013**, *8*, 23. [CrossRef] [PubMed]
15. Rigaud, C.; Lebre, A.-S.; Touraine, R.; Beaupain, B.; Ottolenghi, C.; Chabli, A.; Ansquer, H.; Ozsahin, H.; Di Filippo, S.; De Lonlay, P.; et al. Natural history of Barth syndrome: A national cohort study of 22 patients. *Orphanet J. Rare Dis.* **2013**, *8*, 70. [CrossRef] [PubMed]
16. Huhta, J.C.; Pomerance, H.H.; Barness, E.G. Clinicopathologic conference: Barth Syndrome. *Fetal Pediatr. Pathol.* **2005**, *24*, 239–254. [CrossRef] [PubMed]
17. Engelen, M.; Barbier, M.; Dijkstra, I.M.; Schür, R.; de Bie, R.M.; Verhamme, C.; Dijkgraaf, M.G.; Aubourg, P.A.; Wanders, R.J.; van Geel, B.M.; et al. X-linked adrenoleukodystrophy in women: A cross-sectional cohort study. *Brain* **2014**, *137*, 693–706. [CrossRef]
18. Wang, S.; Li, Y.; Xu, Y.; Ma, Q.; Lin, Z.; Schlame, M.; Bezzerides, V.J.; Strathdee, D.; Pu, W.T. AAV Gene Therapy Prevents and Reverses Heart Failure in a Murine Knockout Model of Barth Syndrome. *Circ. Res.* **2020**, *126*, 1024–1039. [CrossRef]

19. Ren, M.; Xu, Y.; Erdjument-Bromage, H.; Donelian, A.; Phoon, C.K.L.; Terada, N.; Strathdee, D.; Neubert, T.A.; Schlame, M. Extramitochondrial cardiolipin suggests a novel function of mitochondria in spermatogenesis. *J. Cell Biol.* **2019**, *218*, 1491–1502. [CrossRef]
20. Tomczewski, M.V.; Chan, J.Z.; Campbell, Z.E.; Strathdee, D.; Duncan, R.E. Phenotypic Characterization of Male Tafazzin-Knockout Mice at 3, 6, and 12 Months of Age. *Biomedicines* **2023**, *11*, 638. [CrossRef]
21. Even, P.C.; Nadkarni, N.A. Indirect calorimetry in laboratory mice and rats: Principles, practical considerations, interpretation and perspectives. *Am. J. Physiol. Regul. Integr. Comp. Physiol.* **2012**, *303*, R459–R476. [CrossRef] [PubMed]
22. Lusk, G. ANIMAL CALORIMETRY Twenty-Fourth Paper. Analysis of the oxidation of mixtures of carbohydrate and fat. *J. Biol. Chem.* **1924**, *59*, 41–42. [CrossRef]
23. Virtue, S.; Vidal-Puig, A. GTTs and ITTs in mice: Simple tests, complex answers. *Nat. Metab.* **2021**, *3*, 883–886. [CrossRef] [PubMed]
24. Handschin, C.; Chin, S.; Li, P.; Liu, F.; Maratos-Flier, E.; LeBrasseur, N.K.; Yan, Z.; Spiegelman, B.M. Skeletal Muscle Fiber-type Switching, Exercise Intolerance, and Myopathy in PGC-1α Muscle-specific Knock-out Animals. *J. Biol. Chem.* **2007**, *282*, 30014–30021. [CrossRef] [PubMed]
25. Claghorn, G.C.; Fonseca, I.A.T.; Thompson, Z.; Barber, C.; Garland, T. Serotonin-mediated central fatigue underlies increased endurance capacity in mice from lines selectively bred for high voluntary wheel running. *Physiol. Behav.* **2016**, *161*, 145–154. [CrossRef]
26. Chan, J.Z.; Fernandes, M.F.; Steckel, K.E.; Bradley, R.M.; Hashemi, A.; Groh, M.R.; Sciaini, G.; Stark, K.D.; Duncan, R.E. N-oleoylethanolamide treatment of lymphoblasts deficient in Tafazzin improves cell growth and mitochondrial morphology and dynamics. *Sci. Rep.* **2022**, *12*, 9466. [CrossRef]
27. Schlame, M.; Kelley, R.I.; Feigenbaum, A.; Towbin, J.A.; Heerdt, P.M.; Schieble, T.; Wanders, R.J.; DiMauro, S.; Blanck, T.J. Phospholipid abnormalities in children with Barth syndrome. *J. Am. Coll. Cardiol.* **2003**, *42*, 1994–1999. [CrossRef]
28. Houtkooper, R.H.; Rodenburg, R.J.; Thiels, C.; van Lenthe, H.; Stet, F.; Poll-The, B.T.; Stone, J.E.; Steward, C.G.; Wanders, R.J.; Smeitink, J.; et al. Cardiolipin and monolysocardiolipin analysis in fibroblasts, lymphocytes, and tissues using high-performance liquid chromatography-mass spectrometry as a diagnostic test for Barth syndrome. *Anal. Biochem.* **2009**, *387*, 230–237. [CrossRef]
29. Vernon, H.J.; Sandlers, Y.; McClellan, R.; Kelley, R.I. Clinical laboratory studies in Barth Syndrome. *Mol. Genet. Metab.* **2014**, *112*, 143–147. [CrossRef]
30. Płatek, T.; Sordyl, M.; Polus, A.; Olszanecka, A.; Kroczka, S.; Solnica, B. Analysis of tafazzin and deoxyribonuclease 1 like 1 transcripts and X chromosome sequencing in the evaluation of the effect of mosaicism in the TAZ gene on phenotypes in a family affected by Barth syndrome. *Mutat. Res.* **2023**, *826*, 111812. [CrossRef]
31. Johnston, J.; Kelley, R.I.; Feigenbaum, A.; Cox, G.F.; Iyer, G.S.; Funanage, V.L.; Proujansky, R. Mutation characterization and genotype-phenotype correlation in Barth syndrome. *Am. J. Hum. Genet.* **1997**, *61*, 1053–1058. [CrossRef]
32. Orstavik, K.H.; Orstavik, R.E.; Naumova, A.K.; D'Adamo, P.; Gedeon, A.; Bolhuis, P.A.; Barth, P.G.; Toniolo, D. X chromosome inactivation in carriers of Barth syndrome. *Am. J. Hum. Genet.* **1998**, *63*, 1457–1463. [CrossRef] [PubMed]
33. Bakšienė, M.; Benušienė, E.; Morkūnienė, A.; Ambrozaitytė, L.; Utkus, A.; Kučinskas, V. A novel intronic splice site tafazzin gene mutation detected prenatally in a family with Barth syndrome. *Balkan. J. Med. Genet.* **2016**, *19*, 95–100. [CrossRef] [PubMed]
34. Barth, P.G.; Scholte, H.R.; Berden, J.A.; Van der Klei-Van Moorsel, J.M.; Luyt-Houwen, I.E.; Van't Veer-Korthof, E.T.; Van der Harten, J.J.; Sobotka-Plojhar, M.A. An X-linked mitochondrial disease affecting cardiac muscle, skeletal muscle and neutrophil leucocytes. *J. Neurol. Sci.* **1983**, *62*, 327–355. [CrossRef] [PubMed]
35. Cosson, L.; Toutain, A.; Simard, G.; Kulik, W.; Matyas, G.; Guichet, A.; Blasco, H.; Maakaroun-Vermesse, Z.; Vaillant, M.C.; Le Caignec, C.; et al. Barth syndrome in a female patient. *Mol. Genet. Metab.* **2012**, *106*, 115–120. [CrossRef]
36. Ichida, F.; Tsubata, S.; Bowles, K.R.; Haneda, N.; Uese, K.; Miyawaki, T.; Dreyer, W.J.; Messina, J.; Li, H.; Bowles, N.E.; et al. Novel gene mutations in patients with left ventricular noncompaction or Barth syndrome. *Circulation* **2001**, *103*, 1256–1263. [CrossRef]
37. Alquier, T.; Poitout, V. Considerations and guidelines for mouse metabolic phenotyping in diabetes research. *Diabetologia* **2018**, *61*, 526–538. [CrossRef]
38. Brewer, R.A.; Gibbs, V.K.; Smith, D.L., Jr. Targeting glucose metabolism for healthy aging. *Nutr. Healthy Aging* **2016**, *4*, 31–46. [CrossRef]
39. Orstavik, K.H. X chromosome inactivation in clinical practice. *Hum. Genet.* **2009**, *126*, 363–373. [CrossRef]
40. Schlame, M.; Ren, M.; Xu, Y.; Greenberg, M.L.; Haller, I. Molecular symmetry in mitochondrial cardiolipins. *Chem. Phys. Lipids* **2005**, *138*, 38–49. [CrossRef]
41. Soustek, M.S.; Falk, D.J.; Mah, C.S.; Toth, M.J.; Schlame, M.; Lewin, A.S.; Byrne, B.J. Characterization of a transgenic short hairpin RNA-induced murine model of Tafazzin deficiency. *Hum. Gene Ther.* **2011**, *22*, 865–871. [CrossRef] [PubMed]
42. Zhu, S.; Chen, Z.e.; Zhu, M.; Shen, Y.; Leon, L.J.; Chi, L.; Spinozzi, S.; Tan, C.; Gu, Y.; Nguyen, A.; et al. Cardiolipin Remodeling Defects Impair Mitochondrial Architecture and Function in a Murine Model of Barth Syndrome Cardiomyopathy. *Circ. Heart Fail.* **2021**, *14*, e008289. [CrossRef]
43. Powers, C.; Huang, Y.; Strauss, A.; Khuchua, Z. Diminished Exercise Capacity and Mitochondrial bc1 Complex Deficiency in Tafazzin-Knockdown Mice. *Front. Physiol.* **2013**, *4*, 74. [CrossRef] [PubMed]

44. Bashir, A.; Bohnert, K.L.; Reeds, D.N.; Peterson, L.R.; Bittel, A.J.; de Las Fuentes, L.; Pacak, C.A.; Byrne, B.J.; Cade, W.T. Impaired cardiac and skeletal muscle bioenergetics in children, adolescents, and young adults with Barth syndrome. *Physiol. Rep.* **2017**, *5*, e13130. [CrossRef] [PubMed]
45. Xu, Y.; Phoon, C.K.L.; Ren, M.; Schlame, M. A simple mechanistic explanation for Barth syndrome and cardiolipin remodeling. *J. Inherit. Metab. Dis.* **2022**, *45*, 51–59. [CrossRef]
46. Ozcelik, T. X chromosome inactivation and female predisposition to autoimmunity. *Clin. Rev. Allergy Immunol.* **2008**, *34*, 348–351. [CrossRef]
47. Ostan, R.; Monti, D.; Gueresi, P.; Bussolotto, M.; Franceschi, C.; Baggio, G. Gender, aging and longevity in humans: An update of an intriguing/neglected scenario paving the way to a gender-specific medicine. *Clin. Sci.* **2016**, *130*, 1711–1725. [CrossRef]
48. Avdjieva-Tzavella, D.M.; Todorova, A.P.; Kathom, H.M.; Ivanova, M.B.; Yordanova, I.T.; Todorov, T.P.; Litvinenko, I.O.; Dasheva-Dimitrova, A.T.; Tincheva, R.S. Barth Syndrome in Male and Female Siblings Caused by a Novel Mutation in the Taz Gene. *Genet. Couns.* **2016**, *27*, 495–501.
49. Bachou, T.; Giannakopoulos, A.; Trapali, C.; Vazeou, A.; Kattamis, A. A novel mutation in the G4.5 (TAZ) gene in a Greek patient with Barth syndrome. *Blood Cells Mol. Dis.* **2009**, *42*, 262–264. [CrossRef]
50. Brión, M.; de Castro López, M.J.; Santori, M.; Pérez Muñuzuri, A.; López Abel, B.; Baña Souto, A.M.; Martínez Soto, M.I.; Couce, M.L. Prospective and Retrospective Diagnosis of Barth Syndrome Aided by Next-Generation Sequencing. *Am. J. Clin. Pathol.* **2016**, *145*, 507–513. [CrossRef]
51. Kuijpers, T.W.; Maianski, N.A.; Tool, A.T.; Becker, K.; Plecko, B.; Valianpour, F.; Wanders, R.J.; Pereira, R.; Van Hove, J.; Verhoeven, A.J.; et al. Neutrophils in Barth syndrome (BTHS) avidly bind annexin-V in the absence of apoptosis. *Blood* **2004**, *103*, 3915–3923. [CrossRef] [PubMed]
52. Dutta, S.; Sengupta, P. Men and mice: Relating their ages. *Life Sci.* **2016**, *152*, 244–248. [CrossRef] [PubMed]
53. Ishizaki, M.; Kobayashi, M.; Adachi, K.; Matsumura, T.; Kimura, E. Female dystrophinopathy: Review of current literature. *Neuromuscul. Disord.* **2018**, *28*, 572–581. [CrossRef] [PubMed]
54. Politano, L.; Nigro, V.; Nigro, G.; Petretta, V.R.; Passamano, L.; Papparella, S.; Di Somma, S.; Comi, L.I. Development of cardiomyopathy in female carriers of Duchenne and Becker muscular dystrophies. *Jama* **1996**, *275*, 1335–1338. [CrossRef]
55. Adachi, K.; Kawai, H.; Saito, M.; Naruo, T.; Kimura, C.; Mine, H.; Inui, T.; Kashiwagi, S.; Akaike, M. Plasma levels of brain natriuretic peptide as an index for evaluation of cardiac function in female gene carriers of Duchenne muscular dystrophy. *Intern. Med.* **1997**, *36*, 497–500. [CrossRef]
56. Au, W.Y.; Ma, E.S.; Lam, V.M.; Chan, J.L.; Pang, A.; Kwong, Y.L. Glucose 6-phosphate dehydrogenase (G6PD) deficiency in elderly Chinese women heterozygous for G6PD variants. *Am. J. Med. Genet. A* **2004**, *129a*, 208–211. [CrossRef]
57. Au, W.Y.; Lam, V.; Pang, A.; Lee, W.M.; Chan, J.L.; Song, Y.Q.; Ma, E.S.; Kwong, Y.L. Glucose-6-phosphate dehydrogenase deficiency in female octogenarians, nanogenarians, and centenarians. *J. Gerontol. A Biol. Sci. Med. Sci.* **2006**, *61*, 1086–1089. [CrossRef]
58. Schmidt, S.; Träber, F.; Block, W.; Keller, E.; Pohl, C.; von Oertzen, J.; Schild, H.; Schlegel, U.; Klockgether, T. Phenotype assignment in symptomatic female carriers of X-linked adrenoleukodystrophy. *J. Neurol.* **2001**, *248*, 36–44. [CrossRef]
59. Davis, L.E.; Snyder, R.D.; Orth, D.N.; Nicholson, W.E.; Kornfeld, M.; Seelinger, D.F. Adrenoleukodystrophy and adrenomyeloneuropathy associated with partial adrenal insufficiency in three generations of a kindred. *Am. J. Med.* **1979**, *66*, 342–347. [CrossRef]
60. Heffungs, W.; Hameister, H.; Ropers, H.H. Addison disease and cerebral sclerosis in an apparently heterozygous girl: Evidence for inactivation of the adrenoleukodystrophy locus. *Clin. Genet.* **1980**, *18*, 184–188. [CrossRef]
61. Jangouk, P.; Zackowski, K.M.; Naidu, S.; Raymond, G.V. Adrenoleukodystrophy in female heterozygotes: Underrecognized and undertreated. *Mol. Genet. Metab.* **2012**, *105*, 180–185. [CrossRef]
62. Moser, H.W.; Moser, A.B.; Naidu, S.; Bergin, A. Clinical aspects of adrenoleukodystrophy and adrenomyeloneuropathy. *Dev. Neurosci.* **1991**, *13*, 254–261. [CrossRef]
63. Costello, D.J.; Eichler, A.F.; Eichler, F.S. Leukodystrophies: Classification, diagnosis, and treatment. *Neurologist* **2009**, *15*, 319–328. [CrossRef] [PubMed]
64. Dooley, J.M.; Wright, B.A. Adrenoleukodystrophy mimicking multiple sclerosis. *Can. J. Neurol. Sci.* **1985**, *12*, 73–74. [CrossRef] [PubMed]
65. Stöckler, S.; Millner, M.; Molzer, B.; Ebner, F.; Körner, E.; Moser, H.W. Multiple sclerosis-like syndrome in a woman heterozygous for adrenoleukodystrophy. *Eur. Neurol.* **1993**, *33*, 390–392. [CrossRef] [PubMed]
66. O'Neill, B.P.; Moser, H.W.; Saxena, K.M.; Marmion, L.C. Adrenoleukodystrophy: Clinical and biochemical manifestations in carriers. *Neurology* **1984**, *34*, 798–801. [CrossRef]
67. van Geel, B.M.; Koelman, J.H.; Barth, P.G.; Ongerboer de Visser, B.W. Peripheral nerve abnormalities in adrenomyeloneuropathy: A clinical and electrodiagnostic study. *Neurology* **1996**, *46*, 112–118. [CrossRef]
68. Horn, M.A.; Retterstøl, L.; Abdelnoor, M.; Skjeldal, O.H.; Tallaksen, C.M. Adrenoleukodystrophy in Norway: High rate of de novo mutations and age-dependent penetrance. *Pediatr. Neurol.* **2013**, *48*, 212–219. [CrossRef]
69. Jung, H.H.; Wimplinger, I.; Jung, S.; Landau, K.; Gal, A.; Heppner, F.L. Phenotypes of female adrenoleukodystrophy. *Neurology* **2007**, *68*, 960–961. [CrossRef]
70. Maier, E.M.; Kammerer, S.; Muntau, A.C.; Wichers, M.; Braun, A.; Roscher, A.A. Symptoms in carriers of adrenoleukodystrophy relate to skewed X inactivation. *Ann. Neurol.* **2002**, *52*, 683–688. [CrossRef]

71. Migeon, B.R.; Moser, H.W.; Moser, A.B.; Axelman, J.; Sillence, D.; Norum, R.A. Adrenoleukodystrophy: Evidence for X linkage, inactivation, and selection favoring the mutant allele in heterozygous cells. *Proc. Natl. Acad. Sci. USA* **1981**, *78*, 5066–5070. [CrossRef] [PubMed]
72. Watkiss, E.; Webb, T.; Bundey, S. Is skewed X inactivation responsible for symptoms in female carriers for adrenoleucodystrophy? *J. Med. Genet.* **1993**, *30*, 651–654. [CrossRef] [PubMed]
73. Flurkey, K.; Currer, J.M.; Harrison, D.E. Chapter 20—Mouse Models in Aging Research. In *the Mouse in Biomedical Research*, 2nd ed.; Fox, J.G., Davisson, M.T., Quimby, F.W., Barthold, S.W., Newcomer, C.E., Smith, A.L., Eds.; Academic Press: Burlington, NJ, USA, 2007; pp. 637–672.

biology MDPI

Article

Formoterol Acting via β2-Adrenoreceptor Restores Mitochondrial Dysfunction Caused by Parkinson's Disease-Related UQCRC1 Mutation and Improves Mitochondrial Homeostasis Including Dynamic and Transport

Jui-Chih Chang [1,*], Huei-Shin Chang [1], Yi-Chun Chao [2], Ching-Shan Huang [1], Chin-Hsien Lin [3], Zhong-Sheng Wu [4], Hui-Ju Chang [1], Chin-San Liu [5,6,7,8] and Chieh-Sen Chuang [5,*]

1 Center of Regenerative Medicine and Tissue Repair, Institute of ATP, Changhua Christian Hospital, Changhua 500, Taiwan
2 Inflammation Research & Drug Development Center, Changhua Christian Hospital, Changhua 500, Taiwan
3 Department of Neurology, National Taiwan University Hospital, Taipei 100, Taiwan
4 Department of General Research Laboratory of Research, Changhua Christian Hospital, Changhua 500, Taiwan
5 Department of Neurology, Changhua Christian Hospital, Changhua 500, Taiwan
6 Vascular and Genomic Center, Institute of ATP, Changhua Christian Hospital, Changhua 500, Taiwan
7 Graduate Institute of Integrated Medicine, College of Chinese Medicine, China Medical University, Taichung 404, Taiwan
8 College of Medicine, National Chung Hsing University, Taichung 402, Taiwan
* Correspondence: 145520@cch.org.tw (J.-C.C.); 83954@cch.org.tw (C.-S.C.); Tel.: +886-4-7238595 (ext. 4751) (J.-C.C. & C.-S.C.)

Simple Summary: Formoterol, an FDA-approved long-acting beta2-adrenergic receptor agonist, has shown potential benefits in various diseases, yet its effectiveness in Parkinson's disease (PD) is uncertain. The lack of a comprehensive understanding of formoterol's mechanism, particularly in mitochondrial remodeling, contributes to this uncertainty. PD involves mitochondrial dysfunction, leading to disruptions in energy production, heightened oxidative stress, and impaired mitochondrial dynamics and turnover. Understanding this link is vital for developing targeted therapies for PD. To explore this, this study used a cell model that mimics a specific genetic form of PD. This model displayed the above problems with mitochondria. The study found that after treating these cells with formoterol, there were positive effects. The medication enhanced the growth and survival of PD-associate mutant cells while protecting against stress. Crucially, it contributed to restoring normal mitochondrial function and machinery, promoting a rebalance in mitochondrial dynamics, including changes in morphology (fusion/fission), movement, and transport. This effect was achieved by influencing specific cell signals and proteins associated with mitochondrial health. This study underscores formoterol's pivotal role as a mitochondrial dynamic balance regulator, positioning it as a promising therapeutic candidate for PD.

Abstract: Formoterol, a β2-adrenergic receptor (β2AR) agonist, shows promise in various diseases, but its effectiveness in Parkinson's disease (PD) is debated, with unclear regulation of mitochondrial homeostasis. This study employed a cell model featuring mitochondrial ubiquinol-cytochrome c reductase core protein 1 (UQCRC1) variants associated with familial parkinsonism, demonstrating mitochondrial dysfunction and dynamic imbalance, exploring the therapeutic effects and underlying mechanisms of formoterol. Results revealed that 24-h formoterol treatment enhanced cell proliferation, viability, and neuroprotection against oxidative stress. Mitochondrial function, encompassing DNA copy number, repatriation, and complex III-linked respiration, was comprehensively restored, along with the dynamic rebalance of fusion/fission events. Formoterol reduced extensive hypertubulation, in contrast to mitophagy, by significantly upregulating protein Drp-1, in contrast to fusion protein Mfn2, mitophagy-related protein Parkin. The upstream mechanism involved the restoration of ERK signaling and the inhibition of Akt overactivity, contingent on the activation of β2-adrenergic receptors. Formoterol additionally aided in segregating healthy mitochondria for distribution and transport, therefore normalizing mitochondrial arrangement in mutant cells. This study provides preliminary evidence that formoterol offers neuroprotection, acting as a mitochondrial dynamic balance regulator, making it a promising therapeutic candidate for PD.

Keywords: formoterol; Parkinson's disease; ubiquinol-cytochrome c reductase core protein 1; mitochondrial function; mitochondrial dynamics

1. Introduction

Formoterol is a long-acting beta2-adrenergic receptor (β2AR) agonist and a type of medication that is used for treating asthma and chronic obstructive pulmonary disease (COPD), as it relaxes the muscles of the airways, thus affording easier breathing [1]. It is also often used in combination with other medications to help control the symptoms of Parkinson's disease (PD), such as tremors, stiffness, and difficulty with movement [2]. The relationship between β2AR agonists and the risk of PD remains a subject of debate. Although some studies have found no significant association between β2AR medications and PD risk [3,4], others have suggested that the chronic use of β2AR blockers has neuroprotective effects [5] and reduces the risk of PD [6–8]. Moreover, their underlying mechanism has been suggested to be related to the regulation of α-synuclein transcription [9], which increases the activity of dopamine, a neurotransmitter, and decreases neuroinflammation in the brain [10]. Furthermore, formoterol stimulates the production of signaling molecules (such as cyclic AMP) that play a key role in many physiological processes, including the regulation of energy metabolism [11]. Recently, the effect of formoterol on mitochondria, the "powerhouses" of cells, was noted, which has been consistently correlated with the restoration of mitochondrial activity, biogenesis, and homeostasis in different cells and tissues, thus potentially contributing to its effects on metabolism and energy production [12,13]. However, the precise molecular mechanisms by which formoterol affects mitochondrial function, especially in regulating mitochondrial dynamics in PD, remain unknown.

Mitochondria are dynamic organelles that undergo continuous processes of fusion and fission. This phenomenon maintains the hemostasis of mitochondria and the integrity of mitochondrial DNA (mtDNA) in many ways. Mitochondrial fusion shares materials to sustain stress-induced damage. In contrast, mitochondrial fission helps to distribute mitochondria evenly within a cell through mitochondrial transport, together with microtubules, to ensure that all parts of the cell have access to the energy required by them [14]. This process can trigger cells to discard damaged mitochondria via mitophagy to control mitochondrial quality [15]. Notably, mitochondrial dynamic dysfunction also implicates the regulation of cell signaling, the cell cycle, and apoptotic mechanisms in stresses caused by genetic and environmental factors and beyond to cellular energy support [16]. Thus, disruptions in the balance of mitochondrial dynamics have been implicated in the development and progression of various diseases, including PD.

Mitochondrial ubiquinol-cytochrome c reductase core protein 1 (UQCRC1)-associated parkinsonism with polyneuropathy is a rare genetic disorder that is caused by a missense mutation, c.941A > C (p.Tyr314Ser) in the UQCRC1 gene [17,18]. The exact underlying mechanisms involve energy deficits, oxidative stress, and loss of the engagement of cytochrome c to trigger neuronal death [17,19,20]; however, the impact on mitochondrial dynamics remains unclear. In particular, a marked dysregulation of mitochondrial dynamics, as revealed by abnormally elongated mitochondria and an irregular shape, is consistently observed in both UQCRC1-mutant neurons and animals [17,19]. Therefore, in the present study, through the exploration of the machinery related to the maintenance of mitochondrial homeostasis (including mitochondrial fission, fusion, transport, and biogenesis) in a cellular model of UQCRC1 parkinsonism, the therapeutic potential of the targeting of mitochondrial dynamics by formoterol for the future therapy of PD was examined.

2. Materials and Methods

2.1. Cell Culture and Treatment

The wild-type (WT) and mutant *UQCRC1* knock-in human neuroblastoma SH-SY5Y cell lines were gifts from the laboratory of Dr Chin-Hsien Lin [18]. The cells were individually transfected with CRISPR/Cas9 plasmids without site mutation (as a control in this experiment, WT) or carried the c.941A > C (p.Tyr314Ser) heterozygous variant of the *UQCRC1* gene identified in patients with PD (*UQCRC1* mutation) and confirmed by PCR amplification and Sanger sequencing for confirmation [17]. All cells were cultured in DMEM/F12 (Life Technologies, GIBCO BRL, Rockville, MD, USA) supplemented with 10% FBS (BIOSER, Buenos Aires, Argentina), 100 U/mL penicillin, and 100 μg/mL streptomycin (Life Technologies, GIBCO BRL), then grown in a humidified atmosphere containing 5% CO_2.

Mutant cells were treated with 1 μM formoterol alone or in combination with 100 μM propranolol, a β2AR antagonist, for 24 h in the presence or absence of 10 μM tert-butylhydroperoxide (tBH)-induced oxidative stress. The effective doses of various compounds were determined following preliminary WST-1 analysis, with none observed to adversely affect WT cell viability (see Supplementary Information, Figure S1).

2.2. GFP-Labeled Mitochondria

Cells at 80% confluency were transfected with 40 μg of plasmid DNA encoding mitochondrial-matrix-localized AcGFP (import targeting sequence of cytochrome c oxidase subunit 8, COX8) (Clontech, Palo Alto, CA, USA) using electroporation (ECM; BTX Harvard Apparatus, Holliston, MA, USA) according to our previous study [21]. Thirty-six hours later, the cells were transferred to a normal growth medium for 48 h, followed by G418 selection (500 mg/mL).

2.3. Cell Number, Cell Viability, and Filopodia Outgrowth

Cell morphology after the various treatments was assessed using a bright-field Olympus BX43 microscope with the CellSens software (Version 3.2) (Olympus, Tokyo, Japan). Subsequently, cell number and viability were analyzed using a Cell Scepter electronic cell counter (EMD Millipore Corporation, Billerica, MA, USA) and the WST-1 assay (Roche Diagnostics, Taipei, Taiwan), respectively; moreover, the percentage of tBH-induced apoptotic cells was examined using 7-amino actinomycin D (7-AAD) (BD Pharmigen, Franklin Lakes, NJ, USA) staining and detected by a NucleoCounter ® NC-3000™ fluorescence image cytometer (ChemoMetec, Alleroed, Denmark). The filopodia lengths of the treated cells were manually quantified using the ImageJ software (Version 1.48) (National Institutes of Health, Bethesda, MD, USA).

2.4. Quantitative Mitochondrial Morphology and Density

To visualize mitochondria, stained cells were mounted onto a perfusion chamber in a culture medium and imaged at 37 °C using an Olympus FluoView FV 1200 confocal microscope (Tokyo, Japan). The subtypes of mitochondrial morphology were quantified using the automatic morphological subtyping software (MicroP) developed by Peng et al. [22]. Briefly, the morphological classifications were made by analyzing the image features of the segmented mitochondrial objects, clustering them based on functional similarity, merging similar clusters, and defining distinct morphological subtypes based on the clustering results in the literature [22]. Finally, six morphological subtypes of mitochondria were identified, consisting of single and swollen globes, straight and twisting tubules, branched tubules, and loops. To calculate the proportion of globe mitochondria, the single globe and swollen globe shapes were summed and contrasted to the proportion of reticular mitochondria (i.e., the combined population of straight tubule, twisting tubule, and branched mitochondria). The analysis was performed on micrographs from three independent areas per group, and approximately 200–350 mitochondria from 6–8 cells in each image were analyzed semi-automatically. The mitochondrial counts were presented as the total number of mitochondria per cell according to data mentioned above.

2.5. Mitochondrial Function

Mitochondrial function was comprehensively assessed by measuring several parameters, including mitochondrial respiratory parameters: basal respiration, ATP-linked oxygen consumption (OCR), complex III-dependent OCR (CIII activity), mitochondrial DNA (mtDNA) copy number, and reactive oxygen species (ROS) generation (as a whole and in mitochondria (mtROS).

Mitochondrial respiration within saponin (1.25 ng/mL)-permeabilized cells were analyzed via high-resolution respirometry (Oxygraph-2k; Oroboros Instruments, Innsbruck, Austria) and expressed as the respiratory oxygen flow (pmol/second/million cells). The analysis started with the measurement of basal respiration (BR), which was defined as that recorded in cells in MiR05 buffer (Oroboros Instruments) in the absence of additional substrates or effectors; in contrast to ATP-linked production, which was defined as the oligomycin (1 μM)-mediated reduction of respiration in the presence of additional substrates [glutamate (G, 10 mM), malate (M, 2 mM), and ADP (2.5 mM)] (Sigma Aldrich, St Louis, MO, USA); and complex III activity, which was defined as the difference in the respiration change between the addition of duroquinone (DuroQ) (0.5 mM) (Sigma Aldrich) and antimycin A (AA, 5 μM) (Sigma Aldrich). Finally, the shutdown of the mitochondrial electron transport was executed by adding an inhibitor of the mitochondrial Complex IV, sodium azide (20 mM).

For the analysis of mtDNA copy number, DNA was extracted from cultured cells using a Qiagen DNeasy kit (Qiagen, Valencia, CA, USA). Next, quantitative PCR was performed using the SYBR Green PCR Master Mix (Roche Applied Science, Indianapolis, IN, USA) and an ABI Prism 7300 system (Applied Biosystems, Foster City, CA) with specific primer pairs to amplify the mtDNA-encoded nicotinamide adenine dinucleotide dehydrogenase subunit 1 (*ND1*) gene (forward primer: 5′–AACATACCCATGGCCAACCT–3′; and reverse primer: 5′–AGCGAAGGGTTGTAGTAGCCC–3′) and the nuclear DNA-encoded β-actin gene (as an internal control; forward primer: 5′–AGAAAATCTGGCACCACACC–3′; and reverse primer: 5′–CACCTTCTACAATGAGCTGCG–3′) from a total of 50 ng of DNA. The mtDNA copy number was determined based on the copy number ratio between these two genes (ND1/β-actin) [23].

ROS production was analyzed by measuring total ROS using the 2,7-dichlorofluorescein diacetate (DCFDA, Life Technologies) probe, whereas mitochondrial superoxide production was assessed using the MitoSox Red (Life Technologies) probe. The cells were incubated in a medium containing 10 μM DCFH-DA and 50 nM MitoSox Red at 37 °C for 15 min for staining in the dark. All stained cells were washed twice with PBS, resuspended in PBS, and kept on ice for immediate detection using a NucleoCounter ® NC-3000™ fluorescence image cytometer.

2.6. Mitochondrial Motility

Mitochondrial transport imaging was carried out according to a previous study, with some modifications [24]. The live time-lapse imaging of cells treated with GFP-labeled mitochondria was performed using an Olympus FV1200 confocal laser scanning microscope at 37 °C with 5% CO_2. The cells were imaged for 10 min with continuous recording. The acquired images were analyzed for mitochondrial motility using the CellSens (Olympus) software. Briefly, based on morphological criteria, for the analysis of the axonal initial segment, including the proximal and hillock regions, a 10–20-μm segment located at least 10 μm away from the soma was selected. The mitochondrial velocity duration time and the directionality of the movement, as obtained by measuring the angle of the slope, were analyzed in the kymographs generated by CellSens. The proportion of motile mitochondria was manually calculated by dividing the number of mitochondria moving faster than average by the total number of mitochondria based on the image sequences of the kymographs. At least 7–10 axons from 3–5 different cells were analyzed in each group. Considering that the axon extension in mutant cells was not obvious compared with that observed in WT cells, the mobility parameter was analyzed exclusively in the proximal region of axons.

2.7. Western Blotting and Protein Phosphorylation Antibody Array

Treated cells were rinsed with PBS and then suspended in RIPA buffer (Thermo Pierce, Rockford, IL, USA) supplemented with a complete protease and phosphatase inhibitor cocktail (EMD Millipore Corporation). The cells were kept on ice for 30 min and then homogenized. The extracts were centrifuged at 14,000× *g* for 20 min at 4 °C, and the supernatants were analyzed using the Bradford assay. Total proteins (20–30 μg) were separated by SDS–PAGE and transferred onto Immobilon-P membranes (EMD Millipore Corporation). The membranes were then incubated with the primary antibodies, as follows: anti-OPA1 (1:1000, BD Biosciences, Franklin Lakes, NJ, USA), anti-mitofusin 2 (Mfn2) (1:1000, NOVUS Biologicals, Littleton, CO, USA), anti-dynamin-related protein 1 (Drp-1) (1:500, EMD Millipore Corporation), anti-phospho-Drp-1-S616 (1:1000, Cell Signaling Technology, Danvers, MA, USA), anti-phospho-Drp-1-S637 (1:1000, Thermo Fisher Scientific, Inc., Waltham, MA, USA), anti-PTEN-induced kinase 1 (Pink1) (1:1000, NOVUS Biologicals), anti-Parkin (1:1000, Abcam, Cambridge, MA, USA), anti-phospho-p44/42 MAPK (ERK1/2) (Thr202/Tyr204) (1:1000, Cell Signaling Technology), anti-phospho-Akt (Ser473) (1:1000, Cell Signaling Technology), and anti-β-actin (1:1000, NOVUS Biologicals). The membranes were subsequently incubated with horseradish peroxidase (HRP)-conjugated secondary antibodies (Jackson ImmunoResearch, West Grove, PA, USA) at a dilution of 1:10,000. The signals were detected using an image-acquisition system (FUSION SL; Viber Lourmat, Marne-la-Vallee, France) and quantified using the Gel-Pro analyzer software (Version 3.0) (Media Cybernetics, Silver Spring, MD, USA).

The Human/Mouse Akt Pathway Phosphorylation Array C1 includes key proteins of interest in the relevant pathways (ERK1, ERK2, PRAS40, GSK3A, PTEN, GSK3B, RAF-1, mTOR, RPS6, Akt, p27, RSK1, AMPKa, p53, RSK2, BAD, P70S6K, 4E-BP1, and PDK1) and was performed according to the manufacturer's instructions (RayBiotech, Norcross, GA, USA) [25]. Briefly, total protein preparation and HRP signal detection were carried out as described above. A total of 100 μg of the protein extracts from three independent cell lysates was added to each well and incubated for 24 h at 4 °C. Subsequently, the antibody array membranes were washed and incubated with the HRP-conjugated anti-rabbit IgG antibody included in the kit at room temperature for 2 h. The membranes were washed extensively before detection using chemiluminescence.

2.8. Protein Kinase A Activity

Protein kinase A (PKA) activity was examined using a PKA Colorimetric Activity Kit (Thermo Fisher Scientific, Waltham, MA, USA), including a PKA substrate-coated 96-well plate(s), a PKA standard, and an anti-phospho-PKA substrate antibody. Briefly, cell lysis was carried out in the presence of the supplied ATP, and phosphorylation was achieved by the immobilized PKA substrate. After a 90-min incubation followed by a wash, a rabbit antibody specific for the phospho-PKA substrate was bound to the modified immobilized substrate. Then, an antibody specific to rabbit IgG labeled with peroxidase was also added to the plate to bind to the rabbit anti-phospho-PKA substrate. After short incubation and wash steps, the substrate was added, and the absorbance was read at 450 nm using a CLARIOstar microplate reader (BMG LabTech, Ortenberg, Germany). The intensity of the color that developed was directly proportional to the amount of PKA in the samples and standards. All samples were read off the standard curve.

2.9. Statistics

The data are presented in the form of the mean ± standard deviation (SD) and were obtained from a minimum of three independent experiments. Associations between groups were assessed by Student's *t*-test, and within-group differences were assessed by Bonferroni corrected post-hoc tests, which were performed using GraphPad Prism (GraphPad Software, La Jolla, CA, USA). Significance was set at $p < 0.05$.

3. Results

3.1. Formoterol Increased the Viability of UQCRC1 Mutant Cells and Protected against Tertiary-Butyl Hydroperoxide-Induced Cell Damage in a β2-Adrenoceptor-Dependent Manner

The mutant cells exhibited hindered outgrowth (Figure 1a), diminished filopodia length (Figure 1b), and lower viability and proliferation compared to WT cells (Figure 1c). Following a 24-h formoterol treatment, there were significant improvements in these parameters, with a notable increase in cell activity and number (1.4-fold and 1.6-fold, respectively) compared to the disease DMSO group (Figure 1c). Filopodia outgrowth also significantly increased by up to 1.7-fold (Figure 1b). However, when formoterol was used in combination with propranolol, these positive effects were completely abolished (Figure 1a–c). No significant differences were observed in cell viability, growth, and filopodia outgrowth between the groups treated with formoterol plus propranolol and the DMSO group. These results indicate that formoterol's response is mediated through the activation of β2AR.

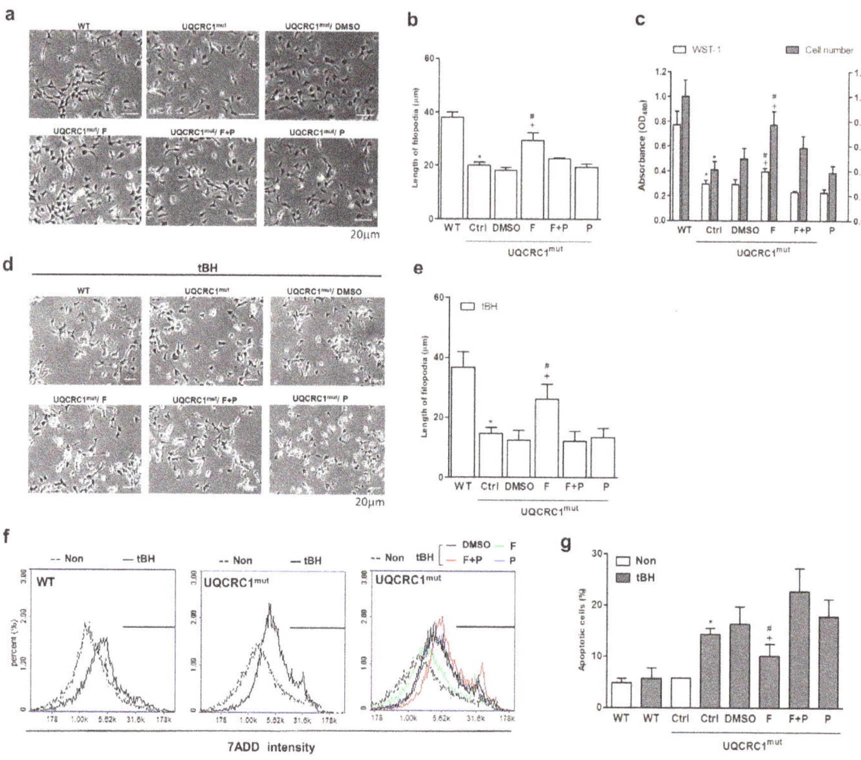

Figure 1. Cell viability and filopodia outgrowth in the absence or presence of tertiary-butyl hydroperoxide (tBH) stimulation. Cell morphology was observed after treatments with or without tBH stimulation for 24 h (10 μM) (**a**,**d**). The filopodia length was quantified by image processing using ImageJ (**b**,**e**). Cell viability and cell proliferation were determined by WST-1 analysis and counted with a Coulter counter (c). The tBH-induced cell death was measured using 7-AAD staining and flow cytometry analysis (**f**), then quantified (**g**). * $p < 0.05$ vs. the WT group or the treated Ctrl group. + $p < 0.05$ vs. the DMSO group. # $p < 0.05$ vs. the F + P group. Data are presented as the mean ± SD. WT: wild-type; Ctrl: control; DMSO, dimethylsulfoxide; F, formoterol; F + P: formoterol plus propranolol; P: propranolol; UQCRC1mut: mutation of the ubiquinol-cytochrome c reductase core protein 1 gene; 7AAD; 7-aminoactinomycin D; tBH: tertiary-butyl hydroperoxide. $N = 6$.

Similar trends were observed in treated mutant cells subjected to tBH-induced oxidative damage (Figure 1d,e). Formoterol, compared to the DMSO group, significantly increased filopodia length by 1.9-fold under oxidative stress conditions through β2AR activation (Figure 1e). While this tBH dosage did not significantly induce cell apoptosis in WT cells, mutant cells showed a substantial 2.6-fold increase in the death rate compared to their non-treated counterparts (Figure 1f,g). Following a 24-h treatment, formoterol effectively reduced tBH-induced cell death by approximately 55% compared to the DMSO control (Figure 1g). Notably, the addition of propranolol nullified this effect, reinforcing the β2AR-dependent nature of formoterol's impact on various cellular responses.

3.2. Formoterol Enhanced mtDNA Copy Number, Reduced ROS Levels, and Restored Mitochondrial Respiration and Complex III Activity, but Not ATP-Linked Respiration

To assess mitochondrial function comprehensively, various parameters were analyzed, including mtDNA copy number, ROS generation, and mitochondrial respiration in WT and mutant cells (Figure 2). Mutant cells exhibited distinct mitochondrial abnormalities compared to WT cells, including a significantly lower number of mtDNA copies (Figure 2a), elevated levels of total and mitochondrial reactive oxygen species (mtROS) generation (Figure 2b,c), and compromised cellular respiratory performance (Figure 2d, left panel). This was evident in markedly reduced basal respiration (BR), electron-transport-linked ATP respiration, and CIII-linked respiration, as depicted in Figure 2e. Formoterol consistently ameliorated these functional losses in mutant cells, enhancing mitochondrial substrate availability, except for ATP-linked respiration (Figure 2d,e). Propranolol addition nullified formoterol's benefits except for mtROS production (Figure 2c), emphasizing the formoterol-mediated regulation of mitochondrial function via β2AR-dependent and independent actions.

3.3. Formoterol Improved the Transition from an Abnormal, Clustered Network to a More Tubular and Globular Mitochondrial Morphology

In contrast to WT cells, where mitochondria were evenly distributed in the cytosol, mutant cells showed abnormalities in both mitochondrial organization and morphology (Figure 3a, left panel). Mutant cells exhibited an excessive clustering of mitochondria in mutant cells, resulting in the formation of large mitochondrial networks around nuclei. It was evidently illustrated in the right panel of Figure 3a, marked by a prevalence of reticular mitochondria exhibiting branching (purple tinge), twisting (orange tinge), and loop structures (red tinge), contrasted with a reduced number of tubular mitochondria (green tinge) and globe mitochondria, including single structures (blue tinge) and swollen structures (yellow tinge). Formoterol effectively rectified this imbalance in mitochondrial morphology, inducing a more even distribution of mitochondria within the cells in mutant cells, resembling the pattern observed in WT cells (Figure 3a). The quantification of clustering mitochondrial morphologies into the reticular network, tubule, and globe subtypes (Figure 3b) revealed that formoterol reduced the fraction of the reticular mitochondria subtype by approximately 50% compared to the DMSO group while increasing the fractions of the tubular and globe mitochondria subtypes. The addition of propranolol negated this effect, indicating that formoterol's actions on mitochondrial morphology were specifically mediated by β2AR activation (Figure 3b).

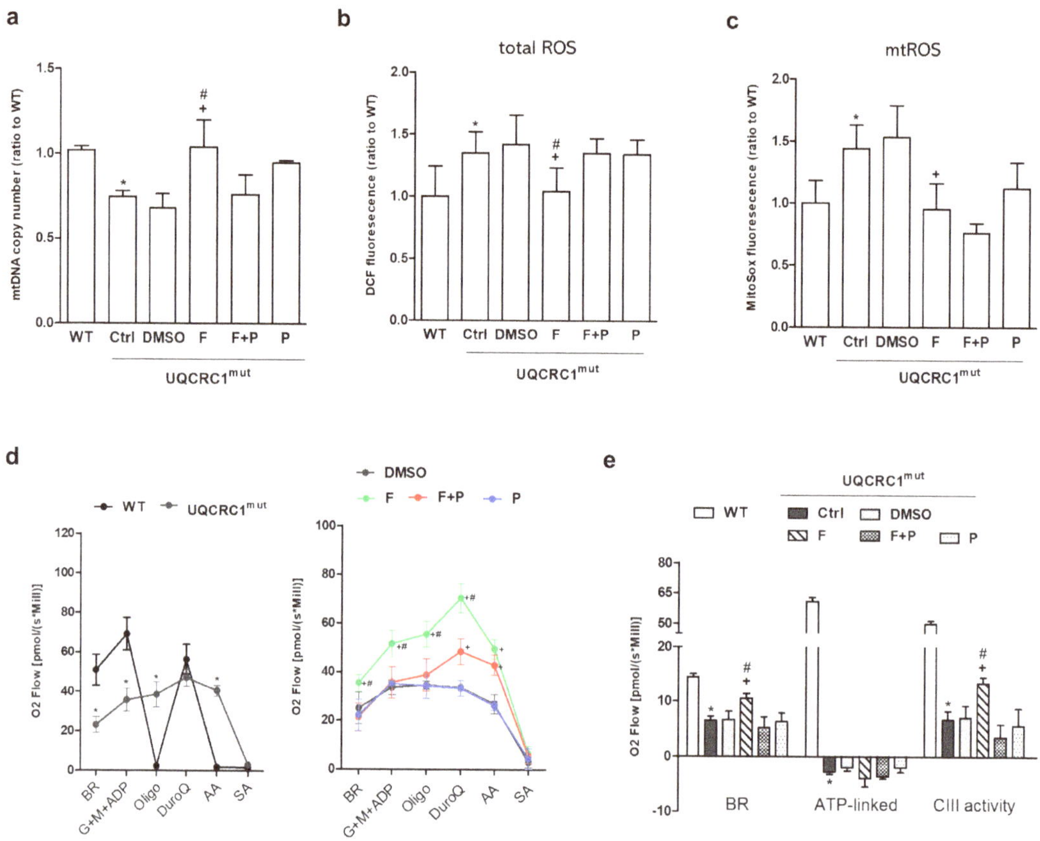

Figure 2. Mitochondrial function and generation of reactive oxygen species. Mitochondrial function was comprehensively assessed after 24h treatments by analyzing the mtDNA content (DNA copy number) (**a**), the level of reactive oxygen species in total (total ROS) (**b**) and in mitochondria (mtROS) (**c**), and mitochondrial respiration (**d**,**e**). Mitochondrial oxygen consumption was measured in permeabilized cells using different substrates and inhibitors of the respiratory chain complexes; the comparison between WT and mutant cells (left panel) or between mutant cells with different treatments (right panel) is shown (**d**). The induced oxygen consumption (oxygen flux) was integrated and quantified according to different approaches to provide an indirect measurement of mitochondrial activity, including basal respiration, ATP−linked respiration (oligomycin-mediated reduction), and CIII−linked respiration (respiratory difference between duroquinone, a CIII substrate, and antimycin A, a CIII inhibitor) (**e**). * $p < 0.05$ vs. the WT group. + $p < 0.05$ vs. the DMSO group. # $p < 0.05$ vs. the F + P group. Data are presented as the mean ± SD. WT: wild-type; Ctrl: control; DMSO, dimethylsulfoxide; F, formoterol; F + P: formoterol plus propranolol; P: propranolol; UQCRC1mut: mutation of the ubiquinol-cytochrome c reductase core protein 1 gene; BR: basal respiration, G: glutamate, M: malate, Oligo: oligomycin; DuroQ: duroquinone, AA: antimycin A, SA: sodium azide. $N = 3$.

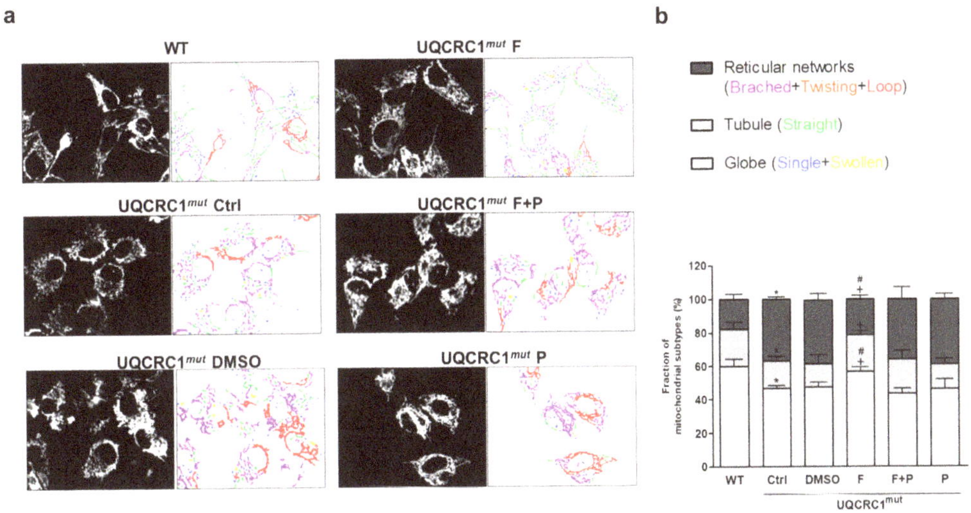

Figure 3. Mitochondrial morphology and distribution. The morphology of GFP-labeled mitochondria was observed after 24-h treatments ((**a**), left panel). The classification of mitochondrial morphology was further analyzed using automatic MicroP software and was presented by the labeling of different color-coded subtypes of mitochondria to show the morphological composition of each group of representative cells ((**a**), right panel). The six distinct mitochondrial subtypes were labeled with different colors ((**a**), right panel) and were classified as class three, as follows: globe, including single (blue) and swollen (yellow); tubule, including straight tubule (green) and reticular networks [including branched tubule (purple), twisting tubule (orange), and loop (red)] (**b**). The percentage of each mitochondrial subtype among the total mitochondrial population was calculated and integrated into the three categories, as described above (**b**). * $p < 0.05$ vs. the WT group. + $p < 0.05$ vs. the DMSO group. # $p < 0.05$ vs. the F + P group. Data are presented as the mean ± SD. WT: wild-type; Ctrl: control; DMSO, dimethylsulfoxide; F, formoterol; F + P: formoterol plus propranolol; P: propranolol; UQCRC1mut: mutation of the ubiquinol-cytochrome c reductase core protein 1 gene.

3.4. Formoterol Regulated Mitochondrial Fusion–Fission Balance through β2-Adrenoreceptor Activation and Was Linked to Counter-Regulation of ERK and Akt Signals

Mutant cells, compared to WT cells, showed a heightened preference for mitochondrial fusion over division, as depicted in Figure 4. The results from Western blot analysis (Figure 4a) and the quantification of proteins associated with mitochondrial dynamics (Figure 4b) showed a substantial elevation in Mfn2 levels (excluding OPA1) and a notable decrease in both Drp-1 expression and its phosphorylation at S616 (Drp-1 S616), a factor recognized for promoting mitochondrial fission. It was accompanied by a distinct dephosphorylation of Drp-1 at S637, a factor recognized for inhibiting mitochondrial fission. Formoterol treatment significantly reversed the aforementioned alterations in Mfn2, Drp-1, and Drp-1 S616 phosphorylation in mutant cells (Figure 4a), showing a significant difference compared to the DMSO control group (Figure 4b). Remarkably, dephosphorylation of Drp-1 at S637 was also distinctly enhanced by formoterol treatment. Furthermore, mutant cells exhibited inhibition of full-length Pink1 (L-form) and no impact on the Parkin protein compared to WT cells (Figure 4a). Formoterol treatment resulted in a significant upregulation of both the full-length Pink1 and the cleaved Pink1 (S-form) proteins, alongside a simultaneous downregulation of the mitophagy-related protein Parkin (Figure 4b). It revealed that the formoterol-induced mitochondrial fission did not result in mitochondrial degradation in mutant cells. Overall, the comprehensive regulation of mitochondrial dynamic-related proteins by formoterol was shown to be mediated through β2AR activation. This was evident from the reversal of these performance actions upon the addition of propranolol, except for Parkin protein, where no significant differences were observed between the formoterol treatments with and without propranolol.

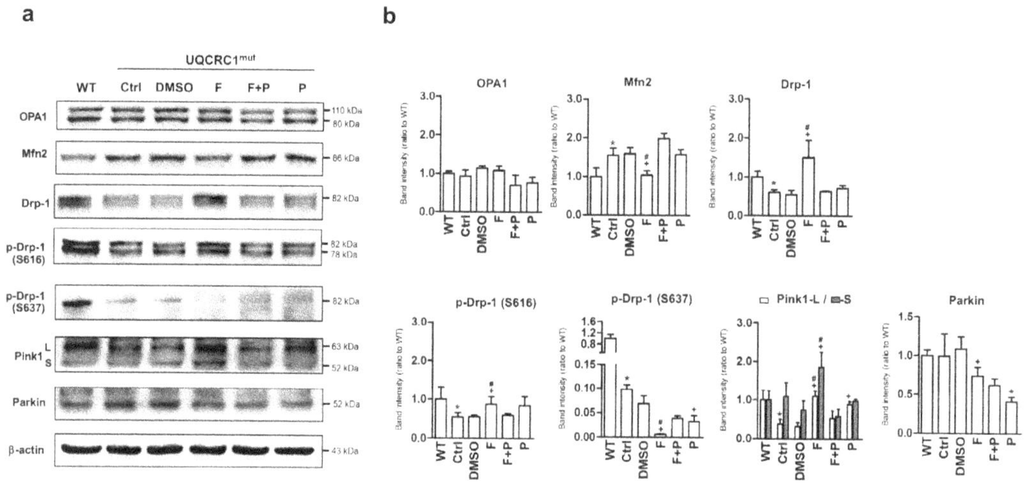

Figure 4. Expression of mitochondrial dynamic-related proteins. The level of mitochondrial fusion-relate (OPA1 and Mfn2), fission-related [total and phosphorylated form of Drp-1 at serine 616 (S616) and 637 (S637)], and mitophagy-related [Long (L) and short form (S) of Pink1 and Parkin)] proteins were analyzed (**a**) by Western blotting and quantified in both WT cells and mutant cells with or without 24-h treatments. Target proteins were quantified by normalizing to β-actin and were presented as the fold change relative to the WT group (**b**). * $p < 0.05$ vs. the WT group. + $p < 0.05$ vs. the DMSO group. # $p < 0.05$ vs. the F + P group. Data are presented as the mean ± SD. WT: wild-type; Ctrl: control; DMSO, dimethylsulfoxide; F, formoterol; F + P: formoterol plus propranolol; P: propranolol; UQCRC1mut: mutation of ubiquinol-cytochrome c reductase core protein 1 gene. N = 3.

To elucidate the downstream pathway of β2AR activation linking the regulation of mitochondrial dynamic, an intercellular signaling array with MAPK phosphorylation antibodies was employed (Figure 5a). Mutant cells displayed elevated levels of Akt phosphorylation at S473, in contrast with the phosphorylation status of ERK1/2 at T202/Y204 and Y185/Y187, compared with WT cells (Figure 5a, left panel). Formoterol effectively counter-regulated the expression of Akt and ERK phosphorylation, and this specific regulation was demonstrated to be dependent on β2AR activation, as demonstrated by the abolished regulation upon cotreatment with propranolol (Figure 5a, left panel). Furthermore, a comparison of pathway-related phosphorylated proteins integrated into the array was conducted for each set of groups. The differences in the expression of the corresponding proteins were listed individually in the right panel of the bar graph depicted in Figure 5a (for the raw data, see Supplementary Information, Table S1). Among the Raf–ERK signaling molecules involved in the positive regulation of formoterol, the induction of 4E-BP1 was even higher than that of ERK1/2. In contrast, formoterol negatively regulated the Akt–RSK–S6-kinase signaling-related molecules (Figure 5a, right panel). Consistent findings of the restoration of ERK signaling and the inhibition of Akt activation in mutant cells by formoterol were confirmed through Western blot analysis (Figure 5b). Furthermore, Furthermore, formoterol treatment showed no effect on the elevated PKA activity in mutant cells when compared to WT cells (Figure 5c).

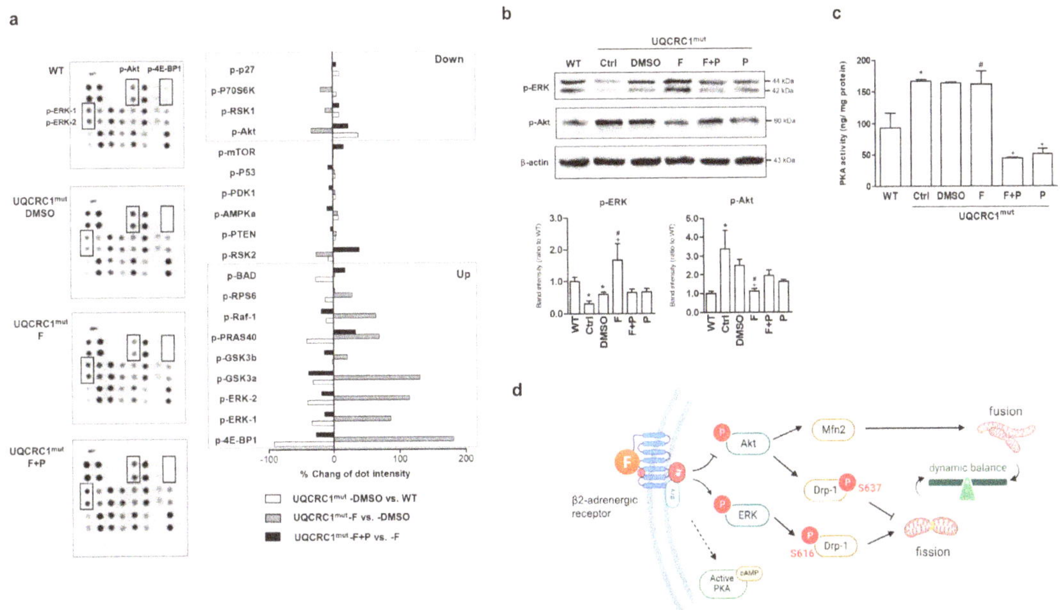

Figure 5. Expression of the downstream related signaling in activation of the β2 adrenergic receptor. T-related regulatory signaling of ERK and Akt phosphorylation was analyzed using a phospho-kinase array of the pools of cell lysates from three independent experiments (**a**). Left panel: immunoblotted membranes (highlighted squares: spots with obvious differences in phosphorylation levels); left panel: quantifications of phosphorylation levels of all spots. The expression differences between different groups were compared (UQCRC1mut−DMSO vs. WT; UQCRC1mut−F vs. UQCRC1mut−DMSO; UQCRC1mut−F + P vs. UQCRC1mut−F), and the reverse regulation direction (up- or downregulation) between inter-groups, UQCRC1mut−DMSO vs. WT; UQCRC1mut−F vs. UQCRC1mut−DMSO, was indicated in the squares (A, right panel). The ERK and Akt phosphorylation was further confirmed by Western blotting, quantified by normalizing to β-actin, and were presented as the fold change relative to the WT group (**b**). The activity of classic protein kinase A (PKA) was measured using a colorimetric activity assay (**c**). A path diagram was constructed based on the above findings to illustrate the regulatory relationship between the mitochondrial dynamic machinery and the activation of the β2 adrenergic receptor by formoterol (**d**). Formoterol treatment rebalanced mitochondrial dynamics by promoting fission and inhibiting abnormal hyperfusion in mutant cells. The regulatory machinery was associated with activating downstream ERK signaling and inhibiting Akt signaling (solid line) rather than being regulated by PKA (dotted line). * $p < 0.05$ vs. the WT group. + $p < 0.05$ vs. the DMSO group. # $p < 0.05$ vs. the F + P group. Data are presented as the mean ± SD. WT: wild-type; Ctrl: control; DMSO, dimethylsulfoxide; F, formoterol; F + P: formoterol plus propranolol; P: propranolol; UQCRC1mut: mutation of ubiquinol-cytochrome c reductase core protein 1 gene; cAMP, cyclic adenosine monophosphate). $N = 3$.

Figure 5d depicts the pathway diagram corresponding to the regulatory relevance of mitochondrial dynamics through the formoterol-induced activation of β2AR. The improvement in the dynamic balance afforded by formoterol was attributed to its simultaneous promotion of the ERK pathway and inhibition of the Akt pathway. This led to an increase in the ratio of Drp-1 S616/Drp-1 S637 in mutant cells, resulting in the favoring of mitochondrial fission over fusion. Simultaneously, the inhibition of Akt overactivation may contribute to the downregulation of Mfn2 expression, therefore further enhancing the manifestation of the aforementioned effects.

3.5. Formoterol Increased the Efficiency of Mitochondrial Anterograde Transportation and Its Mobility

Time-lapse recordings of MitoGFP-labeled mitochondria, together with corresponding kymographs, were utilized to analyze mitochondrial transport in proximal axons between adjacent cells (Figure 6). The representative kymographs provided in Figure 6a illustrated the bidirectional movement of signals as diagonal lines, revealing more active and abrupt movements of mitochondria in WT cells (Supplementary Video S1) compared to mutant cells (Supplementary Video S2). In addition, WT cells also had a higher velocity for anterograde transport (mean velocity: WT cells, 51.2 $\pm$ 0.013 nm/s; vs. UQCRC1 mutant cells, 7.2 $\pm$ 0.002 nm/s; Figure 6b). The rate of mitochondrial retrograde transport was similar in both WT and mutant cells (Figure 6b). Moreover, a substantial decrease in the fraction of motile mitochondria was noted, showing a 52.6% reduction in anterograde transport and a 48.6% reduction in retrograde transport in mutant cells (Figure 6c). Formoterol treatment significantly enhanced mitochondrial mobility (Supplementary Video S3), elevating anterograde movement velocity by 2.1-fold (mean velocity, 25.6 $\pm$ 0.009 nm/s) and increasing the motile ratio by 1.5-fold compared to the DMSO group (Figure 6c). However, formoterol did not exert significant effects on the frequency and rate of mitochondrial retrograde movement (Figure 6b,c). The induction of mitochondrial velocity and mobility by formoterol was consistently nullified by the addition of propranolol (Figure 6a–c) (Supplementary Video S4). Additionally, individual frames from the time-lapse images presented in Figure 6d further illustrated that mitochondria in the WT and formoterol-treated groups displayed significant forward displacement in axons during the time-lapse sequence (the anterograde direction is indicated by the arrow in Figure 6d). In contrast, stationary mitochondria were observed in the mutant cells and those treated with formoterol plus propranolol or propranolol alone (Figure 6d). These findings indicated that the enhancement in mitochondrial velocity and mobility induced by formoterol occurred through β2-adrenoceptor activation.

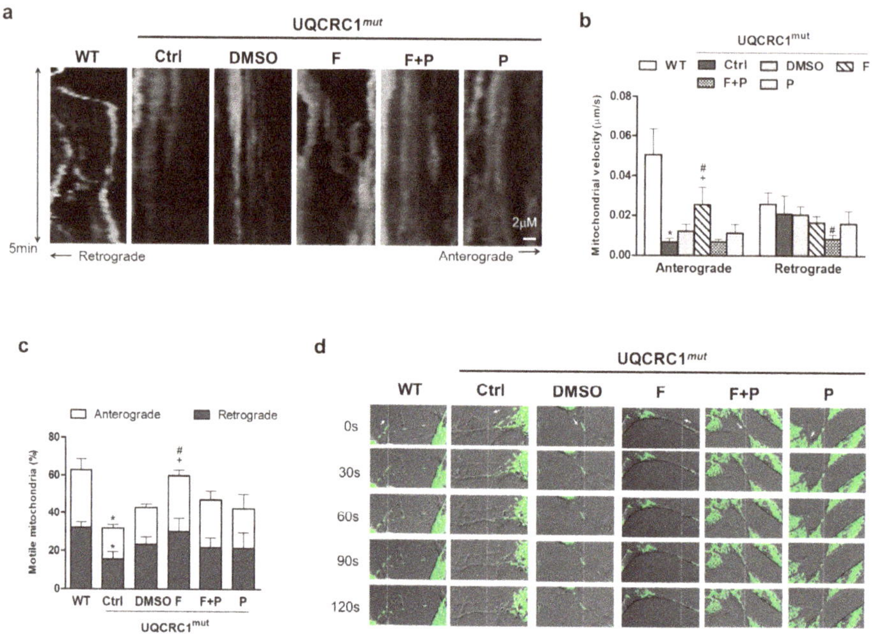

Figure 6. Mitochondrial movement and mobility. Representative kymographs showing the movement of the mitochondria-labeling GFP signal in WT cells or mutant cells with or without 24-h treatments.

Vertical lines were observed for stationary mitochondria, whereas moving mitochondria displayed diagonal lines, indicating their motion in either the anterograde or retrograde direction (**a**). Mitochondrial transport was quantified by measuring mitochondrial velocity (**b**) and calculating the proportion of motile mitochondria exceeding the average velocity in relation to the total mitochondrial population (**c**). Representative time-lapse images specifically showed the mitochondria undergoing anterograde movement (direction indicated by arrows) from their initial position (dashed line, (**d**)). * $p < 0.05$ vs. the WT group. + $p < 0.05$ vs. the DMSO group. # $p < 0.05$ vs. the F + P group. Data are presented as the mean ± SD. WT: wild-type; Ctrl: control; DMSO, dimethylsulfoxide; F, formoterol; F + P: formoterol plus propranolol; P: propranolol; UQCRC1mut: mutation of ubiquinol-cytochrome c reductase core protein 1 gene.

4. Discussion

The effect of formoterol on mitochondrial function has been validated in various diseases, including traumatic brain injury [26], spinal cord injury [27], diabetic kidney disease [28], and acute kidney injury, with those studies providing compelling evidence in support of the use of β2AR ligands for therapeutic mitochondrial biogenesis. This study further demonstrated the therapeutic efficacy of formoterol in PD and explored its impact on mitochondrial dynamics. Abnormalities in fusion and fission processes, crucial in PD pathogenesis [14], are addressed. Formoterol treatment enhanced cell viability, offering protection against ROS-induced cell death. Beyond restoring mitochondrial respiration, it rebalanced mitochondrial dynamics, normalizing the network by segregating healthy mitochondria and facilitating anterograde movement in UQCRC1-mutant cells. Efficacy depended on B2AR activation involving downstream cascades: ERK activation and Akt signaling inhibition. This study underscores formoterol's pivotal role as a mitochondrial dynamic balance regulator, positioning it as a promising therapeutic candidate for PD. On the other hand, understanding the role of mitochondrial homeostasis provides critical insights into the debates surrounding β2AR agonists in PD therapy. By addressing mitochondrial dysregulation, β2AR agonists may offer neuroprotective effects that go beyond symptomatic relief. Clinical trials evaluating β2AR agonists should consider assessing mitochondrial function as a primary outcome measure to elucidate their therapeutic efficacy fully. Moreover, stratifying PD patients based on biomarkers of mitochondrial dysfunction and dynamics dysfunction mitochondrial dysfunction and biomarkers, may help identify subpopulations most likely to benefit from β2AR agonist therapy, therefore resolving uncertainties regarding patient selection and treatment response.

Our study shows that the inhibition of PKA activity by propranolol cotreatment abolished the beneficial effects of formoterol on functional recovery and oxidative stress defense in mutant cells. We propose that the initial PKA activation observed in UQCRC1-mutant cells may serve as a player in neuroprotective mechanisms, as supported by previous research [29,30]. However, restoration of the mitochondrial defects caused by UQCRC1 mutation does not affect PKA activity. It indicates the existence of a mitochondrial function-independent regulation in PKA regulation. For example, calcium ions can activate calmodulin, which subsequently activates adenylate cyclase, leading to elevated cyclic adenosine monophosphate (cAMP) levels and PKA activation. Furthermore, a high level of PKA activity phosphorylates enzymes involved in metabolic pathways and changes metabolic fluxes, which may indirectly affect ATP levels by altering the availability of substrates and intermediates involved in ATP synthesis. Hence, it is plausible that the formoterol treatment had no impact on ATP-linked respiration in mutant cells. Incidentally, although regulating mitochondrial dynamics typically requires significant energy consumption, this is not the case with formoterol's rescue of mitochondrial dynamic abnormalities stemming from mutations in UQCRC1, which impair CIII function in cells. As mitochondrial fragmentation triggered by CIII activity loss operates through energy-independent regulation, it stands in contrast to CV [31]. In particular, our prior research revealed that the mutation in UQCRC1 had minimal effect on the function of CI, CII, or CIV, aside from CIII [17]. This also emphasizes that the relationship between mitochondrial dynamics and mitochondrial oxidative phosphorylation can be dissociated in certain scenarios [32].

PKA activity is primarily regulated by cAMP levels. Elevated cAMP not only boosts PKA activity but also activates adenosine monophosphate-activated protein kinase (AMPK). PKA signaling has been confirmed to induce neuroprotective mitochondrial restructuring into an interconnected network [29]. Otherwise, both PKA and Akt can phosphorylate AMPK to inhibit its activity, resulting in the suppression of mitochondrial fission through Drp-1 phosphorylation [33] and mitochondrial transport in neural axons [34]. Based on our findings, which revealed that formoterol restored mitochondrial fission and anterograde transport by inhibiting Akt phosphorylation while leaving PKA activity unaffected, we propose that the formoterol-mediated inhibition of Akt activation, rather than PKA suppression, plays a pivotal role in regulating the aforementioned mitochondrial dynamics. Further clarification is needed to understand the impact of formoterol on the regulation of AMPK related to mitochondrial dynamics. On the other hand, the consistent finding of extensively interconnected mitochondrial networks observed in UQCRC1-mutant cells is also found in UQCRC2-mutant fibroblasts derived from patients with severe encephalomyopathy [35]. It is well known that UQCRC1 and UQCRC2 are both subunits of CIII that play essential roles in the structure and function of CIII [35]. Unlike UQCRC2-mutant cells, which display an expanded reticular network of mitochondria, more fragmented mitochondria are present [35]. We discovered that UQCRC1 mutation significantly disrupted mitochondrial dynamics, shifting towards hyperfusion, as shown by a notable increase in the reticular network of mitochondria and a decrease in fragmented mitochondria. Reducing mitochondrial stress with formoterol in mutant cells indeed rebalances mitochondrial dynamics and prevents excessive reticular network formation. Indeed, the persistent excessive fusion of mitochondria disrupts both their distribution and turnover, leading to locomotor defects in Drosophila models of Charcot–Marie–Tooth disease type 2A neuropathy [36]. Furthermore, prolonged elongation of mitochondria hinders mitophagy, the process responsible for clearing dysfunctional mitochondria, which in turn diminishes overall mitochondrial function [37,38]. It also disrupts the distribution and transport of mitochondria within cells [32,39], as demonstrated in the present study, and interferes with their interactions with other cellular structures, potentially impacting cellular signaling and response [32].

Formoterol treatment increased Drp-1 activity via phosphorylated Drp1 S616 and dephosphorylated Drp-1 S637 to provide a fine-tuned control of mitochondrial fission and restore an imbalanced mitochondrial dynamic. Drp1, a key regulator of mitochondrial fission, undergoes site-specific phosphorylation. Phosphorylation at Drp1 S616 enhances mitochondrial fission, while phosphorylation at Drp1 Ser637 inhibits this process, triggered by various signaling pathways [40,41]. A current study indicates that the Akt-1 pathway coordinates the concurrent dephosphorylation of Drp1 S616 and phosphorylation of Drp1 S637, leading to the inhibition of mitochondrial fission. Conversely, the promotion of mitochondrial fission through the counter-regulation of Drp1 phosphorylation is mediated by the MEK1-ERK pathway [40]. The two axes of the Akt1–Drp1 and MEK1–ERK-Drp1 pathways can be switched to remodel the mitochondrial dynamics in somatic cell reprogramming [40]. Our finding corroborates this finding: mutant cells with impaired mitochondrial fission exhibit reduced ERK signaling and increased Akt activity compared to WT cells. Formoterol treatment restores mitochondrial dynamics towards fission by concurrently enhancing ERK signaling for Drp-1 S616 phosphorylation and inhibiting Akt signaling for Drp-1 S637 phosphorylation. Furthermore, mutant cells show elevated levels of Mfn2 proteins, in contrast to Drp-1. The physiological levels of Mfn2 expression are strongly correlated with the Akt signaling pathway, to promote mitochondrial fusion [42]. Hence, imbalance in mitochondrial dynamics, favoring fusion over fission, is predominantly attributed to the overactivation of the Akt pathway rather than ERK signals in mutant cells.

Several of the known genes associated with the familial forms of PD are involved in the regulation of mitochondrial function, including Parkin and Pink1 [43]. The downregulation of Pink1 affects the mitochondrial fusion–fission machinery and sensitizes mitochondria to neurotoxins in dopaminergic cells [44]. Pink1 not only phosphorylates Drp-1 S616 to activate mitochondrial fission [45] but also phosphorylates Mfn2 to promote Parkin recruitment for mitophagy, which is a selective process that removes damaged mitochondria [46]. Loss of Pink1 impairs mitochondrial function, leading to mitochondrial dysfunction, increases oxidative stress, and compromises cellular energy production [47]. This is in line with our observation of reduced Pink1 expression in mutant cells. Interestingly, in cells treated with formoterol, both full-length Pink1 and its 52-kDa cleaved form [48] were upregulated, whereas the levels of Parkin and Mfn2 were significantly decreased. We suggest that the formoterol-induced upregulation of Pink1, with consequent mitochondrial fission, does not activate mitophagy. Since Pink1 also regulates mitochondrial fission by phosphorylating Drp1 S616 through a mechanism independent of mitophagy [45]. Moreover, when Pink1 is cleaved at the inner mitochondrial membrane, it retro-translocates to the cytosol, inhibiting Parkin translocation to mitochondria and suppressing mitophagy [49]. Although the precise role of cleaved Pink1, induced by formoterol, in neuronal functions, remains unclear, in healthy mitochondria, it plays vital extramitochondrial roles crucial for neuronal development, survival, synaptogenesis, and plasticity, with significant implications for PD [50,51]. Thus, we suggest that the restoration of Pink1 could play a multifaceted role in supporting neuronal function in the context of the benefits of formoterol.

Formoterol has been shown to decrease the glucose-induced imbalance in mitochondrial dynamics and restore mitochondrial homeostasis in the context of renal proximal tubule cells under diabetic conditions [28]. A similar regulatory role of formoterol was found in the treatment of UQCRC1-mutant cells, resulting in PD, although the specific mechanisms underlying the regulation of mitochondrial homeostasis appear to be dependent on various cellular contexts. Moreover, our findings provide further evidence of the beneficial effects of formoterol, as it significantly promoted anterograde mitochondrial transport and increased mitochondrial mobility. Several studies have explored strategies aimed at enhancing anterograde mitochondrial transport as a means of neuroprotection to manage mitochondrial dysfunction-related neurodegenerative disorders [52–54]. The promotion of mitochondrial anterograde movement facilitates the transport of mitochondria toward axon terminals to support the energy demands required for synaptic transmission and neuronal signaling [53,54], maintain mitochondrial health via the overall quality control of mitochondria within neurons [54], and ensure proper neuronal functions, such as calcium regulation, excitability, and neurotransmission [52,53]. Additionally, the effects of formoterol on healthy SH-SY5Y cells have also been recognized as a crucial factor in neuroprotection and neuroregeneration [55]. This was achieved through the increase in brain-derived neurotrophic factor (BDNF), which is well known for enhancing neuronal survival, differentiation, and synaptic plasticity, along with its receptor TrkB [55]. However, further investigation is necessary to completely understand its mechanisms in neural regulation.

While preclinical evidence indicates promise for formoterol's neuroprotective potential in PD, clinical data regarding the disease-modifying effects of β2AR agonists remains inconclusive. This uncertainty stems from various challenges, including the need to optimize dosing regimens, comprehend the long-term safety profile of formoterol in PD patients, and identify dependable biomarkers for monitoring treatment response and disease progression, which remain unresolved. Further research is essential to uncover the mechanistic basis of formoterol's neuroprotective effects and determine its efficacy as a disease-modifying therapy for PD using human-relevant systems. Patient-derived cell models, such as induced pluripotent stem cells from PD, offer a unique platform for further assessing formoterol's efficacy and safety, closely mirroring the pathophysiological mechanisms of abnormal mitochondrial homeostasis in PD.

5. Conclusions

In summary, by activating B2AR, formoterol not only enhanced mitochondrial function but also corrected the imbalance in mitochondrial dynamics and transportation. This correction contributed to improving the disruption of mitochondrial homeostasis in familial PD caused by mitochondrial genetic defects. The regulatory mechanism involves the restoration of ERK signaling and the inhibition of Akt overactivity, contingent on the activation of β2AR. Formoterol's neuroprotective effects, attributed to its regulation of mitochondrial dynamic balance to uphold mitochondrial homeostasis, suggest promising potential for treating other neurodegenerative diseases with a similar etiology. Moving forward, it is essential to further validate the specificity of formoterol's impact through β2AR on mitochondrial dynamics by integrating experiments involving β2AR knockdown or overexpression, alongside confirming this regulatory mechanism in vivo.

Supplementary Materials: The following supporting information can be downloaded at: https://www.mdpi.com/article/10.3390/biology13040231/s1, Figure S1: Cell viability of wild-type and mutant UQCRC1 knock-in human neuroblastoma SH-SY5Y cells exposed to various doses of formoterol for 24 h; Table S1: Distinct differences in expression of phosphorylated proteins among the compared sets of groups; Video S1: Movement of MitoGFP-labeled mitochondria in wild-type cells; Video S2: Movement of MitoGFP-labeled mitochondria in DMSO-treated UQCRC1-mutant cells; Video S3: Movement of MitoGFP-labeled mitochondria in formoterol-treated UQCRC1-mutant cells; Video S4: Movement of MitoGFP-labeled mitochondria in formoterol plus Propranolol-treated UQCRC1-mutant cells.

Author Contributions: J.-C.C.: Investigation, Methodology, Writing—original draft, Writing—review and editing, Project administration. H.-S.C.: Investigation, Methodology, Validation. Y.-C.C.: Investigation, Validation. C.-S.H.: Investigation, Validation. C.-H.L.: Resources, Methodology, Funding acquisition. Z.-S.W.: Investigation. H.-J.C.: Investigation. C.-S.L.: Resources, Supervision. C.-S.C.: Conceptualization, Supervision, Funding acquisition, Writing—review and editing. All authors have read and agreed to the published version of the manuscript.

Funding: This research was funded by the National Science and Technology Council (MOST 108-2321-B-002-060-MY2) and granted from Changhua Christine Hospital (110-CCH-IRP-097, 111-CCH-IRP-065).

Institutional Review Board Statement: Not applicable.

Informed Consent Statement: Not applicable.

Data Availability Statement: The datasets generated during and/or analyzed during the current study are not publicly available as consent for publication of raw data was not obtained from study participants, but they are available from the corresponding author upon reasonable request.

Acknowledgments: The authors would like to thank Chin-Hsien Lin (National Taiwan University Hospital, Taiwan) for their valuable contributions to cell lines and research support.

Conflicts of Interest: The authors declare no conflicts of interest.

References

1. Billington, C.K.; Penn, R.B.; Hall, I.P. β_2 Agonists. In *Pharmacology and Therapeutics of Asthma and COPD*; Springer: Cham, Switzerland, 2017; pp. 23–40.
2. Bello, F.D.; Giannella, M.; Giorgioni, G.; Piergentili, A.; Quaglia, W. Receptor ligands as helping hands to L-DOPA in the treatment of Parkinson's disease. *Biomolecules* **2019**, *9*, 142. [CrossRef] [PubMed]
3. Chen, W.; Sadatsafavi, M.; Tavakoli, H.; Samii, A.; Etminan, M. Effects of β_2-Adrenergic Agonists on Risk of Parkinson's Disease in COPD: A Population-Based Study. *Pharmacother. J. Hum. Pharmacol. Drug Ther.* **2020**, *40*, 408–415. [CrossRef] [PubMed]
4. Ton, T.G.; Heckbert, S.R.; Longstreth, W., Jr.; Rossing, M.A.; Kukull, W.A.; Franklin, G.M.; Swanson, P.D.; Smith-Weller, T.; Checkoway, H. Calcium channel blockers and β-blockers in relation to Parkinson's disease. *Park. Relat. Disord.* **2007**, *13*, 165–169. [CrossRef] [PubMed]
5. Peterson, L.; Ismond, K.P.; Chapman, E.; Flood, P. Potential benefits of therapeutic use of β_2-adrenergic receptor agonists in neuroprotection and Parkinson's disease. *J. Immunol. Res.* **2014**, *2014*. [CrossRef] [PubMed]
6. Koren, G.; Norton, G.; Radinsky, K.; Shalev, V. Chronic Use of β-Blockers and the Risk of Parkinson's Disease. *Clin. Drug Investig.* **2019**, *39*, 463–468. [CrossRef] [PubMed]

7. Gronich, N.; Abernethy, D.R.; Auriel, E.; Lavi, I.; Rennert, G.; Saliba, W. β_2-adrenoceptor agonists and antagonists and risk of Parkinson's disease. *Mov. Disord.* **2018**, *33*, 1465–1471. [CrossRef]
8. Chen, C.-L.; Wang, S.-Y.; Chen, T.-C.; Chuang, C.-S. Association between β_2-adrenoreceptor medications and risk of Parkinson's disease: A meta-analysis. *Medicina* **2021**, *57*, 1006. [CrossRef] [PubMed]
9. Mittal, S.; Bjørnevik, K.; Im, D.S.; Flierl, A.; Dong, X.; Locascio, J.J.; Abo, K.M.; Long, E.; Jin, M.; Xu, B.; et al. β_2-Adrenoreceptor is a regulator of the α-synuclein gene driving risk of Parkinson's disease. *Science* **2017**, *357*, 891–898. [CrossRef] [PubMed]
10. O'Neill, E.; Yssel, J.D.; McNamara, C.; Harkin, A. Pharmacological targeting of β_2-adrenoceptors is neuroprotective in the LPS inflammatory rat model of Parkinson's disease. *Br. J. Pharmacol.* **2020**, *177*, 282–297. [CrossRef] [PubMed]
11. Anderson, G.P. Current issues with β_2-adrenoceptor agonists: Pharmacology and molecular and cellular mechanisms. *Clin. Rev. Allergy Immunol.* **2006**, *31*, 119–130. [CrossRef] [PubMed]
12. Azevedo Voltarelli, V.; Coronado, M.; Gonçalves Fernandes, L.; Cruz Campos, J.; Jannig, P.R.; Batista Ferreira, J.C.; Fajardo, G.; Chakur Brum, P.; Bernstein, D. β_2-Adrenergic signaling modulates mitochondrial function and morphology in skeletal muscle in response to aerobic exercise. *Cells* **2021**, *10*, 146. [CrossRef] [PubMed]
13. Chen, N.; Ge, M.-M.; Li, D.-Y.; Wang, X.-M.; Liu, D.-Q.; Ye, D.-W.; Tian, Y.-K.; Zhou, Y.-Q.; Chen, J.-P. β_2-adrenoreceptor agonist ameliorates mechanical allodynia in paclitaxel-induced neuropathic pain via induction of mitochondrial biogenesis. *Biomed. Pharmacother.* **2021**, *144*, 112331. [CrossRef] [PubMed]
14. Chen, H.; Chan, D.C. Mitochondrial dynamics–fusion, fission, movement, and mitophagy–in neurodegenerative diseases. *Hum. Mol. Genet.* **2009**, *18*, R169–R176. [CrossRef] [PubMed]
15. Zheng, Y.R.; Zhang, X.N.; Chen, Z. Mitochondrial transport serves as a mitochondrial quality control strategy in axons: Implications for central nervous system disorders. *CNS Neurosci. Ther.* **2019**, *25*, 876–886. [CrossRef] [PubMed]
16. Cho, D.-H.; Nakamura, T.; Lipton, S.A. Mitochondrial dynamics in cell death and neurodegeneration. *Cell. Mol. Life Sci.* **2010**, *67*, 3435–3447. [CrossRef]
17. Lin, C.-H.; Tsai, P.-I.; Lin, H.-Y.; Hattori, N.; Funayama, M.; Jeon, B.; Sato, K.; Abe, K.; Mukai, Y.; Takahashi, Y.; et al. Mitochondrial UQCRC1 mutations cause autosomal dominant parkinsonism with polyneuropathy. *Brain* **2020**, *143*, 3352–3373. [CrossRef] [PubMed]
18. Lin, C.H.; Chen, P.L.; Tai, C.H.; Lin, H.I.; Chen, C.S.; Chen, M.L.; Wu, R.M. A clinical and genetic study of early-onset and familial parkinsonism in Taiwan: An integrated approach combining gene dosage analysis and next-generation sequencing. *Mov. Disord.* **2019**, *34*, 506–515. [CrossRef] [PubMed]
19. Hung, Y.-C.; Huang, K.-L.; Chen, P.-L.; Li, J.-L.; Lu, S.H.-A.; Chang, J.-C.; Lin, H.-Y.; Lo, W.-C.; Huang, S.-Y.; Lee, T.-T.; et al. UQCRC1 engages cytochrome c for neuronal apoptotic cell death. *Cell Rep.* **2021**, *36*, 109729. [CrossRef]
20. Li, J.-L.; Lin, T.-Y.; Chen, P.-L.; Guo, T.-N.; Huang, S.-Y.; Chen, C.-H.; Lin, C.-H.; Chan, C.-C. Mitochondrial function and Parkinson's disease: From the perspective of the electron transport chain. *Front. Mol. Neurosci.* **2021**, *14*, 797833. [CrossRef]
21. Chang, J.-C.; Wu, S.-L.; Liu, K.-H.; Chen, Y.-H.; Chuang, C.-S.; Cheng, F.-C.; Su, H.-L.; Wei, Y.-H.; Kuo, S.-J.; Liu, C.-S. Allogeneic/xenogeneic transplantation of peptide-labeled mitochondria in Parkinson's disease: Restoration of mitochondria functions and attenuation of 6-hydroxydopamine–induced neurotoxicity. *Transl. Res.* **2016**, *170*, 40–56.e3. [CrossRef]
22. Peng, J.-Y.; Lin, C.-C.; Chen, Y.-J.; Kao, L.-S.; Liu, Y.-C.; Chou, C.-C.; Huang, Y.-H.; Chang, F.-R.; Wu, Y.-C.; Tsai, Y.-S.; et al. Automatic morphological subtyping reveals new roles of caspases in mitochondrial dynamics. *PLoS Comput. Biol.* **2011**, *7*, e1002212. [CrossRef] [PubMed]
23. Wu, H.-C.; Fan, X.; Hu, C.-H.; Chao, Y.-C.; Liu, C.-S.; Chang, J.-C.; Sen, Y. Comparison of mitochondrial transplantation by using a stamp-type multineedle injector and platelet-rich plasma therapy for hair aging in naturally aging mice. *Biomed. Pharmacother.* **2020**, *130*, 110520. [CrossRef] [PubMed]
24. Suh, B.K.; Lee, S.; Park, C.; Suh, Y.; Kim, S.J.; Woo, Y.; Nhung, T.T.M.; Lee, S.B.; Mun, D.J.; Goo, B.S.; et al. Schizophrenia-associated dysbindin modulates axonal mitochondrial movement in cooperation with p150glued. *Mol. Brain* **2021**, *14*, 14. [CrossRef] [PubMed]
25. Hussain, S.A.; Venkatesh, T. YBX1/lncRNA SBF2-AS1 interaction regulates proliferation and tamoxifen sensitivity via PI3K/AKT/MTOR signaling in breast cancer cells. *Mol. Biol. Rep.* **2023**, *50*, 3413–3428. [CrossRef] [PubMed]
26. Vekaria, H.J.; Hubbard, W.B.; Scholpa, N.E.; Spry, M.L.; Gooch, J.L.; Prince, S.J.; Schnellmann, R.G.; Sullivan, P.G. Formoterol, a β_2-adrenoreceptor agonist, induces mitochondrial biogenesis and promotes cognitive recovery after traumatic brain injury. *Neurobiol. Dis.* **2020**, *140*, 104866. [CrossRef] [PubMed]
27. Cameron, R.B.; Gibbs, W.S.; Miller, S.R.; Dupre, T.V.; Megyesi, J.; Beeson, C.C.; Schnellmann, R.G. Proximal tubule β_2-adrenergic receptor mediates formoterol-induced recovery of mitochondrial and renal function after ischemia-reperfusion injury. *J. Pharmacol. Exp. Ther.* **2019**, *369*, 173–180. [CrossRef] [PubMed]
28. Cleveland, K.H.; Brosius, F.C., III; Schnellmann, R.G. Regulation of mitochondrial dynamics and energetics in the diabetic renal proximal tubule by the β_2-adrenergic receptor agonist formoterol. *Am. J. Physiol.-Ren. Physiol.* **2020**, *319*, F773–F779. [CrossRef] [PubMed]
29. Merrill, R.A.; Dagda, R.K.; Dickey, A.S.; Cribbs, J.T.; Green, S.H.; Usachev, Y.M.; Strack, S. Mechanism of neuroprotective mitochondrial remodeling by PKA/AKAP1. *PLoS Biol.* **2011**, *9*, e1000612. [CrossRef] [PubMed]

30. Zhang, J.; Feng, J.; Ma, D.; Wang, F.; Wang, Y.; Li, C.; Wang, X.; Yin, X.; Zhang, M.; Dagda, R.K.; et al. Neuroprotective mitochondrial remodeling by AKAP121/PKA protects HT22 cell from glutamate-induced oxidative stress. *Mol. Neurobiol.* **2019**, *56*, 5586–5607. [CrossRef] [PubMed]
31. van der Stel, W.; Yang, H.; le Dévédec, S.E.; van de Water, B.; Beltman, J.B.; Danen, E.H. High-content high-throughput imaging reveals distinct connections between mitochondrial morphology and functionality for OXPHOS complex I, III, and V inhibitors. *Cell Biol. Toxicol.* **2022**, *39*, 415–433. [CrossRef] [PubMed]
32. Huang, D.; Chen, S.; Xiong, D.; Wang, H.; Zhu, L.; Wei, Y.; Li, Y.; Zou, S. Mitochondrial Dynamics: Working with the Cytoskeleton and Intracellular Organelles to Mediate Mechanotransduction. *Aging Dis.* **2023**, *14*, 1511–1532. [CrossRef] [PubMed]
33. Toyama, E.Q.; Herzig, S.; Courchet, J.; Lewis, T.L., Jr.; Losón, O.C.; Hellberg, K.; Young, N.P.; Chen, H.; Polleux, F.; Chan, D.C.; et al. AMP-activated protein kinase mediates mitochondrial fission in response to energy stress. *Science* **2016**, *351*, 275–281. [CrossRef] [PubMed]
34. Tao, K.; Matsuki, N.; Koyama, R. AMP-activated protein kinase mediates activity-dependent axon branching by recruiting mitochondria to axon. *Dev. Neurobiol.* **2014**, *74*, 557–573. [CrossRef] [PubMed]
35. Burska, D.; Stiburek, L.; Krizova, J.; Vanisova, M.; Martinek, V.; Sladkova, J.; Zamecnik, J.; Honzik, T.; Zeman, J.; Hansikova, H.; et al. Homozygous missense mutation in UQCRC2 associated with severe encephalomyopathy, mitochondrial complex III assembly defect and activation of mitochondrial protein quality control. *Biochim. Biophys. Acta Mol. Basis Dis.* **2021**, *1867*, 166147. [CrossRef]
36. El Fissi, N.; Rojo, M.; Aouane, A.; Karatas, E.; Poliacikova, G.; David, C.; Royet, J.; Rival, T. Mitofusin gain and loss of function drive pathogenesis in Drosophila models of CMT 2A neuropathy. *EMBO Rep.* **2018**, *19*, e45241. [CrossRef] [PubMed]
37. Yoon, Y.S.; Yoon, D.S.; Lim, I.K.; Yoon, S.H.; Chung, H.Y.; Rojo, M.; Malka, F.; Jou, M.J.; Martinou, J.C.; Yoon, G. Formation of elongated giant mitochondria in DFO-induced cellular senescence: Involvement of enhanced fusion process through modulation of Fis1. *J. Cell. Physiol.* **2006**, *209*, 468–480. [CrossRef] [PubMed]
38. Vasileiou, P.V.S.; Evangelou, K.; Vlasis, K.; Fildisis, G.; Panayiotidis, M.I.; Chronopoulos, E.; Passias, P.-G.; Kouloukoussa, M.; Gorgoulis, V.G.; Havaki, S. Mitochondrial homeostasis and cellular senescence. *Cells* **2019**, *8*, 686. [CrossRef] [PubMed]
39. Picard, M.; Shirihai, O.S.; Gentil, B.J.; Burelle, Y. Mitochondrial morphology transitions and functions: Implications for retrograde signaling? *Am. J. Physiol. Regul. Integr. Comp. Physiol.* **2013**, *304*, R393–R406. [CrossRef] [PubMed]
40. Cha, Y.; Kim, T.; Jeon, J.; Jang, Y.; Kim, P.B.; Lopes, C.; Leblanc, P.; Cohen, B.M.; Kim, K.-S. SIRT2 regulates mitochondrial dynamics and reprogramming via MEK1-ERK-DRP1 and AKT1-DRP1 axes. *Cell Rep.* **2021**, *37*, 110155. [CrossRef] [PubMed]
41. Ren, L.; Chen, X.; Chen, X.; Li, J.; Cheng, B.; Xia, J. Mitochondrial dynamics: Fission and fusion in fate determination of mesenchymal stem cells. *Front. Cell Dev. Biol.* **2020**, *8*, 580070. [CrossRef] [PubMed]
42. Yi, S.; Cui, C.; Huang, X.; Yin, X.; Li, Y.; Wen, J.; Luan, Q. MFN2 silencing promotes neural differentiation of embryonic stem cells via the Akt signaling pathway. *J. Cell. Physiol.* **2020**, *235*, 1051–1064. [CrossRef] [PubMed]
43. Gasser, T. Update on the genetics of Parkinson's disease. *Mov. Disord.* **2007**, *22*, S343–S350. [CrossRef] [PubMed]
44. Rojas-Charry, L.; Cookson, M.R.; Niño, A.; Arboleda, H.; Arboleda, G. Downregulation of Pink1 influences mitochondrial fusion–fission machinery and sensitizes to neurotoxins in dopaminergic cells. *Neurotoxicology* **2014**, *44*, 140–148. [CrossRef] [PubMed]
45. Han, H.; Tan, J.; Wang, R.; Wan, H.; He, Y.; Yan, X.; Guo, J.; Gao, Q.; Li, J.; Shang, S.; et al. PINK 1 phosphorylates Drp1S616 to regulate mitophagy-independent mitochondrial dynamics. *EMBO Rep.* **2020**, *21*, e48686. [CrossRef] [PubMed]
46. Chen, Y.; Dorn, G.W. PINK1-phosphorylated mitofusin 2 is a Parkin receptor for culling damaged mitochondria. *Science* **2013**, *340*, 471–475. [CrossRef] [PubMed]
47. Gautier, C.A.; Kitada, T.; Shen, J. Loss of PINK1 causes mitochondrial functional defects and increased sensitivity to oxidative stress. *Proc. Natl. Acad. Sci. USA* **2008**, *105*, 11364–11369. [CrossRef] [PubMed]
48. Liu, Y.; Guardia-Laguarta, C.; Yin, J.; Erdjument-Bromage, H.; Martin, B.; James, M.; Jiang, X.; Przedborski, S. The ubiquitination of PINK1 is restricted to its mature 52-kDa form. *Cell Rep.* **2017**, *20*, 30–39. [CrossRef] [PubMed]
49. Fedorowicz, M.A.; de Vries-Schneider, R.L.; Rüb, C.; Becker, D.; Huang, Y.; Zhou, C.; Alessi Wolken, D.M.; Voos, W.; Liu, Y.; Przedborski, S. Cytosolic cleaved PINK1 represses Parkin translocation to mitochondria and mitophagy. *EMBO Rep.* **2014**, *15*, 86–93. [CrossRef] [PubMed]
50. Soman, S.K.; Dagda, R.K. Role of Cleaved PINK1 in Neuronal Development, Synaptogenesis, and Plasticity: Implications for Parkinson's Disease. *Front. Neurosci.* **2021**, *15*, 769331. [CrossRef]
51. Wang, N.; Zhu, P.; Huang, R.; Wang, C.; Sun, L.; Lan, B.; He, Y.; Zhao, H.; Gao, Y. PINK1: The guard of mitochondria. *Life Sci.* **2020**, *259*, 118247. [CrossRef] [PubMed]
52. Norat, P.; Soldozy, S.; Sokolowski, J.D.; Gorick, C.M.; Kumar, J.S.; Chae, Y.; Yağmurlu, K.; Prada, F.; Walker, M.; Levitt, M.R.; et al. Mitochondrial dysfunction in neurological disorders: Exploring mitochondrial transplantation. *npj Regen. Med.* **2020**, *5*, 22. [CrossRef] [PubMed]
53. Sheng, Z.-H.; Cai, Q. Mitochondrial transport in neurons: Impact on synaptic homeostasis and neurodegeneration. *Nat. Rev. Neurosci.* **2012**, *13*, 77–93. [CrossRef] [PubMed]

54. Mandal, A.; Drerup, C.M. Axonal transport and mitochondrial function in neurons. *Front. Cell. Neurosci.* **2019**, *13*, 373. [CrossRef] [PubMed]
55. Ishida, A.; Ohta, T.; Toda, A.; Murata, K.; Usui, C.; Narita, N.; Tanaka, T.; Otani, H. Formoterol, a Long-Acting Beta2 Adrenergic Agonist, Improves Cognitive Function and Promotes Dendritic Complexity in a Mouse Model of Down Syndrome. *J. Alzheimer's Dis.* **2013**, *37*, 557–570.

biology

MDPI

Review

Double-Edged Sword: Exploring the Mitochondria–Complement Bidirectional Connection in Cellular Response and Disease

Jingfei (Carly) Lin [1,2,†], Sinwoo (Wendy) Hwang [1,2,†], Honglin Luo [1,2,*] and Yasir Mohamud [1,2,*]

1 Centre for Heart Lung Innovation, St. Paul's Hospital, Vancouver, BC V6Z 1Y6, Canada
2 Department of Pathology and Laboratory Medicine, University of British Columbia, Vancouver, BC V6Z 1Y6, Canada
* Correspondence: honglin.luo@hli.ubc.ca (H.L.); yasir.mohamud@hli.ubc.ca (Y.M.)
† These authors contributed equally to this work.

Simple Summary: Complement system is an ancient immune pathway that protects us against harmful invaders. Meanwhile, mitochondria, widely known as the powerhouse of the cell, are essential for producing energy and maintaining healthy cells. Bridging past and present studies, this review aims to elucidate an underexplored yet essential connection between the complement system and mitochondria. These interactions are implicated in different diseases across various tissues and organs, such as Alzheimer's disease and cancer, that are in critical need of cure. Mitochondria release signals that impact the activation of the complement system, leading to tissue damage and inflammation; while the complement system alters mitochondrial functions, forming a vicious cycle. This cycle exacerbates disease progression and health outcomes. We hope to highlight potential targets to alleviate societal healthcare burdens by bringing scientists' attention to this novel bidirectional interaction.

Abstract: Mitochondria serve an ultimate purpose that seeks to balance the life and death of cells, a role that extends well beyond the tissue and organ systems to impact not only normal physiology but also the pathogenesis of diverse diseases. Theorized to have originated from ancient proto-bacteria, mitochondria share similarities with bacterial cells, including their own circular DNA, double-membrane structures, and fission dynamics. It is no surprise, then, that mitochondria interact with a bacterium-targeting immune pathway known as a complement system. The complement system is an ancient and sophisticated arm of the immune response that serves as the body's first line of defense against microbial invaders. It operates through a complex cascade of protein activations, rapidly identifying and neutralizing pathogens, and even aiding in the clearance of damaged cells and immune complexes. This dynamic system, intertwining innate and adaptive immunity, holds secrets to understanding numerous diseases. In this review, we explore the bidirectional interplay between mitochondrial dysfunction and the complement system through the release of mitochondrial damage-associated molecular patterns. Additionally, we explore several mitochondria- and complement-related diseases and the potential for new therapeutic strategies.

Keywords: mitochondria; complement system; innate immunity; cell signaling; damage-associated molecular patterns (DAMPs)

1. Introduction

Mitochondria are dynamic organelles critical for key processes, including cellular energy production through oxidative phosphorylation (OXPHOS), metabolism, homeostasis, and cell signaling. Hence known as the powerhouse of the cell, mitochondrial dysfunction can lead to severe consequences. Impaired mitochondria have a causal relationship with several diseases, such as neurodegenerative disorders, metabolic syndromes, and cardiovascular diseases [1–3].

Interestingly, the endosymbiotic theory proposes that mitochondria share an evolutionary ancestry with bacteria. Hence, as remnants of ancient bacteria within host cells, the immune system may perceive mitochondria as foreign entities. Among the diverse immune responses, the complement pathway is widely recognized as a first-line defense against microbial infections. Comprised of over 30 secreted and membrane-bound proteins, the complement system serves diverse functions in both innate immunity and adaptive immune responses [4,5]. The complement system can detect pathogens by three main pathways to trigger a cascade of reactions, leading to inflammation, cell death, and pathogen elimination. In the last decade, advances in complement research have revealed novel functions of the complement system, including the intracellular complement system, known as the complosome [6,7]. The complosome has been found to play a central role in metabolism and cellular homeostasis, modulating essential processes in mitochondria such as glycolysis, ATP generation, and OXPHOS [8–11]. Considering the revelations, further investigation of the implications in cellular mechanisms and disease is needed. While the term "complosome" is specifically employed to denote intracellular complement, this review refrains from making a clear differentiation between intracellular and extracellular complement elements. Given the recent establishment of the complosome concept, distinctions between these compartments remain to be further characterized.

In the past 30 years, novel insights have revealed a tight relationship between the complement system and mitochondria. The complement system employs pattern recognition receptors to detect damage-associated molecular patterns (DAMPs) released from infected, injured, or stressed cells, signaling an immune response [12–15]. Under stress, mitochondria release DAMPs, triggering activation of the innate immune system, which can result in heightened oxidative stress and additional damage to mitochondria, leading to a destructive cycle [16–19]. However, the impact of this interaction on disease pathogenesis is underexplored. Exploring the complex relationship between the complement system and mitochondria in various diseases will help reveal potential therapeutic targets. This review aims to provide an in-depth examination of the reciprocal relationship between mitochondrial dysfunction and the complement system, with a particular focus on their implications in immune signaling and their role in disease pathogenesis.

2. Mitochondria

Mitochondria play pivotal roles in diverse cellular processes, including ion homeostasis and programmed cell death/apoptosis. When subjected to stressors such as genetic mutations, viral infections, or aging, mitochondria are damaged and activate quality control mechanisms to maintain homeostasis. Mitochondria are constantly under dynamic changes through fission and fusion processes, allowing for the removal of damaged mitochondrial segments and the exchange of components [20–22]. Mitophagy is another important pathway whereby autophagosomes selectively remove damaged or dysfunctional mitochondria [23]. Alternatively, the mitochondrial unfolded protein response induces protein folding and eliminates damaged components [24,25].

Mitochondria release DAMPs in response to cellular distress. Under ideal circumstances, quality control processes effectively mitigate stressors, so mitochondrial release of DAMPs would be minimized. However, under extreme stress, when quality control processes prove insufficient, mitochondria release DAMPs such as cytochrome c, reactive oxygen species (ROS), mitochondrial DNA (mtDNA), cardiolipin, and ATP [26–28]. DAMPs can also induce numerous innate immune responses [29]. Furthermore, extracellular accumulation of ATP can lead to loss of mitochondrial membrane potential, disrupting ion homeostasis and cellular bioenergetics [26]. This impairment affects processes reliant on energy availability, such as active transport, cellular signaling, and maintenance of membrane potential [26,29]. Additionally, the release of mtDNA can be recognized by cyclic GAMP-AMP synthase/cGAS, triggering inflammation through the type-I interferon (IFN) pathway [30]. In summary, while mitochondria employ quality control processes to maintain homeostasis, profound mitochondrial damage leads to disrupted ATP production, overproduction of ROS, and cell death. This results in DAMP release to induce innate immune responses. Hence, understanding the ramifications of mitochondrial dysfunction is crucial for developing targeted therapies.

3. Complement System

The complement system is part of the innate immune system. The extracellular complement system is activated through three main pathways: classical, alternative, and lectin pathways. Although each pathway is initiated by different signaling processes, they all converge on the formation of complement component 3 (C3) convertase, which activates C3 by cleavage. Activation of C3 produces building blocks for complement component 5 (C5) convertase, which in turn activates C5. Additionally, activation of complement proteins produces opsonins (e.g., complement component 1q (C1q), C3b, inactivated C3b (iC3b), C3d) and anaphylatoxins (e.g., C3a and C5a) that opsonize pathogens for phagocytosis and recruit immune cells to the site of activation, respectively [4,31]. Ultimately, activation of the complement system leads to the formation of a membrane attack complex (MAC), a pore structure on the cell membrane that causes osmotic imbalance, leading to cell lysis. Recent discoveries of the complosome have demonstrated non-canonical functions of the complement system apart from its canonical functions in immune defense, including opsonization, inflammation, and cell lysis. A summary of the intracellular and extracellular complement system is shown in Figure 1.

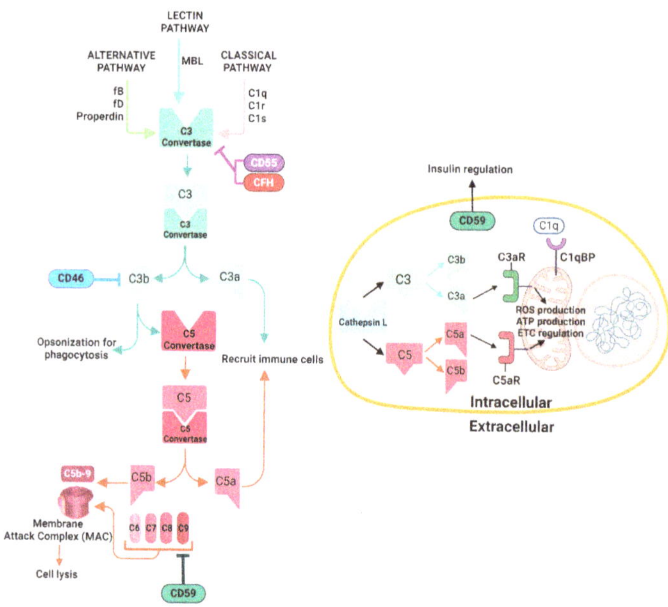

Figure 1. The extracellular and intracellular complement system. The complement system is activated by three main pathways: the classical pathway via C1q, C1s, and C1r forming the C1 complex; the lectin pathway via mannose-binding lectin (MBL); and the alternative pathway via spontaneous hydrolysis of C3, involving factor B (fB), factor D (fD), and properdin. All three pathways converge on the formation of the C3 convertase, which activates C3 by cleaving it into C3a and C3b. C3b, along with other complement components, forms the C5 convertase, which activates C5 by cleaving it into C5a and C5b. The cascade of reactions leads to the formation of the membrane attack complex (MAC). Regulators of the complement system (such as complement factor H (CFH), CD55, CD59, CD46) inhibit different steps of the cascade as indicated. Intracellular CD59 also has a role in insulin regulation. C1q, C3a, and C5a bind to receptors located on mitochondria, regulating mitochondrial functions.

3.1. Internalization Mechanisms of Complement Proteins

Complement proteins are not only produced intracellularly but can also be re-ingested and retro-translocated into the cell. For instance, King et al. found that C3 contains alternative ATG start codons, enabling its translation in the cytosol [32]. They discovered that this form of C3 loses the ability to be secreted and can rescue autophagy in cells with C3 knockout, whereas uptake of extracellular C3 does not achieve this. Additionally, C3 can be produced and secreted, then taken up again by the same cell. For example, Kremlitzka et al. demonstrated that alternative translation start sites of C3 result in the production of the cytosolic form of C3 without glycosylation, exhibiting distinct functions compared to the serum form [33]. The same study also showed that intracellular C3 is retro-translocated from the ER to the cytosol [33]. Similarly, Golec et al. suggested that CD59 is retro-translocated from the ER to the cytosol, and that cytosolic CD59 lacks a glycosylphosphatidylinositol (GPI) anchor [34]. While silencing CD59 resulted in dysregulated insulin production, removing the GPI anchor did not do so, suggesting the existence of an intracellular, non-GPI-anchored pool of CD59 that functions in insulin secretion [34]. Together, this evidence suggests that intracellular complement proteins such as C3 and CD59 have unique genetic and functional profiles, involving intracellular production, retro-translocation, and distinct roles in cellular processes, diverging significantly from their extracellular counterparts.

3.2. Intracellular Complement System

The complement system is predominantly recognized as a liver-derived and serum-circulating extracellular system. Although most complement factors are produced in the liver and secreted, C3 and C5 can also be produced and secreted by T cells [6,9]. Serum complement components can bind to receptors on the surface of T cells to induce effector function and intracellular C3 and C5 production [35,36]. Additionally, C3 and C5 can be activated intracellularly in T cells [9,37]. While the majority of complement is systemic, local production by specific cell types serves specific functions [37]. For example, C1q is mostly/only produced by immune cells including macrophages and dendritic cells [37–39]. Furthermore, C3a receptor (C3aR) and C5a receptor (C5aR) are present on intracellular lysosomal membranes and mitochondrial membranes [6,8,40,41]. These recent insights call for further research into cellular and mechanistic consequences of the complosome within intracellular processes.

Ample evidence demonstrates the presence of diverse complement proteins intracellularly, such as complement factor H (CFH), CD59 (also known as protectin), C3, and C5. CFH is a complement regulator that accelerates the decay of the C3 convertase and serves as a cofactor in the inactivation of C3. CFH was found to localize to lysosomes and acts as a cofactor for cathepsin L (CTSL) in cleavage of C3 into iC3b [42]. In addition, CD59, a GPI-anchored negative regulator of MAC, was found to have intracellular functions in insulin secretions [34].

Complement proteins such as C3 have been discovered intracellularly and can activate immune responses, such as flagging viruses for degradation, mitochondrial antiviral signaling (MAVS), and cytokine production [43]. Cytosolic C3 was reported to interact with cytosolic proteins, such as ATG16L, a component of the autophagy mechanism that converts LC3-I to LC3-II, resulting in an autophagy-dependent restriction of bacterial growth [32,44]. Liszewski et al. demonstrated that C3 is activated intracellularly by CTSL, independent of C3 convertases in T cells [6]. It has also been suggested that C3 is stored in the endoplasmic reticulum and lysosomes in T cells, and the cleavage fragment C3a has a receptor on the lysosome. Upon C3a binding to C3aR, lysosomes can activate glycolysis and OXPHOS, leading to IFN production and activation of both T helper and cytotoxic T cells [6,8]. Additionally, significant levels of intracellular C5 and C5a have been shown by Niyonzima et al. [45]. The distinct localization of C5 and C5a may indicate that C5 activation occurs in post-Golgi compartments [45,46]. Furthermore, Daugan et al. revealed a novel intracellular function of C1s, a proteolytic enzyme that activates C4 and initiates the classical complement pathway in tumor progression and T-cell activation [47]. While silencing C1s decreases cancer cell proliferation and increases T-cell activation, extracellular C1s does not affect the same parameters, suggesting an intracellular role of C1s in tumor cells [47]. Together, these findings strongly support the existence of an intracellular complement system and the broad range of novel functions of the complement system.

3.3. *Interaction of Complosome with Mitochondria*

Exploration of the intracellular complement system has unveiled a wide range of novel functions, particularly its interactions with cellular components. Recent evidence has demonstrated that complosome can mediate cellular homeostatic and metabolic processes, as well as immune cell activation through its interaction with mitochondria. For example, C3 cleavage fragments, such as C3a and C3b, can bind to their respective receptors, C3aR and CD46, to induce mitochondrial processes such as glycolysis and OXPHOS, which are needed for T-cell activation [6,8,48]. Furthermore, the C5 fragment, C5a, has a receptor on mitochondrial membranes, known as mitochondrial C5aR. This receptor was found to play a role in modulating mitochondrial function, such as reducing ATP production in favor of interleukin (IL)-1β generation [45]. This finding was supported by the observation that IL-1β levels decrease after inhibition of intracellular C5aR. Most notably, C1q, one of the initiators of the classical complement pathway, binds directly to C1q binding protein (C1qBP) on mitochondrial membranes [1,49]. Interaction between C1q and C1qBP enhances the expression of mitochondrial biogenesis genes, optimizing respiratory function and oxygen consumption [50]. C1qBP has been identified as a key regulator in tumor progression, apoptosis, phagocytosis, and autoimmunity [1,51–53]. Evidently, diverse interactions between mitochondria and the complement system warrant further investigation. Uncovering these interactions will provide essential insights into their role in disease pathogenesis.

4. Role of Mitochondrial DAMPs in Complement Response

This section will explore how mitochondrial DAMPs activate the complement system, linking mitochondrial damage with complement cascade as shown in Figure 2 and Table 1.

4.1. *Intracellular Interactions and Impacts*

Cytochrome C, Apoptosis, and Complement System

Cytochrome c, a molecule produced in mitochondria, facilitates ATP generation in the electron transport chain and regulates apoptosis [27]. It is widely recognized that under cellular stress, cytochrome c, which is initially localized on inner mitochondrial membranes, is released to the cytosol as a pro-apoptotic signal, triggering apoptosis through the activation of caspases [27]. Intriguingly, C3 and C5, which can also induce cell death, have been found to interact with cytochrome c intracellularly to modulate apoptosis [54,55]. For example, in the context of cardiac ischemia/reperfusion (I/R) injury, Fang et al. detected the presence of cytochrome c within the C3 complex inside cells [54]. Furthermore, under oxidative stress, direct interaction between C3 and cytochrome c in the cytosol was observed in the mouse model [54]. Conversely, in humans, Fang et al. found that C3 does not directly interact with intracellular cytochrome c. Instead, C3 binds to downstream elements of apoptosis, which is triggered by cytochrome c [54]. Additionally, the precursor of C3 was found to bind pro-caspase 3, an inactive component of apoptosis, to reduce apoptosis [54]. Despite the observed reduction in apoptosis by C3 and its precursor, it was noted that the interaction of C3 with the apoptotic pathway can promote necrosis, another type of cell death [54]. Therefore, this interaction between C3, cytochrome c, and apoptosis exerts opposing effects on cell death, increasing necrosis while decreasing apoptosis. Since I/R injuries can result from both necrosis and apoptosis, further understanding the degree of modulation of these two pathways by C3 will provide insights to mitigate damage.

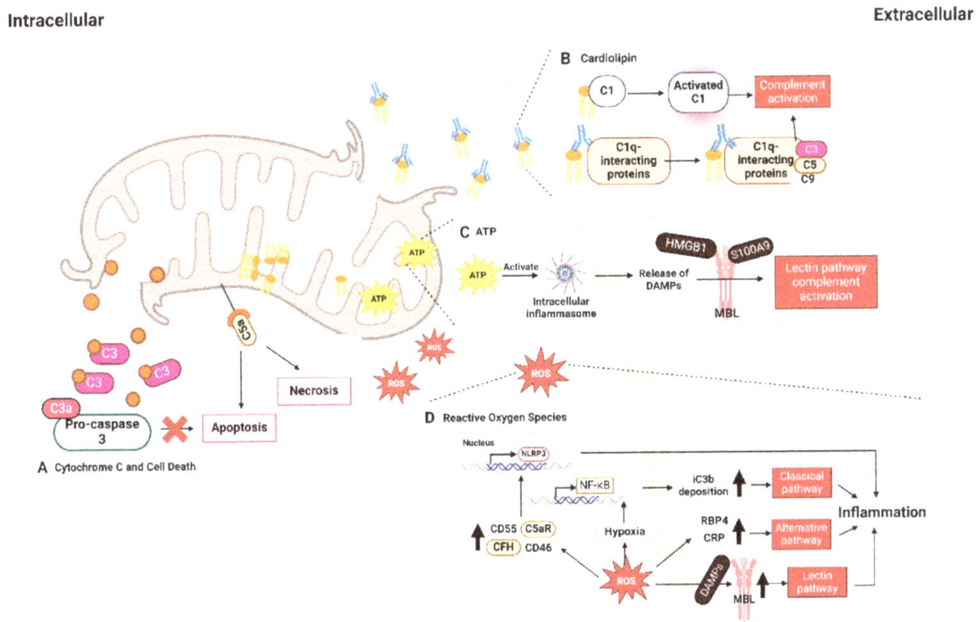

Figure 2. Interactions between mitochondrial damage-associated molecular patterns (DAMPs) and the complement system. Upon cellular stresses, mitochondrial DAMPs become mislocalized and are released from the mitochondria. (**A**) Cytochrome c interacts with C3, leading to the binding of C3a to pro-caspase 3, thereby inhibiting apoptosis. Conversely, binding of C5a to its mitochondrial receptor can induce apoptosis and necrosis. (**B**) Mislocalized cardiolipins from the inner mitochondrial membranes can bind to and activate C1, initiating complement activation. Anti-cardiolipin antibodies can also bind to C1q-binding proteins, providing a platform for the assembly of complement components, further resulting in complement activation. (**C**) ATP released into the cytosol activates intracellular inflammasomes, leading to further release of DAMPs, high molecular group box 1 (HMGB1), and S100 calcium-binding protein A9 (S100A9), which can be recognized by mannose-binding lectin (MBL) to activate the lectin pathway. (**D**) Reactive oxygen species (ROS) activate all three pathways of the complement system. Increased ROS levels elevate the expression of MBL, which recognizes DAMPs to activate the lectin pathway. ROS also induces elevated levels of inflammatory biomarkers such as retinol-binding protein 4 (RBP4) and C-reactive protein (CRP), which in turn activate the alternative pathway. Additionally, ROS enhances inactivated C3b deposition through the hypoxia-induced nuclear factor kappa B (NF-κB) pathway and promotes the expression of complement regulators and receptors, leading to inflammasome gene expressions and classical pathway activation. Receptors in the complement system, C5a receptor (C5aR), CD46, CD55, and complement factor H (CFH), are upregulated to promote the expression of NOD-, LRR-, and pyrin domain-containing protein 3 (NLRP3) to release proinflammatory substances.

In contrast, numerous studies have demonstrated that activated C5a anaphylatoxin exerts pro-apoptotic effects in myocardial I/R [55,56]. The use of anti-C5 treatment antagonizes C5 and decreases the formation of both C5a and MAC, effectively reducing the extent of necrosis and apoptosis in myocardial I/R by decreasing leukocyte infiltration and ROS generation [56]. Similarly, De Hoog et al. observed that the use of C5aR inhibitors leads to improved outcomes in myocardial I/R, evidenced by a decrease in the extent of heart tissue damage and a reduction in apoptosis [55]. Moreover, when C5aR is blocked or its expression is suppressed, leukocyte infiltration into the myocardial infarct area is decreased, thus reducing myocardial damage [55]. Hence, the protective benefits of C5aR inhibitors may result from preventing the binding of intracellular C5a to its mitochondrial receptor and subsequently blocking complement system activation, although the protective effects can also be a result of blocking the plasma membrane C5aR. Future studies are required to distinguish the effects.

4.2. Extracellular Interactions and Impacts

Cardiolipin and Complement System

Under cellular stresses, such as those encountered during ischemic events, cardiolipin, a phospholipid predominantly located in inner mitochondrial membranes, becomes accessible and/or mislocalized [57]. This results in structural and functional alterations to mitochondria, potentially triggering immunological responses including complement activation. Early investigations identified that cardiolipin located on mitoplasts (mitochondria lacking outer membranes) mediates activation of C1 extracellularly [58]. In instances of heart cell death, such as in ischemic heart disease, Rossen et al. discovered that the integrity of mitochondrial outer membranes is compromised, exposing inner membranes to the extracellular complement system [57]. These studies demonstrated that cardiolipin can bind to extracellular C1 and initiate the complement cascade, facilitated by negatively charged phosphate groups present in cardiolipin [57,58].

Furthermore, anti-cardiolipin antibodies were found to specifically accumulate in distinct regions of mitochondria, which are exposed to the extracellular space due to membrane ruptures in injured cardiac cells [57]. These antibodies were found to interact with over 15 mitochondrial components, several of which are proteins that bind to C1q [57]. Additionally, a specific group of C1q-interacting proteins was demonstrated to serve as stable sites for subsequent MAC formation [58]. Conversely, when mitochondria remain undamaged and unexposed to complement components, this interaction does not trigger a physiological response or further complement activation [58]. Therefore, cardiolipin released from the cell likely contributes to the propagation of complement-mediated inflammatory responses by binding to C1 and facilitating the assembly of subsequent complement components, underscoring its significant role in complement activation.

4.3. Intracellular and Extracellular Interactions and Impacts

4.3.1. ATP and Complement System

Beyond its role as the energy currency of cells, ATP has an established role in immune modulation through its direct interaction with cells of the immune system. Studies have revealed that ATP, mostly generated in mitochondria via OXPHOS, can be released as a DAMP. ATP accumulates both intracellularly and extracellularly to trigger inflammation, particularly the lectin pathway of the complement system [5].

For hematopoietic stem/progenitor cells to be mobilized from the bone marrow into the bloodstream, mobilization is initiated by pro-mobilizing stimuli. Upon stimulation by these molecules, ATP produced in mitochondria is released to the cytosol, activating intracellular NOD-, LRR-, and pyrin domain-containing protein 3 (NLRP3) inflammasomes [59]. Ratajczak et al. discovered that ATP-induced inflammasome activation leads to the release of DAMPs, particularly extracellular high molecular group box 1/HMGB1 and S100 calcium-binding protein A9/S100A9. These released DAMPs were observed to bind to extracellularly circulating MBL, resulting in complement activation [59]. Following lectin pathway activation, pro-mobilizing stimuli also cause C5 activation, releasing C5 cleavage fragments, which can optimize the mobilization of stem cells from the bone marrow into peripheral blood [59,60]. The exact same mechanism of MBL-dependent complement activation was observed in microglia cells as well [61]. Hence, ATP not only plays a crucial role in energy supply but also acts as a potent activator of inflammation, through the activation of the lectin pathway in the complement system.

4.3.2. ROS and Complement System

Mitochondria continuously generate ROS as byproducts of aerobic respiration. While ROS can serve as signaling molecules to activate the host defense system against pathogens, excessive ROS production can lead to oxidative damage [62]. Several prior studies indicate that oxidative stress damages cells, leading to the release of DAMPs which activates the extracellular complement system through all three pathways [17,63,64]. It was demonstrated that exposure of urban particulate matter to human umbilical vein endothelial cells enhances ROS production and subsequent activation of the complement system via the alternative pathway [64]. This observation was confirmed by inhibiting ROS production, which suppresses expression of retinol-binding protein 4/RBP4 and c-reactive protein/CRP, which are biomarkers of inflammation, indicating inhibited complement activation [64].

Interestingly, Collard et al. demonstrated that the process of hypoxia and reoxygenation in human endothelial cells triggers activation of the classical complement pathway, resulting in a notable increase in iC3b deposition [17]. Additionally, intracellular ROS can be released as an outcome of different types of cell death, including apoptosis, ferroptosis, and necroptosis, to stimulate extracellular complement activation and iC3b deposition [18,65]. In contrast, antioxidants and inhibition of nuclear factor kappa B (NF-κB) reduce iC3b deposition [18,65]. These findings suggest that iC3b deposition may be regulated by intracellular ROS-induced activation of NF-κB and activation of the classical complement pathway.

Furthermore, in vivo studies demonstrated elevated levels of rat mannose-binding lectin (MBL) and C3 deposition after myocardial reperfusion [63]. Conversely, following oxidative stress in endothelial cells in vitro, preventing accumulation of human MBL reduced complement system activation [63]. It is likely that stressed cardiac cells release DAMPs, which can bind to MBL, resulting in activation of the lectin pathway [66]. Increased expression of MBL also enables a higher possibility of complement activation upon release of DAMPs. Collectively, these findings demonstrate that the deposition of MBL and potential ROS-induced release of DAMPs can mediate the lectin complement pathway.

Dysregulation of oxidative species also leads to hypoxia and reoxygenation inside cells, resulting in increased expression of complement protective factors CD46 and CD55 on the surface of human umbilical vein endothelial cells [17]. Similarly, oxidatively stressed retinal pigment epithelial cells demonstrate elevated levels of complement receptors, such as C5aR, and complement component regulators such as CFH and properdin [67]. These regulators were observed to accumulate along with enhanced NLRP3 expression in retinal pigment epithelial cells under oxidative stress, leading to increased release of proinflammatory substances, regardless of external sources of complement [67].

4.4. Complement System Damages Mitochondria: A Vicious Cycle

As discussed earlier, mitochondria release DAMPs in response to cellular stress, modulating the activation of the complement system. Conversely, complement system activation can induce mitochondrial damage, leading to increased release of DAMPs. Thus, this interplay creates a self-perpetuating cycle that enhances complement system activation and amplifies immune responses. Activation of the complement system has been shown to trigger the production of ROS, causing tissue damage, highlighting the detrimental role of ROS [18]. Chronic ROS levels are known to induce oxidative damage to mitochondrial components, while acute ROS exposure can impair mitochondrial energy production, suggesting that complement-induced ROS likely disrupts mitochondrial structure and bioenergetic functions [16].

Furthermore, as discussed earlier, the pro-inflammatory effects of the complement system are well recognized. C3a and C5a induce the expression of inflammatory cytokines in immune cells, while sublytic MAC triggers the generation of additional inflammatory cytokines. Conversely, Choi et al. demonstrated that the presence of inflammatory cytokines, such as IL-1β or interferon-γ, leads to elevated levels of C3aR on the surface of human umbilical vein endothelial cells [64]. Additionally, complement activation on human umbilical vein endothelial cells following exposure to urban particulate matter stimulates the release of inflammation-inducing proteins, including c-reactive protein and retinol-binding protein 4, associated with the development of atherosclerosis and various cardiovascular diseases [64].

Beyond its known pro-inflammatory effects, recent studies have suggested a potential role of the complement system in metabolism and mitochondrial damage, particularly in regulating C3a and C5a. Nord et al. showed that blocking C3a signaling inhibits complement-induced inflammation and prevents mitochondrial damage, improving recovery from ischemic injury [68]. Similarly, Tsai et al. demonstrated that administration of C5a in kidney endothelial cells activates C5aR, resulting in ROS generation and apoptosis [69]. Inhibiting C5a reduces ROS production, cytochrome c release, and formation of apoptotic cells, suggesting that C5a-induced apoptosis is mediated through C5aR and directly impacts mitochondrial function.

The intricate interplay between mitochondria and the complement system underscores a self-perpetuating cycle wherein mitochondria release DAMPs, triggering complement system activation, and leading to further mitochondrial impairment. Understanding this interaction is crucial for developing treatments for mitochondria-related disorders.

Table 1. **Interactions between mitochondrial DAMPs and complement components.**

Mitochondrial DAMPs	Interactions with Complement	Reference
Cytochrome c	C3	[54]
	C5a	[55,56]
Cardiolipin	C1	[57,58]
ATP	MBL	[59,60]
ROS	iC3b	[17]
	MBL	[63]
	C5a	[69]

DAMPs: damaged-associated molecular patterns; MBL: mannose-binding lectin; ROS: reactive oxygen species.

5. Interplay of Complement and Mitochondria in Human Diseases

In addition to the mitochondrial release of DAMPs, diseases can result from diverse interactions between mitochondria and the complement system, particularly affecting high-energy-demanding organs. Interruptions in bioenergetics profoundly impact these vital areas. This section will explore how complement–mitochondrial damage interplay contributes to disease pathogenesis in localized and systemic conditions. The discussion on organ-specific diseases is summarized in Figure 3.

5.1. Alzheimer's Disease

Alzheimer's disease (AD) is the most diagnosed form of dementia and neurodegenerative disorder worldwide, yet effective treatments remain limited. Amyloid beta (Aβ), a crucial biomarker of AD, is known to damage mitochondria and activate the complement system, creating an intricate loop that propels the disease progression [70].

Numerous studies underscore mitochondrial dysfunction as a significant contributor to AD pathogenesis. For example, it has been observed that Aβ infiltration into mitochondria disrupts energy production at synapses, impeding neuron communication and resulting in cognitive decline [3]. Additionally, Aβ was demonstrated to interact with dynamin-related protein 1/DRP1, a mitochondrial protein responsible for mitochondrial fission. This interaction induces mitochondrial fragmentation and impairs mitophagy, leading to cognitive impairment in AD neurons [71]. Concurrently, Crivelli et al. found that Aβ triggers the release of proinflammatory factors, including C1q, which potentially activates the classical complement pathway in AD neurons [70]. They also observed that these proinflammatory factors induce the generation of extracellular vesicles enriched with ceramide, which plays a role in stimulating ROS production and disrupting mitochondrial membrane potential, thereby causing impairment of mitochondrial respiration [70,72]. Moreover, elevated C1q levels were shown to exacerbate mitochondrial damage through the induction of fatal oxidative stress in neurons [73]. Therefore, both Aβ and Aβ-induced C1q significantly impact mitochondrial functions, jeopardizing the energy supply required for proper neuronal functioning.

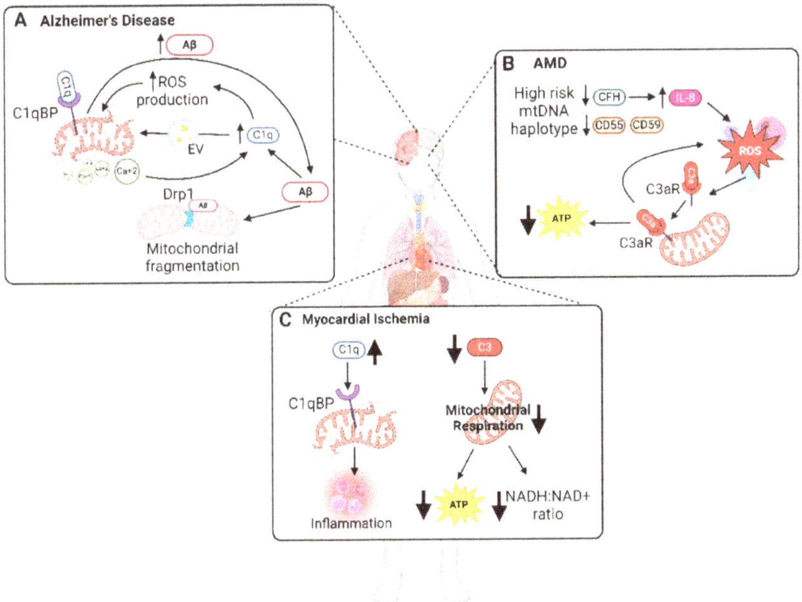

Figure 3. Interactions between the complement system and mitochondria in localized diseases. Complement system and mitochondria exhibit distinct interactions in various localized diseases, contributing to mitochondrial damage and complement dysregulation, thereby impacting disease progression. (**A**) In Alzheimer's disease, amyloid-beta (Aβ) contributes to mitochondrial fragmentation via interaction with dynamin-related protein 1 (Drp1). Additionally, Aβ increases C1q levels, leading to the generation of ceramide-containing extracellular vesicles (EVs) and ROS, both of which contribute to mitochondrial impairments. Calcium overload resulting from mitochondrial damage further induces elevation in C1q levels. Subsequent binding of C1q to its mitochondrial receptor, C1q-binding protein (C1qBP), exacerbates Aβ levels, forming a vicious loop of dysfunction. (**B**) Age-related macular degeneration (AMD) is characterized by lower levels of complement regulators complement factor H (CFH), CD55, and CD59 in mtDNA haplotypes associated with high disease risk. Increased ROS leads to relocation of C3aR to mitochondria, leading to further ROS increase and ATP decrease. (**C**) Accumulated C1q at myocardial ischemic regions binds to mitochondrial protein C1qBP.

Reciprocally, in the early stages of AD, mitochondria damaged by Aβ were observed to subsequently induce increased Aβ accumulation [74]. This perpetuates a vicious cycle where elevated Aβ levels further impair mitochondrial functions, sustaining the progression of AD. Additionally, dysmorphic mitochondria often exhibit impaired or complete loss of homeostasis, including dysregulation of calcium signaling [75]. Datta et al. discovered that an overload of calcium can enhance C1q aggregation near dysmorphic mitochondria [76]. This phenomenon is likely due to the ability of calcium ions to stabilize C1q-like domains, thereby enhancing the accumulation of C1q around regions with elevated calcium concentrations [77]. Moreover, they showed that heightened C1q levels, resulting from calcium homeostasis disruption, trigger subsequent caspase-3 activation, leading to cell death [76,78].

Collectively, these studies support a disease model of AD pathogenesis characterized by the accumulation of Aβ, which damages mitochondria, leading to further Aβ accumulation and subsequent mitochondrial dysfunction. Therefore, given the current evidence from the literature, this cycle is likely to perpetuate the activation of C1q, thereby exacerbating mitochondrial damage and severe neurological symptoms. Escaping this detrimental cycle necessitates treatments that maintain mitochondrial functions and mitigate C1q and Aβ levels.

5.2. Age-Related Macular Degeneration

Age-related macular degeneration (AMD) is one of the major causes of irreversible vision loss in older age groups, impacting one in eight people 60 years of age or older [79]. The roles of complement proteins in retinal health and disease have been implicated. Trakkides et al. demonstrated that adult retinal pigment epithelial cells, or ARPE-19 cells, can produce complement proteins following oxidative stress [67]. Exposure to H_2O_2-induced oxidative stress results in elevated expression of complement receptors CR3 and C5aR1, as well as CFH in ARPE-19 cells [67]. Notably, CFH has been linked to an increased risk of AMD [80]. Furthermore, Kenney et al. concluded that the mtDNA haplotype protective against AMD expresses elevated levels of CFH compared to the haplotype at higher risk of AMD, suggesting a protective function of CFH in AMD [80]. Given that CFH inhibits C3 activation and degrades C3b, it may protect against AMD by lowering downstream complement activation, inflammation, and oxidative stress. This is further supported by enhanced CFH levels after exposure to T cells and oxidative stress [81,82]. In contrast to CFH, other inhibitors of the complement system, such as CD55 and CD59, were found to be downregulated after oxidative stress in ARPE-19 cells, making the cells more susceptible to complement-mediated damage [82]. This highlights intricate interactions between the complement system and oxidative stress in AMD, where CFH functions to inhibit upstream C3 activation and inactivate C3b, while CD55 and CD59 prevent downstream MAC formation.

Furthermore, the susceptible haplotype had decreased levels of ATP, suggesting differences in mitochondrial function, which plays an important role in AMD-associated retinal damage [80]. Together with the evidence that susceptible haplotypes had higher levels of CFH and C3, the complement proteins may play a role in altering mitochondrial processes, resulting in differences in ROS, ATP, and levels of inflammatory markers (i.e., IL-6, IL-1β, and tumor necrosis factor receptor 2/TNFR2) [83]. The production of IL-1β can be caused by C5aR and C3aR signaling via modulation of mitochondrial function and ROS production [45,84]. Notably, upon ROS exposure, C3aR relocates to mitochondria in APRE-19 cells, affecting calcium intake and ATP production [40]. Binding of C3a to mitochondrial C3aR results in decreased ATP production and increased calcium uptake and subsequently elevating ROS levels [85]. Collectively, these findings suggest that inhibiting C3 activation, and thus the formation of C3a offers protection to retinal pigment epithelial cells, at least in part through the mitochondrial C3aR mechanism.

Collectively, this evidence supports a connection between the complement system and mitochondria in AMD, especially through alterations of regulators of complement activation by oxidative stress. Understanding the intricate balance between complement regulation and mitochondrial ROS production is crucial for developing novel therapeutic interventions for AMD.

5.3. Myocardial Ischemia

Myocardial infarction (MI), occlusion of blood flow to the heart, is one of the main causes of cardiovascular mortality. MI-induced heart failure is associated with high morbidity and mortality [86,87]. Due to the large energy demand of the heart, mitochondria comprise a third of cardiomyocytes and provide 95% of ATP in the myocardium [88]. Both mitochondria and the complement system have been implicated in myocardial infarction. As early as 1975, Pinckard et al. identified the release of subcellular fragments in the heart that activate the complement system, triggering inflammation and diseases associated with MI [89]. This study revealed that these subcellular fragments responsible are likely mitochondria in origin, as supported by activation of C1, C2, C3, and C4 by the human heart mitochondria, and an interaction between complement C1 and mitochondrial membrane [89]. Subsequent studies have confirmed this mitochondria–complement protein interaction, especially between C1q and mitochondrial proteins [90–94]. In contrast, Torp et al. found that intracellular C3 protects the heart against I/R injury by promoting mitochondrial respiration [93]. Mice deficient in C3 show reduced mitochondrial respiration, as evidenced by lower levels of ATP and decreased NADH/NAD+ ratio compared to wild-type mice [93]. Furthermore, acute MI can induce biochemical and metabolic disruptions that trigger a series of reactions in mitochondria, resulting in calcium overload and mitochondrial dysfunction [95]. I/R injury could be attributed to the release of mitochondrial DAMPs, activating immune systems such as complement pathway [8,93].

The interplay between mitochondrial function and complement regulation extends to have broader implications, influencing systemic diseases that span across multiple organ systems. A summary of the cross-talk in systematic diseases is depicted in Figure 4.

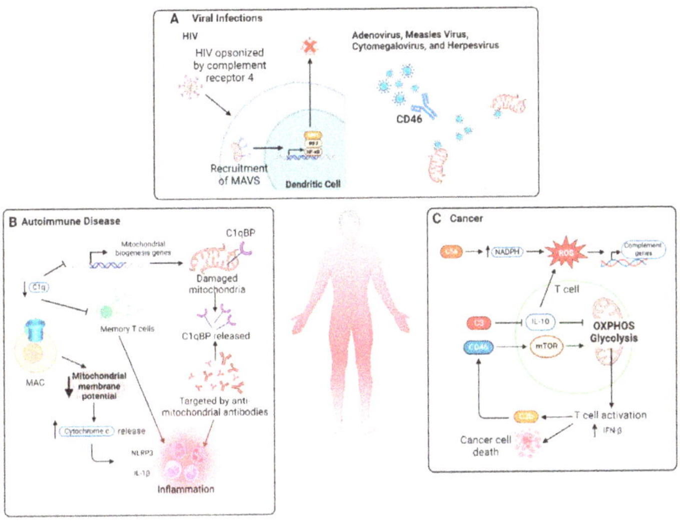

Figure 4. Interactions between the complement system and mitochondria in systemic diseases. Complement system and mitochondria interact across various systemic diseases through mitochondrial DAMPs, influencing immune responses and contributing to inflammation, host protection, and defense. (**A**) Human immunodeficiency virus (HIV), when opsonized by complement receptor 4, recruits mitochondrial antiviral-signaling protein (MAVS), triggering the activation of inflammatory pathways, including TANK-binding kinase 1 (TBK1), interferon regulatory factor 3 (IRF3), and nuclear factor kappa B (NF-κB), ultimately aiding elimination of non-opsonized HIV. Several viruses, such as adenovirus, measles virus, cytomegalovirus, herpesvirus, and coxsackievirus utilize CD46 or CD55 as a receptor to enter host cells, resulting in mitochondrial damage. (**B**) C1q deficiency is associated with autoimmune diseases, as C1q can activate mitochondrial biogenesis genes and sustain memory T-cell activity. Functional consequences of C1q deficiency include damaged mitochondria and the release of mitochondrial proteins such as C1qBP, leading to the formation of anti-mitochondrial antibodies and inflammation. Moreover, the formation of membrane attack complex (MAC) in autoimmune diseases has been linked to a lower mitochondrial membrane potential and release of cytochrome c, contributing to NOD-, LRR-, and pyrin domain-containing protein 3 (NLRP3) activation and interleukin (IL)-1β responses. (**C**) In T cells, CD46 can activate the mammalian target of rapamycin (mTOR) and mitochondrial processes such as oxidative phosphorylation (OXPHOS) and glycolysis, both of which are necessary for T-cell activation and subsequent IFN-β response, leading to protective functions of T cells against cancer. Furthermore, C5a has been found to increase ROS by generating NADPH and activating complement genes by oxidative damage.

5.4. Viral Infections

Complement, as a crucial pathway for innate immunity, is undoubtedly important for pathogen clearance in combating viral infections. Its intricate interactions with host cells during such infections involve various components, including complement receptor 4, MAVS, CD46, and CD55.

Human immunodeficiency virus (HIV) caused over half a million deaths and over 35 million infections in 2019 [96]. HIV clearance relies on the interplay between the complement system and MAVS, located on mitochondrial outer membranes. Posch et al. demonstrated that HIV, when opsonized by the complement system and recognized through complement receptor 4, facilitates the recruitment of MAVS [97]. Initiation of the antiviral recognition pathway is further enhanced by opsonized HIV downregulating the MAVS-suppressive RAF-1/PLK1 pathway [97]. Furthermore, they showed that aggregation of MAVS activates the TBK1/IRF3/NF-κB signaling pathway in dendritic cells, a process essential for the elimination of complement-opsonized HIV [97]. Thus, the complement system, in conjunction with MAVS, is essential for the activation of immune responses and effective clearance of HIV, underscoring the importance of mitochondria in complement system-mediated immune activation.

Moreover, complement inhibitor CD46 is known to be an entry receptor for diverse viruses, including adenoviruses, measles virus, cytomegalovirus, and herpes virus [98]. Similarly, complement regulator CD55 acts as a co-receptor for the cardiotropic coxsackievirus B3 [99]. All aforementioned viruses were found to compromise mitochondrial functions, either by disrupting mitochondrial biogenesis or by inducing apoptotic pathways in a mitochondria-mediated fashion [23,100–103]. As previously discussed, activation of the complement system commonly leads to inhibition of infection; thus, it is likely that CD46, by acting as an inhibitor of the complement system, facilitates viral infections beyond its roles in viral entry. Although no studies have directly linked CD46 with mitochondrial dysfunction during viral infections, the observation that viruses use CD46 as a receptor to invade host cells, leading to subsequent mitochondrial damage, implies that CD46 plays a role in viral mechanisms that impair mitochondrial function. Elucidating whether interactions between viruses and CD46 affect complement regulation and/or mitochondrial function, and understanding the mechanisms involved, is essential in developing treatments to preserve mitochondrial integrity and inhibit viral replication.

In summary, understanding these intricate interactions could help uncover innovative therapeutic interventions targeting both the complement system and mitochondria, offering new avenues to effectively combat viral infections.

5.5. Autoimmune Diseases

Autoimmune diseases occur when the immune system erroneously targets the body's own cells, causing a range of complications such as inflammation and tissue damage. Examples of common autoimmune diseases include systemic lupus erythematosus (SLE), type 1 diabetes, and multiple sclerosis [104]. As part of the immune system, the complement system is a major player in the progression of several autoimmune diseases. However, its involvement in autoimmunity presents a paradox. For example, C1qdeficient individuals are at a higher risk of autoimmune diseases such as SLE and rheumatoid arthritis. Decreases in C1q and formation of anti-C1q-antibodies are observed in patients with SLE [105]. C1q, part of the initiator complex C1 in the classical pathway, along with C1s, C1r, and C4 deficiency (all early complement components), have been associated with SLE [106,107]. Conversely, terminal complement components such as MAC have been implicated in rheumatoid arthritis, glomerulonephritis, and dermatomyositis [106,108–113]. Early complement components appear to be decreased or deficient in SLE, while later complement constituents are present. This paradox may be explained by intracellular complement activation such as C3 and C5 activation by CTSL independent of the canonical pathway, allowing for the formation of MAC without early complement components.

The link between mitochondrial DAMPs and autoimmune diseases is underscored by the fact that the release of mitochondrial DAMPs prompts responses from the complement system. For example, the presence of anti-cardiolipin antibodies, prompted by the release of mitochondrial cardiolipin, is a hallmark of SLE and antiphospholipid syndrome/APS [114–116]. Notably, the hypothesis that impaired mitochondrial quality control is linked to C1q deficiency gains credence, given the vital role of C1q in the removal of apoptotic cells and immune complexes [52]. Furthermore, C1q is known to activate mitochondrial biogenesis genes and support the maintenance of memory T cells, suggesting a cycle where C1q deficiency leads to mitochondrial dysfunction, which in turn exacerbates immune responses in autoimmunity [50].

This vicious cycle ensues in different ways. Studies have found overproduction of ROS in SLE, rheumatoid arthritis, and multiple sclerosis [117–122]. Perl et al. demonstrated increased ROS generation, altered mitochondrial membrane potential, and depleted ATP production in T cells of patients with SLE, indicative of mitochondrial dysfunction [123]. Additionally, Becker et al. reported the release of C1qBP from mitochondrial membranes following mitochondrial damage, which can be targeted by anti-mitochondrial antibodies in SLE [124]. This is important as C1qBP acts as a receptor for C1q and regulates many critical processes such as ATP and ROS generation; thus, the release of C1qBP could potentially lead to dysregulation of ATP and ROS, resulting in mitochondrial dysfunction observed in SLE patients [51,125].

In addition, the presence of MAC in SLE in combination with research findings linking MAC to disruptions in mitochondrial membrane potential suggests another important connection between mitochondria and the complement system in autoimmunity [126]. Specifically, MAC is shown to increase calcium levels and reduce mitochondrial membrane potential, leading to increased cytochrome c release and subsequent increase in NLRP3 inflammasome activation, IL-18 release, and apoptosis [126]. Although the current evidence demonstrates promising links between mitochondrial dysfunction and complement activation, there is a need for more extensive research.

5.6. Cancer

Cancer is an ever-growing concern globally, with lung, colorectal, and stomach cancers being the top 3 leading causes of cancer-related deaths worldwide [126]. Cancer cells can divide uncontrollably, evade apoptosis, escape immune detection, and even exploit the immune system to their advantage [127].

T cells are important in cancer immunotherapy research. Notably, the complement system plays a pivotal role in T-cell activation and homeostasis, acting as a mediator bridging innate and adaptive immune responses. Specifically, C3 and C5, which are found in T cells, are activated by a noncanonical protease, CTSL [6,128]. The resulting cleavage fragments, such as C3a and C5a, bind to their respective receptors to regulate immune cell functions [8,129]. Importantly, C3aR and C5aR are located on lysosomal and mitochondrial membranes, contributing to cell homeostasis [9,40,45,46]. This suggests that intracellular complement activity plays a significant role in cancer immune responses, affecting T-cell activation directly or indirectly by potentially altering mitochondrial functions.

In addition to C3, other complement factors have been shown to regulate anti-tumor immunity. For example, activation of complement regulator CD46 was demonstrated to promote the assembly of lysosomal mTOR in T cells, inducing glycolysis and OXPHOS in mitochondria, which are necessary for T-helper cell induction and IFN-β production [10,130,131]. Through its complement regulatory functions, CD46 can also inactivate C3b produced by T cells [6,10,132]. Collectively, these studies underscore a feedback loop involving complement activation, alterations in mitochondrial activity, and T-cell activation. A shift towards OXPHOS and glycolysis to support T-cell induction may result in reduced ATP production, potentially impairing other crucial cellular functions. Further research is needed to unravel the complex interplay between complement systems, mitochondrial dynamics, and T-cell biology.

Beyond the direct effects on anti-tumor immunity, oncogenic cells may induce mitochondrial damage and complement activation through mitochondrial-derived DAMPs. For example, cytochrome c, a mitochondrial DAMP, has been found to be released in breast cancer cells, leading to the induction of immune responses and apoptosis [133,134]. Increased ROS production and mtDNA release have also been observed in cancer cells [135–137]. Moreover, C5a has been found to activate ROS-generating NADPH oxidases, resulting in a feedback loop [138–140]. Additionally, ROS can induce inflammatory signaling and immune responses, specifically increasing the expression of complement genes [141].

Heat shock proteins (HSPs) also play a role in mitochondrial function and modulating complement response. Mitochondrial HSP70 is expressed highly in tumor cells, and mitochondrial HSP90 exhibits an inhibitory role in C5b-9 or MAC formation [142,143]. This highlights a potential therapeutic direction by targeting HSPs to reduce the immune evasion capabilities of cancer cells.

6. Therapeutic Potential of Targeting Mitochondria and Complement System in Disease Intervention

Mitochondria and the complement system, while established fields of study individually, are understudied areas for therapeutic potential due to the complexity of their interactions and lack of understanding of their connections. The bidirectional nature of this interaction should be noted as a promising avenue for therapeutic intervention. Targeting mitochondria can impact corresponding complement responses, especially through regulation of mitochondrial DAMPs as discussed above, whilst targeting the complement system can both directly and indirectly regulate mitochondrial dysfunction. Currently available drugs, such as eculizumab and pozelimab, target the complement system by inhibiting C5 cleavage [144,145]. Eculizumab has been shown to effectively treat paroxysmal nocturnal hemoglobinuria/PNH and CHAPLE disease, both characterized by a deficiency of negative regulators of complement activation [144,145]. Moreover, C1q presents a potential therapeutic target to address complement–mitochondria interactions in disease progression. For example, the binding of C1q to mitochondrial C1qBP enhanced the expression of mitochondrial biogenesis genes [50]. Drugs targeting C1q, such as C1q inhibitors and anti-C1q antibodies, are currently in the early stages of development [146]. However, further studies are needed to investigate the effect of complement-targeting drugs on mitochondrial function to explore the potential in treating mitochondrial disease, which has limited treatments available.

For interventions directly targeting mitochondria, one of the only existing drugs is antioxidant target ROS to mitigate mitochondrial damage [2]. Studies have shown that antioxidants can restore complement-mediated damage. For example, in cerebral ischemia, antioxidant treatment suppresses C3, reducing neurological damage and infarct volume [147]. Additionally, HSPs represent promising targets, particularly in cancer, where mitochondrial dysfunction and complement dysregulation converge. Particularly, inhibiting HSPs, including mitochondria-localized proteins in the HSP family, leads to strong anti-cancer activity [148]. Increased cytotoxicity of HSP inhibitors may be due to increased complement-mediated cytotoxicity, as HSPs were shown to inhibit MAC formation in cancer cells [143]. Furthermore, modulating CD46 activity in T cells may rescue anti-tumor T-cell responses, which, in combination with other therapeutics, may prove effective in destroying cancer cells [149]. Moreover, targeting specific complement receptors such as C3aR and C5aR holds the potential to modulate inflammatory processes across various diseases. For example, blockade of C5aR improves anti-tumor effects of T cells [150]. However, the efficacy of complement-targeting cancer therapy needs further investigation.

In conclusion, the intersection of mitochondria and the complement system presents a rich landscape for therapeutic innovation. The targeting of multiple components within the complement–mitochondria interaction may yield synergistic effects and overcome the limitations of individual therapies.

7. Conclusions

Proven by various studies across different diseases, the complement system and mitochondria are indeed intricately linked. Both systems respond to stress, whereby the release of mitochondrial DAMPs due to stress and physical membrane damage can trigger activation of the complement system. Beyond mitochondrial DAMP signaling, the interaction also includes T-cell activation, direct binding of complement proteins to mitochondrial proteins, and modulation of mitochondrial processes by complement proteins. Furthermore, mitochondrial functions may rely on other essential organelles. These synergistic mechanisms between organelles and the mitochondria–complement system interactions need further research. This bidirectional interplay creates a cycle between the complement system and mitochondria, yet further studies of these interactions may help uncover novel avenues for therapeutic research and identify potential targets for the treatment of various diseases.

Author Contributions: Conceptualization, J.F.C.L., S.W.H., H.L. and Y.M.; writing—review and editing, J.F.C.L., S.W.H., H.L. and Y.M.; supervision, H.L. and Y.M.; funding acquisition, H.L. All authors have read and agreed to the published version of the manuscript.

Funding: This work was funded by the Natural Sciences and Engineering Research Council (RGPIN-2022-02979) and the Canadian Institutes of Health Research (PJT-173318, PJT-186101, and MM1-174898). Y.M. is a recipient of the Postdoctoral Fellowship co-funded by the Michael Smith Health Research BC, the St. Paul's Foundation, and the Centre for Heart Lung Innovation and the Canadian Institutes of Health Research REDI Early Career Transition Award. J.F.C.L. is recipient of the Natural Sciences and Engineering Research Council of Canada Under-graduate Student Research Awards.

Acknowledgments: We thank members of the Luo Laboratory for their thoughtful contributions. All diagrams are created with BioRender.com (accessed on 14 February 2024).

Conflicts of Interest: The authors declare no competing interests.

Abbreviations

OXPHOS	Oxidative phosphorylation
DAMP	Damage-associated molecular pattern
ROS	Reactive oxidative species
mtDNA	Mitochondrial DNA
IFN	Interferon
C3	Complement component 3
C5	Complement component 5
C1q	Complement component 1q
iC3b	Inactivated C3b
MAC	Membrane attack complex
GPI	Glycosylphosphatidylinositol
C3aR	C3a receptor
C5aR	C5a receptor
CFH	Complement factor H
CTSL	Cathepsin L
MAVS	Mitochondrial antiviral signaling
IL	Interleukin
C1qBP	C1q-binding protein
I/R	Ischemia/reperfusion
NLRP3	NOD-, LRR-, and pyrin domain-containing protein 3
NF-κB	Nuclear factor kappa B
MBL	Mannose-binding lectin
AD	Alzheimer's disease
Aβ	Amyloid beta
AMD	Age-related macular degeneration
MI	Myocardial infarction
HIV	Human immunodeficiency virus
SLE	Systemic lupus erythematosus
HSP	Heat shock protein

References

1. Fogal, V.; Richardson, A.D.; Karmali, P.P.; Scheffler, I.E.; Smith, J.W.; Ruoslahti, E. Mitochondrial p32 protein is a critical regulator of tumor metabolism via maintenance of oxidative phosphorylation. *Mol. Cell Biol.* **2010**, *30*, 1303–1318. [CrossRef]
2. Mohamud, Y.; Li, B.Z.; Bahreyni, A.; Luo, H.L. Mitochondria dysfunction at the heart of viral myocarditis: Mechanistic insights and therapeutic implications. *Viruses* **2023**, *15*, 351. [CrossRef]
3. Guan, P.P.; Ge, T.Q.; Wang, P. As a potential therapeutic target, C1q induces synapse loss via inflammasome-activating apoptotic and mitochondria impairment mechanisms in Alzheimer's disease. *J. Neuroimmune Pharm.* **2023**, *18*, 267–284. [CrossRef] [PubMed]
4. Dunkelberger, J.R.; Song, W.C. Complement and its role in innate and adaptive immune responses. *Cell Res.* **2010**, *20*, 34–50. [CrossRef]
5. Lo, M.R.W.; Woodruff, T.M. Complement: Bridging the innate and adaptive immune systems in sterile inflammation. *J. Leukoc. Biol.* **2020**, *108*, 339–351. [CrossRef]
6. Liszewski, M.K.; Kolev, M.; Le Friec, G.; Leung, M.; Bertram, P.G.; Fara, A.F.; Subias, M.; Pickering, M.C.; Drouet, C.; Meri, S.; et al. Intracellular complement activation sustains T cell homeostasis and mediates effector differentiation. *Immunity* **2013**, *39*, 1143–1157. [CrossRef] [PubMed]
7. Kolev, M.; Le Friec, G.; Kemper, C. Complement—tapping into new sites and effector systems. *Nat. Rev. Immunol.* **2014**, *14*, 811–820. [CrossRef] [PubMed]
8. Rahman, J.; Singh, P.; Merle, N.S.; Niyonzima, N.; Kemper, C. Complement's favourite organelle-Mitochondria? *Brit J. Pharmacol.* **2021**, *178*, 2771–2785. [CrossRef]
9. West, E.E.; Kemper, C. Complosome—The intracellular complement system. *Nat. Rev. Nephrol.* **2023**, *19*, 426–439. [CrossRef]
10. Kolev, M.; Dimeloe, S.; Le Friec, G.; Navarini, A.; Arbore, G.; Povoleri, G.A.; Fischer, M.; Belle, R.; Loeliger, J.; Develioglu, L.; et al. Complement regulates nutrient influx and metabolic reprogramming during Th1 cell responses. *Immunity* **2015**, *42*, 1033–1047. [CrossRef]
11. Hess, C.; Kemper, C. Complement-mediated regulation of metabolism and basic cellular processes. *Immunity* **2016**, *45*, 240–254. [CrossRef] [PubMed]
12. Vijay, K. Toll-like receptors in immunity and inflammatory diseases: Past, present, and future. *Int. Immunopharmacol.* **2018**, *59*, 391–412. [CrossRef] [PubMed]
13. Reis, E.S.; Mastellos, D.C.; Hajishengallis, G.; Lambris, J.D. New insights into the immune functions of complement. *Nat. Rev. Immunol.* **2019**, *19*, 503–516. [CrossRef] [PubMed]
14. Li, D.Y.; Wu, M.H. Pattern recognition receptors in health and diseases. *Signal Transduct. Tar.* **2021**, *6*, 291. [CrossRef] [PubMed]
15. Odendall, C.; Kagan, J.C. Activation and pathogenic manipulation of the sensors of the innate immune system. *Microbes Infect.* **2017**, *19*, 229–237. [CrossRef] [PubMed]
16. Guo, C.Y.; Sun, L.; Chen, X.P.; Zhang, D.S. Oxidative stress, mitochondrial damage and neurodegenerative diseases. *Neural Regen. Res.* **2013**, *8*, 2003–2014. [CrossRef] [PubMed]
17. Collard, C.D.; Vakeva, A.; Bukusoglu, C.; Zund, G.; Sperati, C.J.; Colgan, S.P.; Stahl, G.L. Reoxygenation of hypoxic human umbilical vein endothelial cells activates the classic complement pathway. *Circulation* **1997**, *96*, 326–333. [CrossRef]
18. Collard, C.D.; Agah, A.; Stahl, G.L. Complement activation following reoxygenation of hypoxic human endothelial cells: Role of intracellular reactive oxygen species, NF-κB and new protein synthesis. *Immunopharmacology* **1998**, *39*, 39–50. [CrossRef]
19. West, A.P.; Shadel, G.S. Mitochondrial DNA in innate immune responses and inflammatory pathology. *Nat. Rev. Immunol.* **2017**, *17*, 363–375. [CrossRef]
20. Ryan, M.T.; Hoogenraad, N.J. Mitochondrial-nuclear communications. *Annu. Rev. Biochem.* **2007**, *76*, 701–722. [CrossRef]
21. McBride, H.M.; Neuspiel, M.; Wasiak, S. Mitochondria: More than just a powerhouse. *Curr. Biol.* **2006**, *16*, R551–R560. [CrossRef] [PubMed]
22. Youle, R.J.; van der Bliek, A.M. Mitochondrial fission, fusion, and stress. *Science* **2012**, *337*, 1062–1065. [CrossRef] [PubMed]
23. Mohamud, Y.; Xue, Y.C.; Liu, H.T.; Ng, C.S.; Bahreyni, A.; Luo, H.L. Autophagy receptor protein Tax1-binding protein 1/TRAF6-binding protein is a cellular substrate of enteroviral proteinase. *Front. Microbiol.* **2021**, *12*, 647410. [CrossRef] [PubMed]
24. Ding, W.X.; Yin, X.M. Mitophagy: Mechanisms, pathophysiological roles, and analysis. *Biol. Chem.* **2012**, *393*, 547–564. [CrossRef]
25. Mohamud, Y.; Shi, J.; Tang, H.; Xiang, P.; Xue, Y.C.; Liu, H.; Ng, C.S.; Luo, H. Coxsackievirus infection induces a non-canonical autophagy independent of the ULK and PI3K complexes. *Sci. Rep.* **2020**, *10*, 19068. [CrossRef]
26. Nakahira, K.; Hisata, S.; Choi, A.M.K. The roles of mitochondrial damage-associated molecular patterns in diseases. *Antioxid. Redox Sign* **2015**, *23*, 1329–1350. [CrossRef] [PubMed]
27. Wan, J.M.; Kalpage, H.A.; Vaishnav, A.; Liu, J.; Lee, I.; Mahapatra, G.; Turner, A.A.; Zurek, M.P.; Ji, Q.Q.; Moraes, C.T.; et al. Regulation of respiration and apoptosis by cytochrome c threonine 58 phosphorylation. *Sci. Rep.* **2019**, *9*, 15815. [CrossRef] [PubMed]
28. Murphy, M.P. How mitochondria produce reactive oxygen species. *Biochem. J.* **2009**, *417*, 1–13. [CrossRef]
29. Banoth, B.; Cassel, S.L. Mitochondria in innate immune signaling. *Transl. Res.* **2018**, *202*, 52–68. [CrossRef]
30. Mohamud, Y.; Fu, C.; Fan, Y.M.; Zhang, Y.L.; Lin, J.F.C.; Hwang, S.W.; Wang, Z.C.; Luo, H. Activation of cGAS-STING suppresses coxsackievirus replication via interferon-dependent signaling. *Antivir. Res.* **2024**, *222*, 105811. [CrossRef]

31. Janeway, C.A., Jr.; Travers, P.; Walport, M.; Shlomchik, M.J. The complement system and innate immunity. In *Immunobiology: The Immune System in Health and Disease*, 5th ed.; Garland Science: New York, NY, USA, 2001.
32. King, B.C.; Kulak, K.; Krus, U.; Rosberg, R.; Golec, E.; Wozniak, K.; Gomez, M.F.; Zhang, E.M.; O'Connell, D.J.; Renström, E.; et al. Complement component C3 is highly expressed in human pancreatic islets and prevents β cell death via ATG16L1 interaction and autophagy regulation. *Cell Metab.* **2019**, *29*, 202–210. [CrossRef] [PubMed]
33. Kremlitzka, M.; Colineau, L.; Nowacka, A.A.; Mohlin, F.C.; Wozniak, K.; Blom, A.M.; King, B. Alternative translation and retrotranslocation of cytosolic C3 that detects cytoinvasive bacteria. *Cell Mol. Life Sci.* **2022**, *79*, 291. [CrossRef] [PubMed]
34. Golec, E.; Rosberg, R.; Zhang, E.M.; Renström, E.; Blom, A.M.; King, B. A cryptic non-GPI-anchored cytosolic isoform of CD59 controls insulin exocytosis in pancreatic β-cells by interaction with SNARE proteins. *FASEB J.* **2019**, *33*, 12425–12434. [CrossRef] [PubMed]
35. Strainic, M.G.; Liu, J.B.; Huang, D.P.; An, F.; Lalli, P.N.; Muqim, N.; Shapiro, V.S.; Dubyak, G.R.; Heeger, P.S.; Medof, M.E. Locally produced complement fragments C5a and C3a provide both costimulatory and survival signals to naive CD4 T cells. *Immunity* **2008**, *28*, 425–435. [CrossRef] [PubMed]
36. Kolev, M.; Le Friec, G.; Kemper, C. The role of complement in CD4 T cell homeostasis and effector functions. *Semin. Immunol.* **2013**, *25*, 12–19. [CrossRef] [PubMed]
37. Lubbers, R.; van Essen, M.F.; van Kooten, C.; Trouw, L.A. Production of complement components by cells of the immune system. *Clin. Exp. Immunol.* **2017**, *188*, 183–194. [CrossRef] [PubMed]
38. Morgan, B.P.; Gasque, P. Extrahepatic complement biosynthesis: Where, when and why? *Clin. Exp. Immunol.* **1997**, *107*, 1–7. [CrossRef] [PubMed]
39. Tenner, A.J.; Volkin, D.B. Complement subcomponent-C1q secreted by cultured human-monocytes has subunit structure identical with that of serum-C1q. *Biochem. J.* **1986**, *233*, 451–458. [CrossRef] [PubMed]
40. Ishii, M.; Beeson, G.; Beeson, C.; Rohrer, B. Mitochondrial C3a receptor activation in oxidatively stressed epithelial cells reduces mitochondrial respiration and metabolism. *Front. Immunol.* **2021**, *12*, 628062. [CrossRef] [PubMed]
41. Arbore, G.; West, E.E.; Spolski, R.; Robertson, A.A.B.; Klos, A.; Rheinheimer, C.; Dutow, P.; Woodruff, T.M.; Yu, Z.X.; O'Neill, L.A.; et al. T Helper 1 immunity requires complement-driven NLRP3 inflammasome activity in CD4 T Cells. *Science* **2016**, *352*, aad1210. [CrossRef]
42. Martin, M.; Leffler, J.; Smolag, K.I.; Mytych, J.; Björk, A.; Chaves, L.D.; Alexander, J.J.; Quigg, R.J.; Blom, A.M. Factor H uptake regulates intracellular C3 activation during apoptosis and decreases the inflammatory potential of nucleosomes. *Cell Death Differ.* **2016**, *23*, 903–911. [CrossRef] [PubMed]
43. Tam, J.C.H.; Bidgood, S.R.; McEwan, W.A.; James, L.C. Intracellular sensing of complement C3 activates cell autonomous immunity. *Science* **2014**, *345*, 1256070. [CrossRef] [PubMed]
44. Sorbara, M.T.; Foerster, E.G.; Tsalikis, J.; Abdel-Nour, M.; Mangiapane, J.; Sirluck-Schroeder, I.; Tattoli, I.; van Dalen, R.; Isenman, D.E.; Rohde, J.R.; et al. Complement C3 drives autophagy-dependent restriction of cyto-invasive bacteria. *Cell Host Microbe* **2018**, *23*, 644–652. [CrossRef] [PubMed]
45. Niyonzima, N.; Rahman, J.; Kunz, N.; West, E.E.; Freiwald, T.; Desai, J.; Merle, N.S.; Gidon, A.; Sporsheim, B.; Lionakis, M.S.; et al. Mitochondrial C5aR1 activity in macrophages controls IL-1β production underlying sterile inflammation. *Sci. Immunol.* **2021**, *6*, eabf2489. [CrossRef] [PubMed]
46. Ding, P.; Xu, Y.; Li, L.; Lv, X.; Li, L.; Chen, J.; Zhou, D.; Wang, X.; Wang, Q.; Zhang, W.; et al. Intracellular complement C5a/C5aR1 stabilizes beta-catenin to promote colorectal tumorigenesis. *Cell Rep.* **2022**, *39*, 110851. [CrossRef] [PubMed]
47. Daugan, M.V.; Revel, M.; Russick, J.; Dragon-Durey, M.A.; Gaboriaud, C.; Robe-Rybkine, T.; Poillerat, V.; Grunenwald, A.; Lacroix, G.; Bougouin, A.; et al. Complement C1s and C4d as prognostic biomarkers in renal cancer: Emergence of noncanonical functions of C1s. *Cancer Immunol. Res.* **2021**, *9*, 891–908. [CrossRef] [PubMed]
48. West, E.E.; Kolev, M.; Kemper, C. Complement and the regulation of T cell responses. *Annu. Rev. Immunol.* **2018**, *36*, 309–338. [CrossRef] [PubMed]
49. Jiang, J.Z.; Zhang, Y.; Krainer, A.R.; Xu, R.M. Crystal structure of human p32, a doughnut-shaped acidic mitochondrial matrix protein. *Proc. Natl. Acad. Sci. USA* **1999**, *96*, 3572–3577. [CrossRef] [PubMed]
50. Weyand, C.M.; Goronzy, J.J. A mitochondrial checkpoint in autoimmune disease. *Cell Metab.* **2018**, *28*, 185–186. [CrossRef] [PubMed]
51. Chowdhury, A.R.; Ghosh, O.; Datta, K. Excessive reactive oxygen species induces apoptosis in fibroblasts: Role of mitochondrially accumulated hyaluronic acid binding protein 1 (HABP1/p32/gC1qR). *Exp. Cell Res.* **2008**, *314*, 651–667. [CrossRef]
52. Galvan, M.D.; Greenlee-Wacker, M.C.; Bohlson, S.S. C1q and phagocytosis: The perfect complement to a good meal. *J. Leukoc. Biol.* **2012**, *92*, 489–497. [CrossRef]
53. McGee, A.M.; Douglas, D.L.; Liang, Y.Y.; Hyder, S.M.; Baines, C.P. The mitochondrial protein C1qbp promotes cell proliferation, migration and resistance to cell death. *Cell Cycle* **2011**, *10*, 4119–4127. [CrossRef] [PubMed]
54. Fang, Z.; Lee, H.K.Y.; Liu, J.Y.; Wong, K.A.; Brown, L.M.; Li, X.; Xiaoli, A.M.; Yang, F.J.; Zhang, M. Complement C3 reduces apoptosis via interaction with the intrinsic apoptotic pathway. *Cells* **2023**, *12*, 2282. [CrossRef]
55. De Hoog, V.C.; Timmers, L.; Van Duijvenvoorde, A.; De Jager, S.C.A.; Van Middelaar, B.J.; Smeets, M.B.; Woodruff, T.M.; Doevendans, P.A.; Pasterkamp, G.; Hack, C.E.; et al. Leucocyte expression of complement C5a receptors exacerbates infarct size after myocardial reperfusion injury. *Cardiovasc. Res.* **2014**, *103*, 521–529. [CrossRef]

56. Vakeva, A.P.; Agah, A.; Rollins, S.A.; Matis, L.A.; Li, L.; Stahl, G.L. Myocardial infarction and apoptosis after myocardial ischemia and reperfusion—Role of the terminal complement components and inhibition by anti-C5 therapy. *Circulation* **1998**, *97*, 2259–2267. [CrossRef] [PubMed]
57. Rossen, R.D.; Michael, L.H.; Hawkins, H.K.; Youker, K.; Dreyer, W.J.; Baughn, R.E.; Entman, M.L. Cardiolipin-protein complexes and initiation of complement activation after coronary artery occlusion. *Circ. Res.* **1994**, *75*, 546–555. [CrossRef]
58. Peitsch, M.C.; Tschopp, J.; Kress, A.; Isliker, H. Antibody-independent activation of the complement-system by mitochondria is mediated by cardiolipin. *Biochem. J.* **1988**, *249*, 495–500. [CrossRef]
59. Ratajczak, M.Z.; Adamiak, M.; Thapa, A.; Bujko, K.; Brzezniakiewicz-Janus, K.; Lenkiewicz, A.M. NLRP3 inflammasome couples purinergic signaling with activation of the complement cascade for the optimal release of cells from bone marrow. *Leukemia* **2019**, *33*, 815–825. [CrossRef]
60. Ratajczak, M.Z.; Adamiak, M.; Plonka, M.; Abdel-Latif, A.; Ratajczak, J. Mobilization of hematopoietic stem cells as a result of innate immunity-mediated sterile inflammation in the bone marrow microenvironment-the involvement of extracellular nucleotides and purinergic signaling. *Leukemia* **2018**, *32*, 1116–1123. [CrossRef] [PubMed]
61. Ratajczak, M.Z.; Mack, A.; Bujko, K.; Domingues, A.; Pedziwiatr, D.; Kucia, M.; Ratajczak, J.; Ulrich, H.; Kucharska-Mazur, J.; Samochowiec, J. ATP-Nlrp3 inflammasome-complement cascade axis in sterile brain inflammation in psychiatric patients and its impact on stem cell trafficking. *Stem Cell Rev. Rep.* **2019**, *15*, 497–505. [CrossRef]
62. Paiva, C.N.; Bozza, M.T. Are reactive oxygen species always detrimental to pathogens? *Antioxid. Redox Sign* **2014**, *20*, 1000–1037. [CrossRef] [PubMed]
63. Collard, C.D.; Väkevä, A.; Morrissey, M.A.; Agah, A.; Rollins, S.A.; Reenstra, W.R.; Buras, J.A.; Meri, S.; Stahl, G.L. Complement activation after oxidative stress: Role of the lectin complement pathway. *Am. J. Pathol.* **2000**, *156*, 1549–1556. [CrossRef] [PubMed]
64. Choi, M.S.; Jeon, H.; Yoo, S.M.; Lee, M.S. Activation of the complement system on human endothelial cells by urban particulate matter triggers inflammation-related protein production. *Int. J. Mol. Sci.* **2021**, *22*, 3336. [CrossRef] [PubMed]
65. Villalpando-Rodriguez, G.E.; Gibson, S.B. Reactive oxygen species (ROS) regulates different types of cell death by acting as a rheostat. *Oxid. Med. Cell Longev.* **2021**, *2021*, 9912436. [CrossRef] [PubMed]
66. Amarante-Mendes, G.P.; Adjemian, S.; Branco, L.M.; Zanetti, L.C.; Weinlich, R.; Bortoluci, K.R. Pattern recognition receptors and the host cell death molecular machinery. *Front. Immunol.* **2018**, *9*, 2379. [CrossRef] [PubMed]
67. Trakkides, T.O.; Schäfer, N.; Reichenthaler, M.; Kühn, K.; Brandwijk, R.J.M.G.E.; Toonen, E.J.M.; Urban, F.; Wegener, J.; Enzmann, V.; Pauly, D. Oxidative stress increases endogenous complement-dependent inflammatory and angiogenic responses in retinal pigment epithelial cells independently of exogenous complement sources. *Antioxidants* **2019**, *8*, 548. [CrossRef]
68. Nord, D.M. *Activated Complement Products Contribute to Mitochondrial Damage of the Airway Epithelium during Lung Transplantation*; Medical University of South Carolina: Charleston, SC, USA, 2020.
69. Tsai, I.J.; Lin, W.C.; Yang, Y.H.; Tseng, Y.L.; Lin, Y.H.; Chou, C.H.; Tsau, Y.K. High Concentration of C5a-Induced Mitochondria-Dependent Apoptosis in Murine Kidney Endothelial Cells. *Int. J. Mol. Sci.* **2019**, *20*, 4465. [CrossRef]
70. Crivelli, S.M.; Quadri, Z.; Vekaria, H.J.; Zhu, Z.H.; Tripathi, P.; Elsherbini, A.; Zhang, L.P.; Sullivan, P.G.; Bieberich, E. Inhibition of acid sphingomyelinase reduces reactive astrocyte secretion of mitotoxic extracellular vesicles and improves Alzheimer's disease pathology in the 5xFAD mouse. *Acta Neuropathol. Com.* **2023**, *11*, 135. [CrossRef] [PubMed]
71. Morton, H.; Kshirsagar, S.; Orlov, E.; Bunquin, L.E.; Sawant, N.; Boleng, L.; George, M.; Basu, T.; Ramasubramanian, B.; Pradeepkiran, J.A.; et al. Defective mitophagy and synaptic degeneration in Alzheimer's disease: Focus on aging, mitochondria and synapse. *Free Radic. Biol. Med.* **2021**, *172*, 652–667. [CrossRef]
72. Kogot-Levin, A.; Saada, A. Ceramide and the mitochondrial respiratory chain. *Biochimie* **2014**, *100*, 88–94. [CrossRef]
73. Luo, X.G.; Weber, G.A.; Zheng, J.L.; Gendelman, H.E.; Ikezu, T. C1q-calreticulin induced oxidative neurotoxicity: Relevance for the neuropathogenesis of Alzheimer's disease. *J. Neuroimmunol.* **2003**, *135*, 62–71. [CrossRef] [PubMed]
74. Swerdlow, R.H.; Burns, J.M.; Khan, S.M. The Alzheimer's disease mitochondrial cascade hypothesis: Progress and perspectives. *Biochim. Biophys. Acta (BBA) Mol. Basis Dis.* **2014**, *1842*, 1219–1231. [CrossRef] [PubMed]
75. Protasoni, M.; Zeviani, M. Mitochondrial Structure and Bioenergetics in Normal and Disease Conditions. *Int. J. Mol. Sci.* **2021**, *22*, 586. [CrossRef] [PubMed]
76. Datta, D.; Leslie, S.N.; Morozov, Y.M.; Duque, A.; Rakic, P.; van Dyck, C.H.; Nairn, A.C.; Arnsten, A.F.T. Classical complement cascade initiating C1q protein within neurons in the aged rhesus macaque dorsolateral prefrontal cortex. *J. Neuroinflamm* **2020**, *17*, 8. [CrossRef] [PubMed]
77. Holubowicz, R.; Wojtas, M.; Taube, M.; Kozak, M.; Ozyhar, A.; Dobryszycki, P. Effect of calcium ions on structure and stability of the C1q-like domain of otolin-1 from human and zebrafish. *FEBS J.* **2017**, *284*, 4278–4297. [CrossRef] [PubMed]
78. Li, Z.; Jo, J.; Jia, J.M.; Lo, S.C.; Whitcomb, D.J.; Jiao, S.; Cho, K.; Sheng, M. Caspase-3 activation via mitochondria is required for long-term depression and AMPA receptor internalization. *Cell* **2010**, *141*, 859–871. [CrossRef] [PubMed]
79. Vyawahare, H.; Shinde, P. Age-related macular degeneration: Epidemiology, pathophysiology, diagnosis, and treatment. *Cureus J. Med. Sci.* **2022**, *14*, e29583. [CrossRef]
80. Kenney, M.C.; Chwa, M.; Atilano, S.R.; Pavlis, J.M.; Falatoonzadeh, P.; Ramirez, C.; Malik, D.; Hsu, T.; Woo, G.; Soe, K.; et al. Mitochondrial DNA variants mediate energy production and expression levels for CFH, C3 and EFEMP1 genes: Implications for age-related macular degeneration. *PLoS ONE* **2013**, *8*, e54339. [CrossRef]

81. Juel, H.B.; Kaestel, C.; Folkersen, L.; Faber, C.; Heegaard, N.H.H.; Borup, R.; Nissen, M.H. Retinal pigment epithelial cells upregulate expression of complement factors after co-culture with activated T cells. *Exp. Eye Res.* **2011**, *92*, 180–188. [CrossRef]
82. Thurman, J.M.; Renner, B.; Kunchithapautham, K.; Ferreira, V.P.; Pangburn, M.K.; Ablonczy, Z.; Tomlinson, S.; Holers, V.M.; Rohrer, B. Oxidative stress renders retinal pigment epithelial cells susceptible to complement-mediated injury. *J. Biol. Chem.* **2009**, *284*, 16939–16947. [CrossRef]
83. Bellizzi, D.; Cavalcante, P.; Taverna, D.; Rose, G.; Passarino, G.; Salvioli, S.; Franceschi, C.; De Benedictis, G. Gene expression of cytokines and cytokine receptors is modulated by the common variability of the mitochondrial DNA in cybrid cell lines. *Genes. Cells* **2006**, *11*, 883–891. [CrossRef]
84. Asgari, E.; Le Friec, G.; Yamamoto, H.; Perucha, E.; Sacks, S.S.; Köhl, J.; Cook, H.T.; Kemper, C. C3a modulates IL-1β secretion in human monocytes by regulating ATP efflux and subsequent NLRP3 inflammasome activation. *Blood* **2013**, *122*, 3473–3481. [CrossRef]
85. Görlach, A.; Bertram, K.; Hudecova, S.; Krizanova, O. Calcium and ROS: A mutual interplay. *Redox Biol.* **2015**, *6*, 260–271. [CrossRef]
86. Moraes-Silva, I.C.; Rodrigues, B.; Coelho, H.J.; Feriani, D.J.; Irigoyen, M.C. Myocardial infarction and exercise training: Evidence from basic science. *Adv. Exp. Med. Biol.* **2017**, *999*, 139–153. [CrossRef]
87. Salari, N.; Morddarvanjoghi, F.; Abdolmaleki, A.; Rasoulpoor, S.; Khaleghi, A.A.; Hezarkhani, L.A.; Shohaimi, S.; Mohammadi, M. The global prevalence of myocardial infarction: A systematic review and meta-analysis. *BMC Cardiovasc. Disor.* **2023**, *23*. [CrossRef]
88. Nguyen, B.Y.; Ruiz-Velasco, A.; Bui, T.; Collins, L.; Wang, X.; Liu, W. Mitochondrial function in the heart: The insight into mechanisms and therapeutic potentials. *Brit J. Pharmacol.* **2019**, *176*, 4302–4318. [CrossRef]
89. Pinckard, R.N.; Olson, M.S.; Giclas, P.C.; Terry, R.; Boyer, J.T.; O'Rourke, R.A. Consumption of classical complement components by heart subcellular membranes in vitro and in patients after acute myocardial infarction. *J. Clin. Investig.* **1975**, *56*, 740–750. [CrossRef]
90. Kagiyama, A.; Savage, H.E.; Michael, L.H.; Hanson, G.; Entman, M.L.; Rossen, R.D. Molecular-basis of complement activation in ischemic myocardium—Identification of specific molecules of mitochondrial origin that bind human C1q and fix complement. *Circ. Res.* **1989**, *64*, 607–615. [CrossRef]
91. Rossen, R.D.; Michael, L.H.; Kagiyama, A.; Savage, H.E.; Hanson, G.; Reisberg, M.A.; Moake, J.N.; Kim, S.H.; Self, D.; Weakley, S. Mechanism of complement activation after coronary artery occlusion: Evidence that myocardial ischemia in dogs causes release of constituents of myocardial subcellular origin that complex with human C1q in vivo. *Circ. Res.* **1988**, *62*, 572–584. [CrossRef]
92. Rossen, R.D.; Swain, J.L.; Michael, L.H.; Weakley, S.; Giannini, E.; Entman, M.L. Selective accumulation of the first component of complement and leukocytes in ischemic canine heart muscle. A possible initiator of an extra myocardial mechanism of ischemic injury. *Circ. Res.* **1985**, *57*, 119–130. [CrossRef]
93. Torp, M.K.; Ranheim, T.; Schjalm, C.; Hjorth, M.; Heiestad, C.M.; Dalen, K.T.; Nilsson, P.H.; Mollnes, T.E.; Pischke, S.E.; Lien, E.; et al. Intracellular complement component 3 attenuated ischemia-reperfusion injury in the isolated buffer-perfused mouse heart and is associated with improved metabolic homeostasis. *Front. Immunol.* **2022**, *13*, 870811. [CrossRef]
94. Orrem, H.L.; Nilsson, P.H.; Pischke, S.E.; Grindheim, G.; Garred, P.; Seljeflot, I.; Husebye, T.; Aukrust, P.; Yndestad, A.; Andersen, G.O.; et al. Acute heart failure following myocardial infarction: Complement activation correlates with the severity of heart failure in patients developing cardiogenic shock. *Esc. Heart Fail.* **2018**, *5*, 292–301. [CrossRef]
95. Ramachandra, C.J.A.; Hernandez-Resendiz, S.; Crespo-Avilan, G.E.; Lin, Y.H.; Hausenloy, D.J. Mitochondria in acute myocardial infarction and cardioprotection. *EBioMedicine* **2020**, *57*, 102884. [CrossRef]
96. Tian, X.B.; Chen, J.J.; Wang, X.; Xie, Y.W.; Zhang, X.D.; Han, D.T.; Fu, H.J.; Yin, W.P.; Wu, N.P. Global, regional, and national HIV/AIDS disease burden levels and trends in 1990–2019: A systematic analysis for the global burden of disease 2019 study. *Front Public Health* **2023**, *11*, 1068664. [CrossRef]
97. Posch, W.; Bermejo-Jambrina, M.; Steger, M.; Witting, C.; Diem, G.; Hortnagl, P.; Hackl, H.; Lass-Florl, C.; Huber, L.A.; Geijtenbeek, T.B.H.; et al. Complement potentiates immune sensing of HIV-1 and early type I interferon responses. *mBio* **2021**, *12*, e0240821. [CrossRef]
98. Liszewski, M.K.; Atkinson, J.P. Membrane cofactor protein (MCP.; CD46): Deficiency states and pathogen connections. *Curr. Opin. Immunol.* **2021**, *72*, 126–134. [CrossRef]
99. Yanagawa, B.; Spiller, O.B.; Proctor, D.G.; Choy, J.; Luo, H.L.; Zhang, H.F.M.; Suarez, A.; Yang, D.C.; McManus, B.M. Soluble recombinant coxsackievirus and adenovirus receptor abrogates coxsackievirus B3-mediated pancreatitis and myocarditis in mice. *J. Infect. Dis.* **2004**, *189*, 1431–1439. [CrossRef]
100. Morrison, B.J.; Abu-Asab, M.; Morris, J.C.; Steel, J.C. Localization of human recombinant adenoviral vectors to the mitochondria following transduction of human cell lines. *Acta Virol.* **2019**, *63*, 111–116. [CrossRef]
101. Sato, H.; Hoshi, M.; Ikeda, F.; Fujiyuki, T.; Yoneda, M.; Kai, C. Downregulation of mitochondrial biogenesis by virus infection triggers antiviral responses by cyclic GMP-AMP synthase. *PLoS Pathog.* **2021**, *17*, e1009841. [CrossRef]
102. Combs, J.A.; Norton, E.B.; Saifudeen, Z.R.; Bentrup, K.H.Z.; Katakam, P.V.; Morris, C.A.; Myers, L.; Kaur, A.; Sullivan, D.E.; Zwezdaryk, K.J. Human cytomegalovirus alters host cell mitochondrial function during acute infection. *J. Virol.* **2020**, *94*, e01183-19. [CrossRef]

103. Li, L.; Chi, J.; Zhou, F.; Guo, D.; Wang, F.; Liu, G.; Zhang, C.; Yao, K. Human herpesvirus 6A induces apoptosis of HSB-2 cells via a mitochondrion-related caspase pathway. *J. Biomed. Res.* **2010**, *24*, 444–451. [CrossRef] [PubMed]
104. Wang, L.F.; Wang, F.S.; Gershwin, M.E. Human autoimmune diseases: A comprehensive update. *J. Intern. Med.* **2015**, *278*, 369–395. [CrossRef] [PubMed]
105. Orbai, A.M.; Truedsson, L.; Sturfelt, G.; Nived, O.; Fang, H.; Alarcón, G.S.; Gordon, C.; Merrill, J.T.; Fortin, P.R.; Bruce, I.N.; et al. Anti-C1q antibodies in systemic lupus erythematosus. *Lupus* **2015**, *24*, 42–49. [CrossRef] [PubMed]
106. Lintner, K.E.; Wu, Y.L.; Yang, Y.; Spencer, C.H.; Hauptmann, G.; Hebert, L.A.; Atkinson, J.P.; Yu, C.Y. Early components of the complement classical activation pathway in human systemic autoimmune diseases. *Front. Immunol.* **2016**, *7*, 36. [CrossRef]
107. Atkinson, J.P.; Liszewski, M.K.; Yu, C.Y. Clinical aspects of the complement system in systemic lupus erythematosus. In *Systemic Lupus Erythematosus*; Academic Press: Cambridge, MA, USA, 2021; pp. 113–122.
108. Hughes, J.; Nangaku, M.; Alpers, C.E.; Shankland, S.J.; Couser, W.G.; Johnson, R.J. C5b-9 membrane attack complex mediates endothelial cell apoptosis in experimental glomerulonephritis. *Am. J. Physiol.-Ren.* **2000**, *278*, F747–F757. [CrossRef] [PubMed]
109. Oleesky, D.A.; Daniels, R.H.; Williams, B.D.; Amos, N.; Morgan, B.P. Terminal complement complexes and C1/C1 inhibitor complexes in rheumatoid-arthritis and other arthritic conditions. *Clin. Exp. Immunol.* **1991**, *84*, 250–255.
110. Biró, É.; Nieuwland, R.; Tak, P.P.; Pronk, L.M.; Schaap, M.C.L.; Sturk, A.; Hack, C.E. Activated complement components and complement activator molecules on the surface of cell-derived microparticles in patients with rheumatoid arthritis and healthy individuals. *Ann. Rheum. Dis.* **2007**, *66*, 1085–1092. [CrossRef] [PubMed]
111. Makinde, V.A.; Senaldi, G.; Jawad, A.S.M.; Berry, H.; Vergani, D. Reflection of disease-activity in rheumatoid-arthritis by indexes of activation of the classical complement pathway. *Ann. Rheum. Dis.* **1989**, *48*, 302–306. [CrossRef]
112. Mascaro, J.M.; Hausmann, G.; Herrero, C.; Grau, J.M.; Cid, M.C.; Palou, J.; Mascaro, J.M. Membrane attack complex deposits in cutaneous lesions of dermatomyositis. *J. Investig. Dermatol.* **1995**, *104*, 665. [CrossRef]
113. Konttinen, Y.T.; Ceponis, A.; Meri, S.; Vuorikoski, A.; Kortekangas, P.; Sorsa, T.; Sukura, A.; Santavirta, S. Complement in acute and chronic arthritides: Assessment of C3c, C9, and protectin (CD59) in synovial membrane. *Ann. Rheum. Dis.* **1996**, *55*, 888–894. [CrossRef]
114. Abu-Shakra, M.; Gladman, D.D.; Urowitz, M.B.; Farewell, V. Anticardiolipin antibodies in systemic lupus erythematosus: Clinical and laboratory correlations. *Am. J. Med.* **1995**, *99*, 624–628. [CrossRef] [PubMed]
115. Cohen, S.B.; Goldenberg, M.; Rabinovici, J.; Lidor, A.L.; Dulitzky, M.; Gilburd, B.; Shoenfeld, Y.; Schiff, E. Anti-cardiolipin antibodies in fetal blood and amniotic fluid derived from patients with the anti-phospholipid syndrome. *Hum. Reprod.* **2000**, *15*, 1170–1172. [CrossRef] [PubMed]
116. Jiao, Y.H.; Yan, Z.Y.; Yang, A.M. Mitochondria in innate immunity signaling and its therapeutic implications in autoimmune diseases. *Front. Immunol.* **2023**, *14*, 1160035. [CrossRef] [PubMed]
117. Yan, Z.; Chen, Q.; Xia, Y.M. Oxidative stress contributes to inflammatory and cellular damage in systemic lupus erythematosus: Cellular markers and molecular mechanism. *J. Inflamm. Res.* **2023**, *16*, 453–465. [CrossRef]
118. Yevgi, R.; Demir, R. Oxidative stress activity of fingolimod in multiple sclerosis. *Clin. Neurol. Neurosur* **2021**, *202*, 106500. [CrossRef] [PubMed]
119. Tobore, T.O. Oxidative/Nitroxidative stress and multiple sclerosis. *J. Mol. Neurosci.* **2021**, *71*, 506–514. [CrossRef] [PubMed]
120. Smallwood, M.J.; Nissim, A.; Knight, A.R.; Whiteman, M.; Haigh, R.; Winyard, P.G. Oxidative stress in autoimmune rheumatic diseases. *Free Radic. Biol. Med.* **2018**, *125*, 3–14. [CrossRef] [PubMed]
121. Yang, J.; Yang, X.; Zou, H.; Li, M. Oxidative stress and treg and Th17 dysfunction in systemic lupus erythematosus. *Oxid. Med. Cell Longev.* **2016**, *2016*, 2526174. [CrossRef] [PubMed]
122. Hu, C.F.; Zhang, J.D.; Hong, S.Z.; Li, H.C.; Lu, L.; Xie, G.Q.; Luo, W.Q.; Du, Y.; Xie, Z.J.; Han, X.L.; et al. Oxidative stress-induced aberrant lipid metabolism is an important causal factor for dysfunction of immunocytes from patients with systemic lupus erythematosus. *Free Radic. Biol. Med.* **2021**, *163*, 210–219. [CrossRef]
123. Perl, A.; Gergely, P.; Nagy, G.; Koncz, A.; Banki, K. Mitochondrial hyperpolarization: A checkpoint of T-cell life, death and autoimmunity. *Trends Immunol.* **2004**, *25*, 360–367. [CrossRef]
124. Becker, Y.L.C.; Gagné, J.P.; Julien, A.S.; Lévesque, T.; Allaeys, I.; Gougeard, N.; Rubio, V.; Boisvert, F.M.; Jean, D.; Wagner, E.; et al. Identification of mitofusin 1 and complement component 1q subcomponent binding protein as mitochondrial targets in systemic lupus erythematosus. *Arthritis Rheumatol.* **2022**, *74*, 1193–1203. [CrossRef]
125. Saha, P.; Chowdhury, A.R.; Dutta, S.; Chatterjee, S.; Ghosh, I.; Datta, K. Autophagic vacuolation induced by excess ROS generation in HABP1/p32/gC1qR overexpressing fibroblasts and its reversal by polymeric hyaluronan. *PLoS ONE* **2013**, *8*, e78131. [CrossRef]
126. Jimenez-Duran, G.; Kozole, J.; Peltier-Heap, R.; Dickinson, E.R.; Kwiatkowski, C.R.; Zappacosta, F.; Annan, R.S.; Galwey, N.W.; Nichols, E.M.; Modis, L.K.; et al. Complement membrane attack complex is an immunometabolic regulator of NLRP3 activation and IL-18 secretion in human macrophages. *Front. Immunol.* **2022**, *13*, 918551. [CrossRef]
127. Hanahan, D.; Weinberg, R.A. Hallmarks of cancer: The next generation. *Cell* **2011**, *144*, 646–674. [CrossRef]
128. Frade, R.; Rodrigues-Lima, F.; Huang, S.Y.; Xie, K.P.; Guillaume, N.; Bar-Eli, M. Procathepsin-L, a proteinase that cleaves human C3 (the third component of complement), confers high tumorigenic and metastatic properties to human melanoma cells. *Cancer Res.* **1998**, *58*, 2733–2736. [CrossRef]
129. Hajishengallis, G.; Reis, E.S.; Mastellos, D.C.; Ricklin, D.; Lambris, J.D. Novel mechanisms and functions of complement. *Nat. Immunol.* **2017**, *18*, 1288–1298. [CrossRef]

130. Liszewski, M.K.; Kemper, C. Complement in motion: The evolution of CD46 from a complement regulator to an orchestrator of normal cell physiology. *J. Immunol.* **2019**, *203*, 3–5. [CrossRef]
131. Le Friec, G.; Sheppard, D.; Whiteman, P.; Karsten, C.M.; Shamoun, S.A.T.; Laing, A.; Bugeon, L.; Dallman, M.J.; Melchionna, T.; Chillakuri, C.; et al. The CD46-Jagged1 interaction is critical for human TH1 immunity. *Nat. Immunol.* **2012**, *13*, 1213–1221. [CrossRef]
132. Cardone, J.; Le Friec, G.; Vantourout, P.; Roberts, A.; Fuchs, A.; Jackson, I.; Suddason, T.; Lord, G.; Atkinson, J.P.; Cope, A.; et al. Complement regulator CD46 temporally regulates cytokine production by conventional and unconventional T cells. *Nat. Immunol.* **2010**, *11*, 862–871. [CrossRef]
133. Coussens, L.M.; Werb, Z. Inflammation and cancer. *Nature* **2002**, *420*, 860–867. [CrossRef]
134. Abramczyk, H.; Brozek-Pluska, B.; Kopec, M. Double face of cytochrome in cancers by Raman imaging. *Sci. Rep.* **2022**, *12*, 2120. [CrossRef]
135. Maeda, H.; Akaike, T. Nitric oxide and oxygen radicals in infection, inflammation, and cancer. *Biochem. Mosc.* **1998**, *63*, 854–865.
136. Wiseman, H.; Halliwell, B. Damage to DNA by reactive oxygen and nitrogen species: Role in inflammatory disease and progression to cancer. *Biochem. J.* **1996**, *313*, 17–29. [CrossRef]
137. Federico, A.; Morgillo, F.; Tuccillo, C.; Ciardiello, F.; Loguercio, C. Chronic inflammation and oxidative stress in human carcinogenesis. *Int. J. Cancer* **2007**, *121*, 2381–2386. [CrossRef]
138. Nathan, C.; Ding, A. SnapShot: Reactive oxygen intermediates (ROI). *Cell* **2010**, *140*, 951. [CrossRef]
139. Bae, Y.S.; Oh, H.; Rhee, S.G.; Yoo, Y.D. Regulation of reactive oxygen species generation in cell signaling. *Mol. Cells* **2011**, *32*, 491–509. [CrossRef]
140. Markiewski, M.M.; DeAngelis, R.A.; Benencia, F.; Ricklin-Lichtsteiner, S.K.; Koutoulaki, A.; Gerard, C.; Coukos, G.; Lambris, J.D. Modulation of the antitumor immune response by complement. *Nat. Immunol.* **2008**, *9*, 1225–1235. [CrossRef]
141. Oshi, M.; Gandhi, S.; Yan, L.; Tokumaru, Y.; Wu, R.R.; Yamada, A.; Matsuyama, R.; Endo, I.; Takabe, K. Abundance of reactive oxygen species (ROS) is associated with tumor aggressiveness, immune response, and worse survival in breast cancer. *Breast Cancer Res. Tr.* **2022**, *194*, 231–241. [CrossRef]
142. Kang, B.H.; Plescia, J.; Dohi, T.; Rosa, J.; Doxsey, S.J.; Altieri, D.C. Regulation of tumor cell mitochondrial Homeostasis by an organelle-specific Hsp90 chaperone network. *Cell* **2007**, *131*, 257–270. [CrossRef]
143. Rozenberg, P.; Ziporen, L.; Gancz, D.; Saar-Ray, M.; Fishelson, Z. Cooperation between Hsp90 and mortalin/GRP75 in resistance to cell death induced by complement C5b-9. *Cell Death Dis.* **2018**, *9*, 150. [CrossRef]
144. Ozen, A.; Kasap, N.; Vujkovic-Cvijin, I.; Apps, R.; Cheung, F.; Karakoc-Aydiner, E.; Akkelle, B.; Sari, S.; Tutar, E.; Ozcay, F.; et al. Broadly effective metabolic and immune recovery with C5 inhibition in CHAPLE disease. *Nat. Immunol.* **2021**, *22*, 128–139. [CrossRef] [PubMed]
145. Hillmen, P.; Young, N.S.; Schubert, J.; Brodsky, R.A.; Socié, G.; Muus, P.; Röth, A.; Szer, J.; Elebute, M.O.; Nakamura, R.; et al. The complement inhibitor eculizumab in paroxysmal nocturnal hemoglobinuria. *N. Engl. J. Med.* **2006**, *355*, 1233–1243. [CrossRef] [PubMed]
146. West, E.E.; Woodruff, T.; Fremeaux-Bacchi, V.; Kemper, C. Complement in human disease: Approved and up-and-coming therapeutics. *Lancet* **2024**, *403*, 392–405. [CrossRef]
147. Yang, J.; Ahn, H.N.; Chang, M.; Narasimhan, P.; Chan, P.H.; Song, Y.S. Complement component 3 inhibition by an antioxidant is neuroprotective after cerebral ischemia and reperfusion in mice. *J. Neurochem.* **2013**, *124*, 523–535. [CrossRef] [PubMed]
148. Park, H.K.; Yoon, N.G.; Lee, J.E.; Hu, S.; Yoon, S.; Kim, S.Y.; Hong, J.H.; Nam, D.; Chae, Y.C.; Park, J.B.; et al. Unleashing the full potential of Hsp90 inhibitors as cancer therapeutics through simultaneous inactivation of Hsp90, Grp94, and TRAP1. *Exp. Mol. Med.* **2020**, *52*, 79–91. [CrossRef] [PubMed]
149. Bahreyni, A.; Mohamud, Y.; Luo, H.L. Emerging nanomedicines for effective breast cancer immunotherapy. *J. Nanobiotechnol.* **2020**, *18*, 180. [CrossRef] [PubMed]
150. Luan, X.; Lei, T.; Fang, J.; Liu, X.; Fu, H.; Li, Y.; Chu, W.; Jiang, P.; Tong, C.; Qi, H.; et al. Blockade of C5a receptor unleashes tumor-associated macrophage antitumor response and enhances CXCL9-dependent CD8(+) T cell activity. *Mol. Ther.* **2024**, *32*, 469–489. [CrossRef]

MDPI AG
Grosspeteranlage 5
4052 Basel
Switzerland
Tel.: +41 61 683 77 34

Biology Editorial Office
E-mail: biology@mdpi.com
www.mdpi.com/journal/biology

www.ingramcontent.com/pod-product-compliance
Lightning Source LLC
Chambersburg PA
CBHW040743250926
51850CB00007BB/1397
9783725857159